Arthritis Sourcebook

Basic Consumer Health Information about Specific Forms of Arthritis and Related Disorders, Including Rheumatoid Arthritis, Osteoarthritis, Gout, Polymyalgia Rheumatica, Psoriatic Arthritis, Spondyloarthropathies, Juvenile Rheumatoid Arthritis, and Juvenile Ankylosing Spondylitis; Along with Information about Medical, Surgical, and Alternative Treatment Options, and Including Strategies for Coping with Pain, Fatigue, and Stress

Edited by Allan R. Cook. 575 pages. 1998. 0-7808-0201-2. $78.

Back & Neck Disorders Sourcebook

Basic Information about Disorders and Injuries of the Spinal Cord and Vertebrae, Including Facts on Chiropractic Treatment, Surgical Interventions, Paralysis, and Rehabilitation, Along with Advice for Preventing Back Trouble

Edited by Karen Bellenir. 548 pages. 1997. 0-7808-0202-0. $78.

"The strength of this work is its basic, easy-to-read format. Recommended."
— *Reference and User Services Quarterly, Winter '97*

Blood & Circulatory Disorders Sourcebook

Basic Information about Blood and Its Components, Anemias, Leukemias, Bleeding Disorders, and Circulatory Disorders, Including Aplastic Anemia, Thalassemia, Sickle-Cell Disease, Hemochromatosis, Hemophilia, Von Willebrand Disease, and Vascular Diseases; Along with a Special Section on Blood Transfusions and Blood Supply Safety, a Glossary, and Source Listings for Further Help and Information

Edited by Karen Bellenir and Linda M. Shin. 575 pages. 1998. 0-7808-0203-9. $78.

Brain Disorders Sourcebook

Basic Consumer Health Information about Strokes, Epilepsy, Amyotrophic Lateral Sclerosis (ALS/Lou Gehrig's Disease), Parkinson's Disease, Brain Tumors, Cerebral Palsy, Headache, Tourette Syndrome, and More; Along with Statistical Data, Treatment and Rehabilitation Options, Coping Strategies, Reports on Current Research Initiatives, a Glossary, and Resource Listings for Additional Help and Information

Edited by Karen Bellenir. 600 pages. 1999. 0-7808-0229-2. $78.

Burns Sourcebook

Basic Information about Various Types of Burns and Scalds, Including Flame, Heat, Electrical, Chemical, and Sun; Along with Short- and Long-Term Treatments, Tissue Reconstruction, Plastic Surgery, Prevention Suggestions, and First Aid

Edited by Allan R. Cook. 600 pages. 1999. 0-7808-0204-7. $78.

Cancer Sourcebook, 1st Edition

Basic Information on Cancer Types, Symptoms, Diagnostic Methods, and Treatments, Including Statistics on Cancer Occurrences Worldwide and the Risks Associated with Known Carcinogens and Activities

Edited by Frank E. Bair. 932 pages. 1990. 1-55888-888-8. $78.

"Written in nontechnical language. Useful for patients, their families, medical professionals, and librarians."
— *Guide to Reference Books, '96*

"Designed with the non-medical professional in mind. Libraries and medical facilities interested in patient education should certainly consider adding the *Cancer Sourcebook* to their holdings. This compact collection of reliable information . . . is an invaluable tool for helping patients and patients' families and friends to take the first steps in coping with the many difficulties of cancer."
— *Medical Reference Services Quarterly, Winter '91*

"Specifically created for the nontechnical reader . . . an important resource for the general reader trying to understand the complexities of cancer."
— *American Reference Books Annual, '91*

"This publication's nontechnical nature and very comprehensive format make it useful for both the general public and undergraduate students." — *Choice, Oct '90*

New Cancer Sourcebook, 2nd Edition

Basic Information about Major Forms and Stages of Cancer, Featuring Facts about Primary and Secondary Tumors of the Respiratory, Nervous, Lymphatic, Circulatory, Skeletal, and Gastrointestinal Systems, and Specific Organs; Statistical and Demographic Data; Treatment Options; and Strategies for Coping

Edited by Allan R. Cook. 1,313 pages. 1996. 0-7808-0041-9. $78.

"This book is an excellent resource for patients with newly diagnosed cancer and their families. The dialogue is simple, direct, and comprehensive. Highly recommended for patients and families to aid in their understanding of cancer and its treatment."
— *Booklist Health Sciences Supplement, Oct '97*

"The amount of factual and useful information is extensive. The writing is very clear, geared to general readers. Recommended for all levels." — *Choice, Jan '97*

Continues next page

Cancer Sourcebook, 3rd Edition

Basic Information about Major Forms and Stages of Cancer, Featuring Facts about Primary and Secondary Tumors of the Respiratory, Nervous, Lymphatic, Circulatory, Skeletal, and Gastrointestinal Systems, and Specific Organs, Statistical and Demographic Data, Treatment Options, and Strategies for Coping

Edited by Edward J. Prucha. 800 pages. 1999. 0-7808-0227-6. $78.

Cancer Sourcebook for Women

Basic Information about Specific Forms of Cancer That Affect Women, Featuring Facts about Breast Cancer, Cervical Cancer, Ovarian Cancer, Cancer of the Uterus and Uterine Sarcoma, Cancer of the Vagina, and Cancer of the Vulva; Statistical and Demographic Data; Treatments, Self-Help Management Suggestions, and Current Research Initiatives

Edited by Allan R. Cook and Peter D. Dresser. 524 pages. 1996. 0-7808-0076-1. $78.

". . . written in easily understandable, non-technical language. Recommended for public libraries or hospital and academic libraries that collect patient education or consumer health materials."
— *Medical Reference Services Quarterly, Spring '97*

"Would be of value in a consumer health library. . . . written with the health care consumer in mind. Medical jargon is at a minimum, and medical terms are explained in clear, understandable sentences."
— *Bulletin of the MLA, Oct '96*

"The availability under one cover of all these pertinent publications, grouped under cohesive headings, makes this certainly a most useful sourcebook."
— *Choice, Jun '96*

"Presents a comprehensive knowledge base for general readers. Men and women both benefit from the gold mine of information nestled between the two covers of this book. Recommended."
— *Academic Library Book Review, Summer '96*

"This timely book is highly recommended for consumer health and patient education collections in all libraries."
— *Library Journal, Apr '96*

Cancer Sourcebook for Women, 2nd Edition

Basic Information about Specific Forms of Cancer That Affect Women, Featuring Facts about Breast Cancer, Cervical Cancer, Ovarian Cancer, Cancer of the Uterus and Uterine Sarcoma, Cancer of the Vagina, and Cancer of the Vulva, Statistical and Demographic Data, Treatments, Self-Help Management Suggestions, and Current Research Initiatives

Edited by Edward J. Prucha. 600 pages. 1999. 0-7808-0226-8. $78.

Cardiovascular Diseases & Disorders Sourcebook

Basic Information about Cardiovascular Diseases and Disorders, Featuring Facts about the Cardiovascular System, Demographic and Statistical Data, Descriptions of Pharmacological and Surgical Interventions, Lifestyle Modifications, and a Special Section Focusing on Heart Disorders in Children

Edited by Karen Bellenir and Peter D. Dresser. 683 pages. 1995. 0-7808-0032-X. $78.

". . . comprehensive format provides an extensive overview on this subject."
— *Choice, Jun '96*

". . . an easily understood, complete, up-to-date resource. This well executed public health tool will make valuable information available to those that need it most, patients and their families. The typeface, sturdy non-reflective paper, and library binding add a feel of quality found wanting in other publications. Highly recommended for academic and general libraries."
— *Academic Library Book Review, Summer '96*

Communication Disorders Sourcebook

Basic Information about Deafness and Hearing Loss, Speech and Language Disorders, Voice Disorders, Balance and Vestibular Disorders, and Disorders of Smell, Taste, and Touch

Edited by Linda M. Ross. 533 pages. 1996. 0-7808-0077-X. $78.

"This is skillfully edited and is a welcome resource for the layperson. It should be found in every public and medical library."
— *Booklist Health Sciences Supplement, Oct '97*

Congenital Disorders Sourcebook

Basic Information about Disorders Acquired during Gestation, Including Spina Bifida, Hydrocephalus, Cerebral Palsy, Heart Defects, Craniofacial Abnormalities, Fetal Alcohol Syndrome, and More, Along with Current Treatment Options and Statistical Data

Edited by Karen Bellenir. 607 pages. 1997. 0-7808-0205-5. $78.

"Recommended reference source." — *Booklist, Oct '97*

Consumer Issues in Health Care Sourcebook

Basic Information about Health Care Fundamentals and Related Consumer Issues, Including Exams and Screening Tests, Physician Specialties, Choosing a Doctor, Using Prescription and Over-the-Counter Medications Safely, Avoiding Health Scams, Managing Common Health Risks in the Home, Care Options for Chronically or Terminally Ill Patients, and a List of Resources for Obtaining Help and Further Information

Edited by Karen Bellenir. 592 pages. 1998. 0-7808-0221-7. $78.

Continues in back end sheets

Burns
SOURCEBOOK

Health Reference Series

AIDS Sourcebook, 1st Edition

AIDS Sourcebook, 2nd Edition

Allergies Sourcebook

Alternative Medicine Sourcebook

Alzheimer's, Stroke & 29 Other Neurological Disorders Sourcebook

Alzheimer's Disease Sourcebook, 2nd Edition

Arthritis Sourcebook

Back & Neck Disorders Sourcebook

Blood & Circulatory Disorders Sourcebook

Brain Disorders Sourcebook

Burns Sourcebook

Cancer Sourcebook, 1st Edition

New Cancer Sourcebook, 2nd Edition

Cancer Sourcebook, 3rd Edition

Cancer Sourcebook for Women

Cancer Sourcebook for Women, 2nd Edition

Cardiovascular Diseases & Disorders Sourcebook

Communication Disorders Sourcebook

Congenital Disorders Sourcebook

Consumer Issues in Health Care Sourcebook

Contagious & Non-Contagious Infectious Diseases Sourcebook

Death & Dying Sourcebook

Diabetes Sourcebook, 1st Edition

Diabetes Sourcebook, 2nd Edition

Diet & Nutrition Sourcebook, 1st Edition

Diet & Nutrition Sourcebook, 2nd Edition

Domestic Violence Sourcebook

Ear, Nose & Throat Disorders Sourcebook

Endocrine & Metabolic Disorders Sourcebook

Environmentally Induced Disorders Sourcebook

Ethical Issues in Medicine Sourcebook

Fitness & Exercise Sourcebook

Food & Animal Borne Diseases Sourcebook

Forensic Medicine Sourcebook

Gastrointestinal Diseases & Disorders Sourcebook

Genetic Disorders Sourcebook

Head Trauma Sourcebook

Health Insurance Sourcebook

Healthy Aging Sourcebook

Immune System Disorders Sourcebook

Kidney & Urinary Tract Diseases & Disorders Sourcebook

Learning Disabilities Sourcebook

Medical Tests Sourcebook

Men's Health Concerns Sourcebook

Mental Health Disorders Sourcebook

Ophthalmic Disorders Sourcebook

Oral Health Sourcebook

Pain Sourcebook

Physical & Mental Issues in Aging Sourcebook

Pregnancy & Birth Sourcebook

Public Health Sourcebook

Rehabilitation Sourcebook

Respiratory Diseases & Disorders Sourcebook

Sexually Transmitted Diseases Sourcebook

Skin Disorders Sourcebook

Sleep Disorders Sourcebook

Sports Injuries Sourcebook

Substance Abuse Sourcebook

Women's Health Concerns Sourcebook

Workplace Health & Safety Sourcebook

Health Reference Series

First Edition

Burns
SOURCEBOOK

*Basic Consumer Health Information
about Various Types of Burns and
Scalds, Including Flame, Heat, Cold,
Electrical, Chemical, and Sun Burns;
Along with Information on Short-Term
and Long-Term Treatments, Tissue
Reconstruction, Plastic Surgery,
Prevention Suggestions, and First Aid*

Edited by
Allan R. Cook

Omnigraphics, Inc.

Penobscot Building / Detroit, MI 48226

Bibliographic Note

Because this page cannot legibly accommodate all the copyright notices, the Bibliographic Note portion of the Preface constitutes an extension of the copyright notice.

Beginning with books published in 1999, each new volume of the *Health Reference Series* will be individually titled and called a "First Edition." Subsequent updates will carry sequential edition numbers. To help avoid confusion and to provide maximum flexibility in our ability to respond to informational needs, the practice of consecutively numbering each volume will be discontinued.

Edited by Allan R. Cook

Health Reference Series

Karen Bellenir, *Series Editor*
Peter D. Dresser, *Managing Editor*
Joan Margeson, *Research Associate*
Dawn Matthews, *Verification Assistant*
Margaret Mary Missar, *Research Coordinator*
Jenifer Swanson, *Research Associate*

Omnigraphics, Inc.

Matthew P. Barbour, *Vice President, Operations*
Laurie Lanzen Harris, *Vice President, Editorial Director*
Thomas J. Murphy, *Vice President, Finance and Comptroller*
Peter E. Ruffner, *Senior Vice President*
Jane J. Steele, *Marketing Consultant*

Frederick G. Ruffner, Jr., Publisher

© 1999, Omnigraphics, Inc.

Library of Congress Cataloging-in-Publication Data

Burns sourcebook / edited by Allan R. Cook — 1st ed.
  p. cm. — (Health reference series)
  Includes bibliographical references and index.
  ISBN 0-7808-0204-7 (library binding : alk. paper)
  1. Burns and scalds Popular works. 2. Wounds and injuries — Treatment Popular works. I. Cook, Allan R. II. Series. [DNLM 1. Burns Popular Works.
  WO 704 B9675 1999]
RD96.4.B895 1999
617.1'1—dc21
DNLM/DLC   99-24510
for Library of Congress   CIP

∞

This book is printed on acid-free paper meeting the ANSI Z39.48 Standard. The infinity symbol that appears above indicates that the paper in this book meets that standard.

Printed in the United States

Table of Contents

Part VI: Emergency Procedures and First Aid

Part VII: Additional Help and Information

Preface

About this Book

Medical advances in the later half of this century have produced dramatic changes in the care of burn victims. At one time, doctors could not save patients with burns to more than 30 percent of their bodies. Today, patients with burns to more than 90 percent burn of their body have a chance of survival. Doctors have learned much about the how the body reacts to burns of all types and how the skin can be repaired. Even so, each year, fire kills 20 times more people than hurricanes, tornados, floods, and earthquakes combined. For children and young adults, burns are the leading cause of death in the home.

Burn fatalities, numbered annually at about 5,500 in the United States, represent only a small portion of the more than 1.25 million burn injuries reported each year. Of those injured, between 5 and 10 percent require hospitalization, often with a long, painful period of reconstruction and recovery. Although medical science has produced dramatic declines in both burn fatalities and long-term impact of burn injuries, prevention plays a vital role. According to experts, more than half of all burns that occur each year are fully preventable.

This book contains basic information for the layperson on the nature of specific forms of burns, their identification and classification, treatment strategies and advances, and the psychological effects of long-term pain, disfiguring scarring, and the protracted treatment regimens. It also offers first-aid responses to accidental burns and strategies to reduce the risk of burn injury.

How to Use this Book

This book is divided into parts and chapters. Parts focus on broad areas of interest and chapters on specific topics within those areas.

Part I: *Burn Statistics* presents statistical data on the incidence of fires and burn injuries. It describes burn treatment facilities usage and typical burn victims.

Part II: *Types and Degrees of Burns* lists the most common forms of burn injuries and their classifications by degree.

Part III: *Treatment Protocols for Severe Burns* traces the physical treatment of severe burns from initial assessment through reconstruction and replacement of damaged tissue and describes the operation of a modern burn care unit.

Part IV: *Rehabilitation and Coping* discusses rehabilitation and psychological recovery.

Part V: *Safety and Prevention* looks at some common fire and burn hazards and offers suggestions for minimizing their risk.

Part VI: *Emergency Procedures and First Aid* offers strategies for dealing with fire and burn emergencies both at work and in the home. Adequate first aid treatment delivered in a timely manner can often greatly reduce the severity of burn injuries.

Part VII: *Additional Help and Information* lists other sources of information and assistance.

Bibliographic Note

This volume contains individual documents and excerpts from periodic publications issued by the National Institutes of Health (NIH), its sister agencies and subagencies, and the U.S. Consumer Product Safety Commission (CPSC).

It also includes copyrighted articles, reprinted with permission, from American Burn Association, *Burns*; American Physical Therapy Association; Aspen Publishers, *Topics in Emergency Medicine*, *Pain in the Critically Ill: Assessment and Management*; Burn Prevention Foundation; *Clinical Issues in Critical Care Nursing*; *Critical Care*

Nursing Clinics of North America; Burn Science Publishers, *Journal of Burn Care and Rehabilitation*; *Clinical Factors*; Current Science Ltd., *Current Opinion in Surgical Infections*; *Emergency*; *Emergency Medical Services*; J.B. Lippincott Co., *Problems in General Surgery*; Elsevier Science Inc., *Burns, Journal of Emergency Medicine*; Mayo Foundation for Medical Education and Research; National Fire Protection Association (NFPA), *NFPA Journal*; *Parade Magazine*; Phoenix Society for Burn Survivors; *Safety & Health*; Shriners Burn Institute, *Support Line*; *The Coordinator*; W.B. Saunders Company, *Dermatologic Clinics*; Williams and Wilkins, *Hazardous Materials Toxicology, Pediatric Rehabilitation*; *and WNYF*.

All copyrighted material is reprinted with permission. Document numbers where applicable and specific source citations are provided on the appropriate page of each chapter. Every effort has been made to secure all necessary rights to reprint the copyrighted material. If any omissions have been made, please contact Omnigraphics to make corrections for future editions.

Acknowledgements

Many people and organizations have contributed the material in this volume. In addition to the organizations listed above, special thanks are due to Margaret Mary Missar for her patient search for the documents that make up this volume, Maria Franklin for securing reprint permissions, Karen Bellenir for her technical assistance and advice, Bruce the Scanman for his photonic portation processing and David Cook for his text cleaning assistance.

Note from the Editor

This book is part of Omnigraphics' Health Reference Series. The series provides basic information about a broad range of medical concerns. It is not intended to serve as a tool for diagnosing illness, in prescribing treatments, or as a substitute for the physician/patient relationship. All persons concerned about medical symptoms or the possibility of disease are encouraged to seek professional care from an appropriate health care provider.

Our Advisory Board

The *Health Reference Series* is reviewed by an Advisory Board comprised of librarians from public, academic, and medical libraries. We would like to thank the following board members for providing guidance to the development of this series:

Nancy Bulgarelli,
William Beaumont Hospital Library, Royal Oak, MI

Karen Morgan, Mardigian Library,
University of Michigan, Dearborn, MI

Rosemary Orlando,
St. Clair Shores Public Library, St. Clair Shores, MI

Health Reference Series *Update Policy*

The inaugural book in the *Health Reference Series* was the first edition of *Cancer Sourcebook* published in 1992. Since then, the *Series* has been enthusiastically received by libraries and in the medical community. In order to maintain the standard of providing high-quality health information for the lay person, the editorial staff at Omnigraphics felt it was necessary to implement a policy of updating volumes when warranted.

Medical researchers have been making tremendous strides, and the challenge to stay current with the most recent advances is one our editors take seriously. Each decision to update a volume will be made on an individual basis. Some of the considerations will include how much new information is available and the feedback we receive from people who use the books. If there's a topic you would like to see added to the update list, or an area of medical concern you feel has not been adequately addressed, please write to:

Editor
Health Reference Series
Omnigraphics, Inc.
2500 Penobscot Bldg.
Detroit, MI 48226

The commitment to providing on-going coverage of important medical developments has also led to some technical changes in the *Health Reference Series*. Beginning with books published in 1999, each new volume will be individually titled and called a "First Edition." Subsequent updates will carry sequential edition numbers. To help avoid confusion and to provide maximum flexibility in our ability to respond to informational needs, the practice of consecutively numbering each volume will be discontinued.

Part One

Burn Statistics

Chapter 1

Facts and Figures in Brief

Total Burn Incidence in the United States—1.25 Million Injuries per Year (1992).

This figure is a composite estimate drawn from the National Health Interview Survey (NHIS), a continuous household interview survey of the nation's health (1991-93 data) and three other periodic federal surveys,—the National Ambulatory Medical Care Survey, the National Hospital Ambulatory Medical Care Survey and the National Medical Expenditure Survey.

Trend: The incidence of burn injury, in the United States has declined significantly from the two million annual injuries estimated in the first NHIS survey report, drawn from 1957-61 data. Since that time, the rate of medically-attended burn injuries has declined from about 10/10,000 to 4.2/10,000.

Total Fire and Burn Deaths—5,250 per Year (1993)

This estimate includes about 4,000 deaths from housefires and 1,250 from other sources, including motor vehicle and aircraft crashes, contact with electricity, chemicals or hot liquids and substances, and other sources of fire or flames. Since the respective role of flame and smoke in fire deaths is often not determined by autopsy, specific "burn" death totals cannot be distinguished from those, which result from smoke poisoning.

Trend: Fire and burn deaths in the United States declined about 40 percent from 1971 to 1993. Since the U.S. population grew 25 percent during that period, the rate of decline was 50 percent.

Sources: Annual survey of fire departments by the National Fire Protection Association and annual Vital and Health Statistics reports of the National Center for Health Statistics.

Total Hospital and Burn Center Admissions—about 50,000 per Year (1992-94)

Total Hospital Emergency Department Burn Visits—about 400,000 per Year (1992-1994)

Of the 50,000 total estimated hospital and burn center admissions, 23,000 were admitted to specialized burn treatment centers (1993). [note: Burn center hospitals averaged 170 burn admissions per year, other hospitals only five.]

Trend. Total annual acute hospitalizations for burn injury decreased from 90,000 to 51,000 (42 percent) from 1971 to 1993. Some of the decline reflects a decease in repeat hospitalization during acute treatment. Simultaneously, burn center admissions increased from 12,000 to 23,000 Burn center admissions thusgrew from 13 to 45 percent of total acute burn admissions during this period. No trend data are available for hospital emergency department or outpatient visits for burn injury.

Sources: National Hospital Discharge Survey. National Hospital Ambulatory Medical Care Survey (annual) and American Burn Association survey of burn care facilities in the U. S. (triennial).

Severity of Burn Injuries

Among fire and burn injuries admitted to burn centers, the mean size of the burn injury is about 14 percent of total body surface area [percent TBSA] (1991-93). Burns of 10 percent TBSA or less accounted for 54 percent of burn center admissions, while burns of 60 percent

4

TBSA or more accounted for 4 percent of admissions. About 6 percent of burn center admissions do not survive, most of whom have suffered severe inhalation injury in fires.

Trend: Since 1965, burns of 10 percent TBSA or loss have increased from about 26 percent to 54 percent of burn center admissions. Simultaneously, the fraction of very large burns (60 percent TBSA or greater) has declined from 10 to less than 4 percent of total admissions. This mainly reflects increased appreciation of the importance of specialized care in treating burn injury and rehabilitating its survivors.

Sources: A survey of 28 burn centers contributing data to the American Burn Association burn patient registry (1991-93) and data from the National Burn Information Exchange (1965-85.)

Chapter 2

Trends in Burn Injuries

Burn Injuries

Overview

During 1991-93, the U.S. averaged an estimated 1,129,000 burn injuries per year. (See Table 2.1) That is four burn injuries for every 1,000 people in the country per year. These burns arose from contact with hot gases, liquids, or solid objects, or electrical, chemical, or radiation effects. Burn injuries need not involve fire, and fire injuries need not involve burns.

This estimate, like most of the other figures in this section, is taken from the National Health Interview Survey (NHIS), conducted by the National Center for Health Statistics. NHIS is a survey of people in their homes, so it is not subject to the problems of under-reporting that affect statistics based on injuries reported to fire departments, hospital emergency rooms, or some other organization.

NHIS estimates can be subject to substantial variations based on sample size, interviewee recall, and the precise methods used by the survey to help interviewers remember not-so-recent injuries. Also, the range of injuries deemed to be reportable was narrowed in the early 1980s, and this accounts for part of the nearly 50 percent decline since the 1960s.

Although this survey is conducted on a continuous basis with periodic reports, analyses with sufficient detail to isolate burn injuries are done on an irregular basis and usually combine two to three years of data to improve the sample size. Even so, because of the limited sample size (about 50,000 households and 120,000 people per year), many of the estimates are subject to considerable sampling error (i.e., over 30 percent), as shown in the tables of this section. This also makes it impossible, based on the published analyses, to provide annually updated estimates of the nation's burn incidence, even in the form of multi-year rolling averages. Notwithstanding all these limitations, there clearly has been dramatic, real progress in reducing burn injury rates over the past three decades.

Males suffer more burn injuries than females, overall and relative to their shares of the population, and the gap between the two sexes

Table 2.1. U.S. Burn Injuries Estimated Annual Averages

	1957-1961	1965-1967	1980-1981	1985-1987	1991-1993
Total	1,973,000	2,333,000	2,130,000	1,735,000	1,129,000
Rate per 100 people	1.1	1.2	1.0	0.7	0.4
Males	1,082,000	1,297,000	1,026,000	981,000	726,000
Rate per 100 males	1.3	1.4	1.0	0.9	0.6
Females	892,000	936,000	1,104,000	772,000	403,000
Rate per 100 females	1.0	0.9	1.0	0.6	0.3
Children**	NA	NA	571	385,000	376,000
Rate per 100 people	1.1	1.1	1.0	0.6	0.6
Age 45 and up	NA	NA	291,000*	300,000*	155,000*
Rate per 100 people	NA	0.8	0.4*	0.4*	0.2*

NA - Not available

*Relative standard error of estimate exceeds 30%

**Children are defined as under 15 in 1957-1961; under 17 in 1965-1967 and 1980-1981; and under 18 in 1985-1987 and 1991-1993.

Sources: *Types of Injuries, Incidence and Associated Disability, United States*: July 1957-June 1961, Series 10, No. 8, 1964; and July 1965-June 1967, Series 10, No. 57, 1970; *Types of Injuries and Impairments Due to Injuries - United States*, Series 10, No. 159, 1986; *Types of Injuries by Selected Characteristics, 1985-87,* Series 10, No. 175, 1990; and advance data from John Gary Collins, U.S. Department of Health and Human Services, National Center for Health Statistics, author of 1991-93 data analysis (forthcoming) and previous two studies.

was wider in the latest survey analysis than ever before. Older adults tend to have lower burn injury rates than the all-ages average, and this is true even if people age 65 and older are isolated, which cannot be done with available data for three of the five survey analyses. Children show no consistent pattern of burn injury risk relative to the overall population. Unfortunately, the preschool age group, which is known to have high higher risk of fire injury than other children, cannot be isolated.

Burn injury rates per 100 persons are higher for the poor (see Table 2.2) but show only minor differences by race and no consistent patterns by region. Burn injury rates also appear to have increased for the poor, but this conclusion is blurred, by the shifting categories used to define the poorest group. Differences by educational level are not available for all analyses and are not so consistent as differences by income.

The NHIS characterizes the severity of burn injuries in several ways—medically attended injury, injury resulting in restricted activity, and injury resulting in confinement to bed (also called bed-disabling injury). These characterizations are done independently, so there is no guarantee that, for example, a bed-disabling injury was also a restricted-activity burn injury, even though it seems logical that this would be so. There is no information in the NHIS regarding the first, second and third degree scale of burn depth nor the extent of body surface burned.

In 1991-93, 95 percent of estimated injuries were medically attended (see Table 2.3). The large change between 1980-81 and 1985-87 in percentage of burn injuries that were medically attended probably reflects the change in definitions and reporting conventions, which required medical treatment or a half-day of restricted activity to qualify an injury as reportable. Some of the increase may reflect greater geographic and financial access to health care and resulting greater use of it.

More than one-third of all 1991-93 burn injuries (39 percent) resulted in some period of restricted activity, down substantially from earlier percentages. However, the average period of restricted activity with such an injury has been steadily rising. (This was calculated by the author by dividing the number of restricted-activity days by the number of injuries, from the source reports.) In those analyses that provide additional detail, the average length of the restricted-activity periods for females have been shorter. For all of the detailed analyses cited in this paragraph and the next one, however, the large sampling errors in the estimates raise substantial questions about the statistical significance of trends or compliance at this level of detail.

Only one burn injury in nine in 1991-93 resulted in some confinement to bed. The average period of confinement has been rising steadily and dramatically. (This was calculated by the author by dividing the number of days of bed disability by the number of bed-

Table 2.2. Comparative Burn Injury Rates per 100 People Annual Averages

	1957-1961	1965-1967	1980-1981	1985-1987	1991-1993
Overall	1.1	1.2	1.0	0.7	0.4
Males	1.3	1.4	1.0	0.9	0.6
Females	1.0	0.9	1.0	0.6	0.3
Children**	1.1	1.1	1.0	0.6	0.6
Age 45 and up	NA	0.8	0.4*	0.4*	0.2*
White	NA	1.2	1.0	0.7	0.4
Black	NA	1.2	1.1*	0.6*	0.6*
Northeast	1.0	1.0	0.7	0.8	0.3*
North Central	1.0	1.3	0.9	0.6*	0.6
South	1.3	1.3	1.0	0.7	0.5
West	1.2	0.9	1.2	1.0	0.4*
Poorest***	1.2	1.5	1.9	1.8	NA
Most Affluent***	0.9	1.0	1.1	0.8*	NA

NA - Not available or not yet available

*Relative standard error of estimate exceeds 30%

**Children are defined as under 15 in 1957-1961; under 17 in 1965-1967 and 1980-1981; and under 18 in 1985-1987 and 1991-1993.

***Poorest group is defined as family income less than $4,000 in 1957-61, less than $5,000 in 1965-67 and 1980-81, and less than $10,000 in 1985-87. Most affluent group is defined as family income more than $7,000 in 1957-61, more than $10,000 in 1965-67, more than $25,000 in 1980-81, and more than $35,000 in 1985-87.

Sources: *Types of Injuries, Incidence and Associated Disability, United States*: July 1957-June 1961, Series 10, No. 8, 1964; and July 1965-June 1967, Series 10, No. 57, 1970; *Types of Injuries and Impairments Due to Injuries - United States*, Series 10, No. 159, 1986; *Types of Injuries by Selected Characteristics*, 1985-87, Series 10, No. 175, 1990; and advance data from John Gary Collins, U.S. Department of Health and Human Services, National Center for Health Statistics, author of 1991-93 data analysis (forthcoming) and previous two studies.

disabling injuries, from the source reports.) In analyses that provide additional detail, adults over age 44 have had longer average periods of bed-disabling injuries than other age groups, and males with burn injuries have been much more likely to be confined to bed than females.

Table 2.3. Indicators of Burn Injury Severity Annual Averages

	1957-1961	1965-1967	1980-1981	1985-1987	1991-1993
Number of medically attended injuries	1,719,000	1,932,000	1,615,000	1,614,000	1,073,000
Percent of burn injuries that are medically attended	87	87	76	92	95
Number of restricted - activity injuries	NA	NA	1,213,000	810,000	445,000
Percent of burn injuries involving restricted activity	NA	NA	57	46	39
Average number of restricted activity days per injury	3.7	4.0	6.1	8.8	NA
Number of bed-disability injuries	NA	NA	244,000*	399,000	124,000
Percent of burn injuries involving bed disability	NA	NA	11*	23	11
Average number of bed-disability days per injury	1.1	1.5	5.7	8.1	NA

NA - Not available or not yet available

*Relative standard error of estimate exceeds 30%

Sources: *Types of Injuries, Incidence and Associated Disability, United States*: July 1957-June 1961, Series 10, No. 8, 1964; and July 1965-June 1967, Series 10, No. 57, 1970; *Types of Injuries and Impairments Due to Injuries - United States*, Series 10, No. 159, 1986; *Types of Injuries by Selected Characteristics, 1985-87*, Series 10, No. 175, 1990; and advance data from John Gary Collins, U.S. Department of Health and Human Services, author of 1991-93 data analysis (forthcoming) and previous two studies.

Special Data Bases on Burn Injuries

Other data sources capture a smaller fraction of more serious burn injuries, based on their involvement with some part of the health care system. The U.S. Consumer Product Safety Commission (CPSC) tracks injuries that involve a consumer product and are reported to hospital emergency rooms, in the National Electronic Injury Surveillance System (NEISS). Analysis of this data provides the best picture of the relative frequency of different types of burns involving consumer products (see Table 2.4). Table 2.4 shows that electrical burns are a very small fraction of hospital emergency room burn injuries related to consumer products, both overall and for those requiring hospitalization. If burns with no consumer-product involvement were added, estimates derived by Peter Brigham of the Burn Foundation from the National Hospital Ambulatory Medical Care Survey for 1992-1993 indicate that the estimate of total burn injuries receiving emergency room treatment would more than double, with much of the increase being scalds from spills of hot liquids where no consumer product involvement was reported.

Table 2.4. Burn Injuries That Involved a Consumer Product and Were Reported to Hospital Emergency Rooms, 1993

Type of Burn Injury	Number of Emergency Room Injuries		Number of Emergency Room Injuries Admitted to Hospitals	
Thermal (fire or hot object)	151,000	(64%)	11,100	(51%)
Scald	77,700	(33%)	9,700	(45%)
Electrical	6,100	(3%)	600	(3%)
Unknown-type	2,900	(1%)	200	(1%)
Total	237,700	(100%)	21,600	(100%)

Note: Chemical or radiation burns are not captured in this table. Some scalds may be omitted for lack of a consumer product connection. Sums may not equal totals because of rounding error.

Source: Beatrice Harwood, "Common products that cause uncommonly severe burn injuries," *NFPA Journal*, January/February 1996, pp. 79-83.

Beatrice Harwood's analysis of 1993 NEISS data also identified some other notable patterns:

- Hospitalization is much more likely for thermal burns if the victim is age 65 or older.

- Hospitalization is much more likely for scalds if the victim is age 4 or younger.

- Hair curlers and curling irons accounted for more thermal or electrical burns (10 percent of the total) than any other product group, and most (62 percent) of those victims were children under age 15. By contrast, a larger product category—portable appliance designed to produce controlled heat—which includes curling irons, hair curlers, irons, electric blankets, and hair dryers, accounted for only 1 percent of 1988-92 home fires and associated home fire injuries to civilians.*

- Gasoline and clothing were the leading products associated with injuries leading to hospitalization, accounting for 23 percent and 9 percent, respectively.

The 21,600 estimated 1993 consumer, product-related burn injuries involving a hospital emergency room visit followed by admission to the hospital may be seen as the consumer, product-related share of the 1993 injuries within the 51,000 estimated annual average of 1991-93 acute burn injury admissions to hospitals.** Also compare the latter to an estimated 23,000 1992 admissions specifically to burn center hospitals. Both of the latter figures capture burns with or without consumer product involvement.

Deaths Due to Burns

Fatal burn injuries would include the following:

- Fire deaths due to burns, previously estimated in this report at roughly 1,000 per year in recent years, or about one-fourth of fire deaths coded as such on death certificates.

- The burn share of fire deaths, such as motor vehicle post-crash fire deaths or incendiary fire deaths (homicide or suicide), not captured in the first group. There is no consensus way to estimate these deaths, but under a wide range of assumptions, they would number in the low to mid-hundreds.

- Non-fire burn deaths, including deaths due to contact with "hot objects" (see Table 2.5) and, depending on definitional conventions, deaths due to contact with electrical current, which for this report are kept separate, in the next section.

- Delayed deaths for which the link to initial burn injuries is lost by the time the patient dies and a death certificate is completed. This may be the most uncertain part of all.

Table 2.5. Accidental Deaths Involving Contact with Hot Objects or Substances

Year	Total
1980	194
1981	192
1982	154
1983	139
1984	142
1985	176
1986	134
1987	137
1988	122
1989	142
1990	131
1991	125
1992	131
1993	130

Note: Includes corrosive substances and steam

Sources: National Safety Council, *Accident Facts*, 1981-1996 editions, 1121 Spring Lake Drive, Itasca, IL 60143

Safety Recommendations

1. Know the first aid steps to apply if burns occur, including ap-
    plying cool water for 10-15 minutes to carry heat away from
    the burn and seeking medical attention if the burn blisters.

2. Turn pot handles inward so pots cannot be knocked off the
    stove or pulled down by small children.

3. Place hot liquids away from the edge of the table and avoid
    using tablecloths that hang over the edge.

4. Be especially careful with food cooked in a microwave oven,
    which can be dangerously hot. Remove lids or wraps carefully
    to prevent steam burns.

5. Check the temperature setting on the water heater, and be
    sure that undiluted hot tap water is not so hot that it could
    scald. Set it at or below 120°F or 48°C.

6. Learn to stop, drop, and roll if clothes catch fire, and be sure
    all family members, including children, know the technique
    also.

7. Cover unused wall outlets with safety caps to protect children,
    and be sure unattended children do not have access to
    matches, lighters, hot liquids, hot objects (like space heaters),
    or plugged-in electrical cords or devices.

8. Be careful when using flammable or combustible liquids. Use
    them only in well-ventilated areas and away from heat
    sources, including non-obvious heat sources like the pilot
    lights of water heaters and stoves. Avoid use of these liquids
    to start, enhance, or revive a planned fire, such as an outdoor
    grill fire, fireplace fire, or campfire.

9. Be careful when using or working near chemicals, including
    car battery acid. Take steps to avoid splashes. If a burn oc-
    curs, flush the area with cool water immediately and seek
    medical attention.

10. Use caution when burning trash. Discourage very old or very
    young family members from conducting such operations, as
    they may be unable to react quickly if a hazard develops.

11. Wear tight-fitting sleeves when cooking, and be particularly careful when reaching over stove burners.

*Alison L. Miller, *The U.S. Home Product Report*, 1988-1992 (Appliances and Equipment), Quincy, MA: National Fire Protection Association, Fire Analysis & Research Division, August 1994.

**Peter A. Brigham and Elizabeth McLoughlin, "Burn incidence and medical care use in the United States," *Journal of Burn Care and Rehabilitation,* March/April 1996, pp. 95-107.

—by John R Hall, Jr.

Fire Analysis and Research Division, National Fire Protection Association, #1 Batterymarch Park, PO Box 9101, Quincy, MA 02269-9101.

Chapter 3

Profile of a Fire Victim

Injury or death caused by fire is frequent and largely preventable. This study was undertaken to define the populations, locations, times and behaviors associated with fatal fires. Seven hundred and twenty seven fatalities occurring within the State of New Jersey, between the years 1985 and 1991, were examined retrospectively. Most deaths were attributed to a combination of smoke inhalation and burn injury. Five hundred and seventy four fatalities occurred in residential fires. Smoking materials were the most common source of ignition for residential fires. More than half of the fatal residential fires started between the hours of 11 p.m. and 7 a.m. Children and the elderly represented a disproportionate percentage of fire victims. Victims under the age of 11 years or over the age of 70 years constituted 22.1 percent of the state population but 39.5 percent of all fire fatalities. Fire prevention efforts should target home fire safety, and should concentrate on children and the elderly. The development of fire-safe smoking materials should be encouraged.

Introduction

Fire is responsible for substantial morbidity and mortality in the USA. Every year, fire causes 20 times more deaths than hurricanes, tornados, floods and earthquakes combined.[1] Burns and fires are the third leading cause of accidental death in all age groups[1,2], the second

---

leading cause of death in the home for all ages[3] and the leading cause of death in the home for children and young adults[3,4].

Annually in the USA, there are 2.4 million reported fires[3,5] resulting in 7.8 billion dollars of direct property loss, an estimated 30 billion dollars of indirect loss, 29,000 civilian injuries, 101,000 firefighter injuries and 6,000 civilian fatalities[2,3,5,6]. These figures do not include losses from the estimated 90 percent of fires that are not reported to fire departments[7,8,] nor from fire fatalities that result from road traffic accidents, suicide or arson[2]. Fire death rates in the USA and Canada are twice as high as in Western Europe and Japan[3].

Many fires, and most fire-related injuries, are preventable[9]. Fire requires the interaction of fuel, oxygen and a source of ignition, and the union of these elements is frequently a result of human behavior. Prevention can be achieved by eliminating or reducing the risk of ignition, by removing the fuel from the site of potential ignition or by altering the human behavior that brings the fuel and ignition source together[3]. Analysis of human behavior resulting in fire and fire-related injury is hampered by a paucity of data.

Most fire loss-data are collected with the intent of protection of property rather than protection of life. The US Fire Administration National Fire Incident Reporting System (NFIRS) and the databases maintained by the National Fire Protection Association (NFPA) do not reference fire-related injury or death in detail. Likewise, few medical studies of fire fatalities have been published[10-13]. Of an estimated 108,000 fire fatalities occurring in the USA between 1971 and 1989, fewer than 1,000 cases have been reviewed in the medical literature.

To be effective, fire and burn prevention efforts should target the populations at highest risk, and should identify the circumstances most likely to result in injury or death. The following retrospective study was performed to examine the circumstances, causes and contributing factors for 727 fire fatalities that occurred within the State of New Jersey over a 7 year period.

Materials and Methods

Records of the New Jersey State Medical Examiners Office were examined retrospectively for any deaths attributable to fire, burns or smoke inhalation during the 7 year period 1985-91. Reporting sources included local medical examiners, attending physicians, hospital emergency departments and police or fire agencies. Data abstracted included demographic information such as age, sex and race; the location and circumstance of the fire and the date and time of pronouncement of death. The cause of the fire and the time of fire onset (time that the fire was reported to the fire department) was obtained from field reports submitted with blood or tissue samples. It was not logistically possible to examine individual fire department records for each incident. Toxicological analysis of this cohort is described elsewhere[14,15].

Results

Seven hundred and twenty-seven fire fatalities were identified. There were 424 males (59.8 percent) and 285 females (40.2 percent). The race was identified as White in 360 cases, Black in 253 cases and Hispanic in 56 cases. Race, age or sex was undetermined in several cases due to severe charring. The demographics of the study group, compared to the 1990 Census baseline state population, are presented in *Table 3.1*.

The cause of death was attributed to smoke inhalation and burn injury in 471 cases, to smoke inhalation without cutaneous burn in 178 cases, and to fire or burns in 71 victims.

The size of the cutaneous burn injury was documented in 210 cases. Eighty-seven victims were described as 'charred' or 'incinerated' and 18 had burns of 100 percent of the body surface. The remaining 75 victims had an average burn size of 55.8 percent of the total body surface area.

Table 3.1 Comparison of study group with baseline state population

Group	Fire fatality %	1990 Census %
Male	59.8	48.7
Female	40.2	51.3
White	53.3	48.7
Black	37.5	13.4
Hispanic	8.2	9.5
Other	1.0	28.4
Age		
<10yr	21.9	13.2
>70yr	17.6	8.9

Five hundred and seventy-four victims died in structure fires, predominantly in buildings used as permanent or temporary residences. Fifteen victims died in fires occurring in industrial, commercial or non-residential structures. There were 63 vehicle fires, six fatalities from aircraft fires and one electrocution.

Four hundred and eighty-three victims died at the scene of the fire. An additional 71 were dead on arrival at the hospital, or had cardiopulmonary resuscitation performed on scene or en route. Ninety-two victims survived for up to 6 hours following the onset of the fire, with the average survival time being 1.9 hours. Fifty-nine deaths occurring more than 6 hours after the onset of the fire were classified as delayed fire deaths. The average survival time for this group was 8.6 days.

The average age of the victims was 39.4 years, with a range of 0.1 − 97 years (*Figure 3.1*). One hundred and forty-eight victims were under the age of 11 years and 119 were over the age of 70 years. This group constituted 22.1 percent of the baseline state population, but 39.5 percent of the fire fatalities (*Table 3.1*). Children between the ages of 2 and 4 years had the highest fatality rate and these 3 years alone accounted for 10.6 percent of all fatalities in this study.

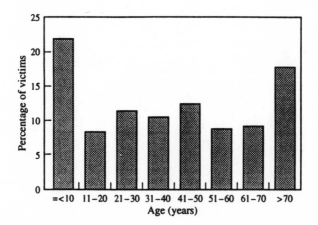

Figure 3.1. *Age Distribution of Fatalities*

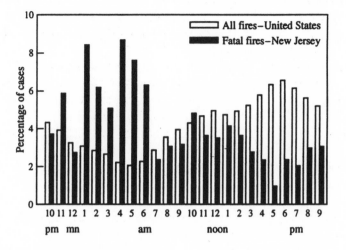

Figure 3.2. Time of onset of fires

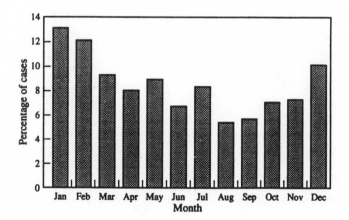

Figure 3.3. Seasonal variation

Table 3.2 Cause of ignition in fatal structure fires

Cause	No.
Smoking or suspected smoking materials	**41**
Smoking in bed	11
Fire in couch	8
Cigarette	7
Smoking in couch	3
Smoking in chair	3
Mattress or bed fire	6
Bedroom fire	3
Homicide or arson	**27**
Kitchen fires	**26**
Heating System	**22**
Kerosene heater	13
Electric heater	4
Wood burning stove	2
Portable oil heater	1
Space heater	1
Furnace	1
Children starting fire	**10**
Playing with matches or lighter	8
Playing with hairdryer	1
Left unsupervised	1
Other	**22**
Suicide	6
Electrical	4
Jumped to escape fire	4
Firefighting	3
Lightning strike to home	2
Gas leak	2
Radio malfunction	1

The majority (51.3 percent) of fatal fires had an onset between the hours of 11 p.m. and 7 a.m. suggesting that fires may be more common at night. In reality, the converse is true. Data on the onset-time of non-fatal fires within the State of New Jersey was not available for comparison, however such information is collected on a national basis by the US Fire Administration[5] and was examined. On a national basis, residential fires requiring fire department response have a peak incidence between the hours of 6 p.m. and 7 p.m., coincident with dinner preparation. Only 21.9 percent of all fires reported to fire departments start between 11 p.m. and 7 a. m.[5]. Fires that start at night are not more common, but are more likely to result in a fatality. *Figure 3.2* compares time of onset of fatal fires within the State of New Jersey to the time of onset of all fires reported to fire departments on a national basis.

The seasonal variation in fires that result in fatality is presented in *Figure 3.3*. Not surprisingly, fatal fires are more common during winter months, reflecting an increased use of central or portable heating systems.

The cause of fires resulting in fatality was known or suspected for 148 of 574 house fires (25.7 percent), and is presented in *Table 3.2*. Within this small sample, smoking materials were the most common cause of ignition, followed by homicide/arson, cooking or kitchen fires and heating systems. As most of the fires had an onset during the late evening hours, it is possible that many of the fires with unassigned cause were started by smoldering smoking materials or by home heating systems, rather than by food preparation activities.

Discussion

This study identified populations and behaviors associated with fatal fires. Most deaths resulted from fires that occurred at night in residential structures. The most commonly reported source of ignition was smoking materials. Nearly 90 percent of the fatalities occurred at the scene or within 6 hours of the onset of the fire, suggesting that primary fire prevention offers the greatest promise of reducing fire deaths.

Children and the elderly were over-represented among fire fatalities compared to the baseline state population. These two populations are also at increased risk of non-fatal burn injury. The increased incidence of burns in children is normally attributed to their dependence upon caretakers[4], although children may be the cause of up to 10 percent of fatal house fires when they play with matches or other ignition sources[2]. Children playing with fire is the sixth leading cause of fire deaths in the USA, and the leading cause of fire death under age 6 years[16]. Likewise, fire poses an increased risk for the elderly. The National Fire Protection Association estimates that those aged 65 years or over have a fire-death rate over twice that of the national average. This risk increases to three times the national average at age 75 years and to 4 times the average at age 85 years[17]. Fire injury among the elderly is thought to be related to an impaired ability to detect or escape from fire, although escape does not guarantee survival as the mortality associated with even minor burn injury rises sharply with increasing age[18,19].

Seventy-nine percent of fatal fires in this study occurred in residential structures. Fire remains a significant hazard in the home, a location that most consider secure and safe from danger. In other studies, residential structure fires comprise only one-quarter of incidents reported to fire departments but are responsible for 64—79 percent of fire-related injuries and 72–80 percent of fire-related deaths[1,2,5,11-13,16,20]. Patients rescued from house fires constitute less than 5 percent of hospital admissions for burns, but up to 45 percent of all burn-center deaths[21,22]. Deaths from house fires have seasonal and hourly variation and are more common in the winter [2,23,24] and in the late evening and early morning hours[5,11]. Overall, mobile homes have fire-death rates more than twice as high as other types of residences[5] and mobile homes without smoke detectors have a fatality risk up to four times higher[1].

Factors contributing to the high rate of fatal residential structure fires include the failure to install or maintain smoke detectors, the intemperate use of alcohol or other intoxicants[7,15] and conditions that impair escape[24]. The major factor, however, appears to be the careless use of tobacco products. Smoking materials are the most common ignition source for fatal residential fires in this and other studies,[15,10,11,16,25,26] and fires started by smoking materials are responsible for 1500—2300 fatalities and 7000 serious injuries each year[11,26]. Many of the victims killed in such fires are not the smokers themselves[11,26]. Tobacco-related fires usually start in upholstered furniture or bedding as the result of smoking in bed, alcohol use or both[1,10,16,17,23]. Birky and colleagues[10] reported that this single scenario was responsible for 47 percent of all fatal fires in Maryland over a 6-year period.

'Fire-safe' cigarettes that cease to burn when left unattended have been advocated by fire-prevention groups, the American Burn Association and the American Medical Association[20,26]. The technical and economic feasibility of fire-safe cigarettes has been demonstrated by research performed by the National Bureau of Standards[26]. Unfortunately, commercial production of such cigarettes has not been undertaken and the federal funding of research designed to prevent 'only 1500 deaths' a year has been questioned in view of the other known health hazards of smoking[27].

The usefulness of smoke detectors was not addressed by this study. Smoke detectors are widely believed to decrease the risk of a fatal home fire by 40–50 percent[17,28,29], however, detection of a fire is not synonymous with successful escape, and at least one study suggests that smoke detectors do not reduce the fire-death rate for those with cognitive or physical disability[13]. Since nearly 40 percent of the fatalities in the present study were at the extremes of age, the efficacy of smoke detectors as a preventive measure is difficult to assess.

Residential fire sprinklers are an evolving technology derived from long-term industrial experience. It is estimated that residential sprinklers in combination with smoke detectors could reduce home fire fatalities by up to 73 percent[1]. In the future, this combination may prove to be particularly useful in protecting the impaired, the young and the elderly from fires in the home[30].

Fire in the home represents a significant hazard. The age groups most likely to be affected include those least likely to survive the physiological challenges of a burn injury. Physicians providing paediatric or geriatric care should stress the dangers of fire in the home and should promote home fire safety. Smoking cessation should be encouraged, both to decrease cardiopulmonary morbidity and mortality and to decrease the likelihood of thermal injury. Patients who continue to smoke should be warned about the dangers of smoking in bed and smoking while intoxicated, as these activities are hazardous to both smoker and to those living in close proximity.

Acknowledgements

The assistance of Mary Ellen Nangle, RN, MS with data collection is greatly appreciated.

References

1. Council on Scientific Affairs. Preventing death and injury from fires with automatic sprinklers and smoke detectors. JAMA 1987, 257: 1618 1620.

2. Baker SP, O'Neill B, Ginsburg Mj, Li G, eds. Fire, burns and lightning. In: The Injury Fact Book, 2nd edn. New York: Oxford University Press, 1992.

3. Hall JR, Cote AE. America's fire problem and fire protection. In: Cote AE, Linville JL, eds. Fire Protection Handbook, 17th edn. Quincy, MA: National Fire Protection Association, 1991.

4. East MK, Jones CA, Feller 1, Saxon MI, Wolfe RA. Epidemiology of burns in children. In: Carvajal HF, Parks DH, eds. Burns in Children: pediatric burn management. Chicago: Year-book Medical Publishers, 1988.

5. United States Fire Administration. Fire in the United States 1983 1987 and Highlights for 1988. Publication no. FA94. Emmitsburg, MD: Federal Emergency Management Agency, US Fire Administration, 1990.

6. Pruitt BA Jr, Mason AD, Goodwin CW. Epidemiology of burn injury and demography of burn care facilities. Prob Gen Surg 1990; 7: 235–251.

7. Barilo Dj, Rush BF, Goode R, Lin RL, Freda A, Anderson E. Is ethanol the unknown toxin in smoke inhalation injury? Am Surg 1986; 52: 641–645.

8. National Household Fire Survey. US Bureau of the Census, 1974.

9. O'Ya H, Ohmori S. Most burns are preventable. Burns 1978; 5: 8–11.

10. Birky MM, Halpin BM, Caplan YH, Fisher RS, McAllister JM, Dixon AM. Fire fatality study. Fire Mater 1979, 3: 211–217.

11. Mierley MC, Baker SP. Fatal house fires in an urban population. JAMA 1983; 249: 1466–1468.

12. Anderson RA, Watson AA, Harland WA. Fire deaths in the Glasgow area: 1 general considerations and pathology. Med Sci Law 1981; 21: 175–183.

13. Runyan CK Bandiwala SI, Linzer MA, Sacks jj, Butts J. Risk factors for residential fires. New Engl J Med 1992; 327: 859–863.

14. Barillo DJ, Goode P, Fitzpatrick J. Cyanide and carbo xyhemoglobin levels in fire fatalities. (publication pending)

15. Barillo DJ, Goode R. Substance abuse in fire victims. J Burn Care Rehabil (in press).

26

16. Bradley HL. One- and two-family dwellings. In: Cote AE, Linville JL, eds. *Fire Protection Handbook,* 17th edn. Quincy, MA: National Fire Protection Association, 1991.

17. Hall JR. Use of fire loss information. In: Cote AE, Linville JL, eds. *Fire Protection Handbook*, 17th edn. Quincy MA: National Fire Protection Association, 1991.

18. Anous MM, Heimbach DM. Causes of death and predictors in burned patients more than 60 years of age. *J Trauma* 1986; 26:135–139.

19. Burge jj, Katz B, Edwards R et al. Surgical treatment of burns in elderly patients. *J Trauma* 1988; 28: 214–217.

20. Patetta Mj, Cole TB. A population-based descriptive study of housefire deaths in North Carolina. *Am J Public Health* 1990; 80: 1116–1117.

21. Demling RH. Medical progress: burns. *New Engl j Med* 1985; 313:1389–1397.

22. Jay KM, Bartlett RH, Danet R, Allyn PA. Burn epidemiology, a basis for burn prevention. J Trauma 1977, 17: 943–947.

23. Centres for Disease Control. Public health surveillance of 1990 injury control objectives for the nation. MMWR 1988; 37 (SS-1): 139–145.

24. Centres for Disease Control. Leads from the MMWR. Regional distribution of deaths from residential fires—United States 197-1984. JAMA 1987; 258: 2355–2356.

25. Baker SP. What keeps the home fires burning? *New Engl j Med* 1992; 327:887–888.

26. Botkin JR. The fire-safe cigarette. JAMA 1986; 260:226–229.

27. Popp Mj. Fleecing the taxpayer to develop a fire-safe cigarette (letter). JAMA 1988; 260: 2664.

28. Hall JR. The US experience with smoke detectors: who has them, how well do they work, when don't they work? *NFPA Journal* 1994; 88: 36–46.

29. Hall HR. A decade of detectors: measuring the effect. *Fire J* 1985; 79:37–43.

30.	Langley J. Deaths to the elderly in residential institutions due to major fires (letter). *New Zealand Med j* 1989, 102:419.

— by D. J. Barillo[1] and R. Goode[2]

[1]Newark Fire Department and [2]Edwin Albano Institute of Forensic Science, Newark, New Jersey, USA

Chapter 4

Trends in
Burn-Care-Facilities Usage

Abstract

Recent estimates related to annual burn incidence and medical care use in the United States include 5500 deaths from fire and burns (1991), 51,000 acute hospital admissions for burn injury (1991 to 1993 average), and 1.25 million total burn injuries (1992). Time trends from 1971 to 1991 reveal significant declines in each estimate. Taking into account the 25 percent increase in the U.S. population during this period, the rates of decline in deaths attributed to fire and burns and acute hospitalization for burn injury are both about 50 percent. The rates of decline are similar in sample statistics for all burns receiving medical care and for all burns above a reportable level of severity. In addition to providing current and time-series estimates, this chapter discusses burn injury coding issues and describes the data sources from which national and state estimates can be derived. The principal objective is to establish and describe a set of burn injury data baselines in a manner that will facilitate future tracking of burn incidence and medical care use at the national and state level by practitioners and researchers. (*J Burn Care Rehabil* 1996;17:95-107).

Accurate and timely statistics are crucial to understanding patterns and trends in burn injury incidence, causes, medical care use, costs, and outcomes.

No single data system at the state or national level captures these aspects of all injuries. Therefore composite statistical profiles for burns and other injuries must be drawn from a variety of data sources and systems, each of which has its own purpose. These sources range from vital statistics registries, which count all births and deaths in the population, to ongoing surveys, whose sample sizes may require combining several years of data to achieve an acceptable level of validity.

Drawing on a historical review of major data sources, we present recent national estimates for deaths from fire and burns, hospital admissions for burn injury (to hospitals with and without burn centers), and total burn incidence. Table 4.1 depicts these estimates and their primary sources.

Sufficient statistics are now available dating back to the early 1970s to enable the tracking of general trends in these estimates. This review reveals significant declines in the national incidence of burn injury and medical care use during the past two decades. This progress coincides with an increased national focus on burn treatment and prevention. During this period regional burn treatment centers have been established in virtually every major population center, smoke detectors have come into widespread use, fire and burn prevention education has expanded substantially, and regulation of consumer product and occupational safety has increased significantly. The lower burn incidence also reflects other societal changes, such as overall declines in smoking[1] and alcohol abuse,[2] changes in home cooking practices,[3] and reduced industrial employment.

Reduced hospitalization for burn injury also reflects a shift in treatment from inpatient to outpatient settings, resulting from upgraded pre-hospital and emergency department treatment and new financial incentives. Hospital admissions overall have declined sharply, reflecting changing technology, the introduction in 1983 of Diagnosis-Related Group—based payment in the federal Medicare program, and the adoption of more stringent reimbursement policies by most other third-party payers.

Table 4.1. Major U.S. Fire/Burn Death and Burn Injury Statistics

Statistic	Annual estimate	Main data source
Fire and burn deaths	5,500 (1991)	Vital Statistics of the United States
Acute hospital admissions for burns	51,000 (1991-1993)	NHDS
Burn center hospitals only	23,000 (1992)	ABA burn center director survey
Total burn incidence	1.25 million (1992)	(Composite estimate derived from four federal surveys)

Material

For this chapter we reviewed available federal government and independent publications and obtained unpublished data from several sources. Most federal burn injury statistics are derived from surveys sponsored by the National Center for Health Statistics (NCHS). Other public agencies or private organizations active in national data collection and analysis relevant to burn injury include the American Burn Association (ABA), the National Fire Protection Association (NFPA), the National Highway Safety Traffic Administration, the U.S. Consumer Product Safety Commission, and the U.S. Fire Administration (USFA). Data were also analyzed from admissions to the Burn Foundation's burn center consortium and from statewide data bases for Pennsylvania and California, two of an increasing number of states with comprehensive hospital discharge data systems.

Coding Systems and Issues

A review of coding systems and related issues is essential as background to a discussion of burn injury statistics. The coding scheme currently used in the United States to classify vital records data is the Ninth Revision of the International Statistical Classification of Diseases, Injuries, and Causes of Death (ICD-9), produced by the World Health Organization. The ICD includes disease and nature of injury codes and a supplementary classification of external cause of injury (E codes).

Deaths attributed to injuries are presented in national vital statistics by E code (e.g., fire, flames) rather than the physical diagnosis (burns, multi-organ failure, pneumonia, etc.), although the latter information is normally part of the death certificate.

Although the vital statistics system captures virtually every death in the United States, the tradition of categorizing deaths with respect to a single, cause is especially problematic for burn injuries, where it can obscure the relationship between external causes and their physical manifestations, the combined impact of burns and other injuries, notably smoke inhalation, and the role of pre-injury conditions.[4-6] This makes it impossible to derive a specific number for "burn deaths," as will be discussed with respect to deaths from fire, electricity, and the late effect of injury. Other issues related to injury coding in general[7] and burn coding in particular[8] have been described in detail by Baker and Langley.

Although the national vital statistics system has always classified *fatal* injuries according to the external cause, the drive to document

31

the causes of *all* injury morbidity only gained momentum in the late 1980s.[9] By the end of 1994, 16 states had mandated that E codes be assigned to all injury-related hospital inpatient records. A broadly endorsed proposal also recently called for the standardization and E coding of injury-related emergency department records.[10]

Coding changes in the Tenth Revision of the ICD provide for improved recording of injury activities and where they took place. The expansion of the code set at what is now E code 924, will also improve the identification of specific vehicles and vectors for burns caused by hot liquids, substances, and objects. Thus our knowledge of particular burn injury scenarios and our ability to develop more precisely targeted prevention strategies should improve after ICD-10 is adopted in the United States by the end of the 1990s.[11]

In assessing the meaning of burn injury statistics, a distinction between treatment and incidence data should also be noted. There is

Table 4.2. Summary of External Causes of Deaths Associated with Fire and Burns

Type	No.
Counts	
Fire and flame	
A. Unintentional	4,120
B. Assault, suicide and undermined intent	516
Hot liquids, substances, and objects (includes caustics and corrosives)	125
Subtotal	4,761
Estimates	
Motor vehicle accidents	600
Electricity, lightning	80
Aircraft crashes	50
Other fire and burn injuries	20
Subtotal	750
Combined counts and estimates	5,511

(*Sources: Vital Statistics of the United States,* 1987 to 1989, and 1991; NFPA surveys, 1985 to 1992; NHTSA data, 1979 to 1986; Pennsylvania vital statistics, 1992; California hospital discharge data, 1992; Burn Foundation burn center registry data, 1987 to 1990.)

minor duplication of injuries in hospital discharge data and moderate duplication in outpatient visit data. Medical care statistics are only approximate indicators of injury severity, because caretakers may seek medical treatment for a burn sustained by a young child that an adult would ignore or self-treat, and the professional decision to treat and release or admit a patient may hinge on social factors such as the availability of caretakers, suspected child abuse, or distance from the patient's residence. Trends in burn treatment statistics also reflect the influence of more general trends in health care management and finance.

Results

Fire and Burn Deaths

Estimates. There were an estimated 5500 deaths in the United States in 1991 in which fire and burn injury played a major role. For that year the NCHS identified 4636 deaths from fire and flames and 125 from hot liquids, substances, and objects. Of the fire and flame deaths, 4120 were classified as "unintentional," and 516 were attributed to suicide, assault, or undetermined intent (Table 4.2).[12]

An estimated 750 additional deaths occurred in 1991 in which fire and burns were partially or totally responsible. These deaths were assigned E codes not limited to fire or burn injury, including motor vehicle and aircraft crashes, boat explosions, contact with electrical current or lightning, and other occupational accidents. Most of the additional fire and burn-related deaths resulted from motor vehicle crashes (about 600, or 1 percent to 2 percent, of all vehicle crash deaths) and electricity or lightning (about 80, or 10 percent, of all such deaths) (Table 4.3).

Combining these counts and estimates produced an estimate of 5511 deaths linked to fire and burns in 1991, which we rounded to 5500.

Trends. Based on U.S. Vital Statistics reports, deaths attributed to fire and flames and hot liquid, substance, or object contact dropped an estimated 40 percent from 1971 to 1991.[13] The 1991 figure is a count of 4761, as noted above. The 1971 figure of 7800 is an estimate developed by the authors because data in some E codes were unavailable before 1979. That year the United States adopted the Ninth Revision of the ICD, which added fourth digits identifying thermal mechanisms to the E codes for otherwise unspecified suicide, assault,

Table 4.3. Estimates of 1991 fire and burn deaths in E codes other than fire and flame or hot object/substance contact

E CODE		Total Deaths (approximate)	% Fire/burn (estimate)	Total fire/burn (approximate)
Description	No.			
Motor vehicle accident	E810-25	40,000	1.5	600
Explosion, fire, or burning in watercraft	E 837	10	50	5
Aircraft crash	E840	1,000	5	50
Lightning	E907	100	5	5
Machinery	E919	1,000	<1	0-5
Explosion of pressure vessel	E921	50	<10	0-5
Explosive materials	E923	200	5	5-10
Electric current	E925	750	10	75
Late effects	E929, 959 969, 989			5
All other, unspecified	Miscellaneous			10
TOTAL				750

(*Sources: Vital Statistics of the United States,* 1987 to 1989; NFPA, 1985 to 1992[motor vehicle accident data only]; Pennsylvania Vital Statistics, 1992; California hospital discharge data, 1992; Burn Foundation burn center registry data, 1987 to 1990.)

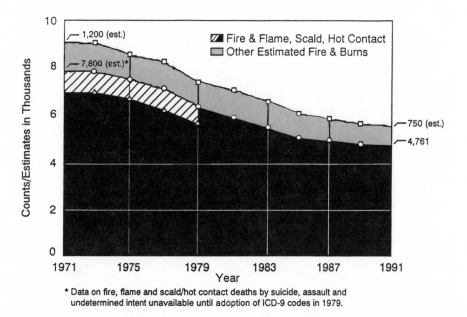

* Data on fire, flame and scald/hot contact deaths by suicide, assault and undetermined intent unavailable until adoption of ICD-9 codes in 1979.

Figure 4.1. *Estimated deaths from fire and burns, 1971 to 1991. Categories shown are: (1) estimates (1971 to 1979) and counts (1979 to 1991) of deaths in E codes specific to fire/flame and hot substance/object contact and (2) estimated deaths in E codes not limited to fire and burns.* (Sources: Vital Statistics of the United States, *Burn Foundation Registry, California hospital discharge, NFPA, NHTSA, and Pennsylvania vital statistics data.)*

34

and undetermined intent. Because the ratio of fire and flame deaths coded "unintentional" to those now assigned to these other categories has remained about 8:1 since 1979, we used the same ratio to derive a more inclusive estimate of total fire and flame deaths for 1971 through 1979.

Based on a 20-year review of vital statistics trends in other E code categories that contain some fire and burn deaths, it appears that deaths from fire and burns in these other categories have dropped at a rate remarkably similar to that of the decline in E codes limited to fire and burns. Accordingly, we estimate that total deaths in the United States related to fire and, burns also declined about 40 percent from 1971 to 1991, from about 9000 to 5500 (Figure 4.1).

To the degree that inhalation injury and burns can be distinguished as causes of fire deaths, it appears that deaths from burns have declined even more rapidly. In tracking national vital statistics data for structure fire deaths from 1979 to 1990, Hall and Harwood[14,15] noted that deaths attributed to burns dropped 51 percent, whereas those coded as smoke inhalation only dropped 12 percent. By 1990 of 3607 deaths in structure fires, 2755 (76.4 percent) were attributed to smoke inhalation and just 730 (20.2 percent) to burns, with the other 122 deaths (3.4 percent) coded "other" or "unknown."

Burn deaths may have declined more rapidly as a result of successful prevention strategies and improved burn care. Smoke inhalation deaths may have declined more slowly because of the vulnerability of the human respiratory system, the prevalence of toxic hazards, and more rapid smoke spread related to changes in the composition of materials in the built environment. Improved coding of fire deaths may also help explain the difference, as suggested by an in-depth study of the medical and physical causes of Maryland fire deaths in the late 1970s, in which only 10 percent of deaths were attributed to burns."

Data Sources.

Vital Statistics. The Vital Statistics Division of NCHS publishes national statistics annually in three volume sets of Vital Statistics of the United States. These statistics are drawn from the birth and death certificate files in the state vital statistics offices that record vital events occurring in the United States. The states obtain mortality data from death certificates filed by funeral directors, who must obtain medical examiner or coroner certification of the causes of any injury-related deaths. NCHS combines state statistics into national totals.

Because of the many steps in this process, the bound volumes of national statistics currently do not appear until several years after the events they record. With the spread of emerging technology, the data from which these statistics are drawn is increasingly accessible through public use data tapes and CD-ROMS, available from the National Technical Information Services and through CDC WONDER, a new multiple database information system from the Centers for Disease Control and Prevention.[17] Additional death certificate data available from electronic sources can be especially useful to reviews of multiple causes, physical effects, and significant conditions related to fire and burn deaths.

The "single cause" limitation of published statistics, identified previously with respect to the roles of flame and smoke in fire deaths, creates similar problems for distinguishing the effects of thermal and kinetic energy in electrical injury trauma.

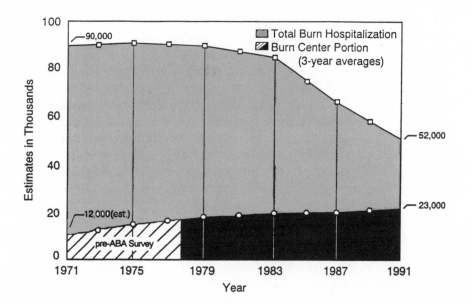

Figure 4.2. Hospital admissions for burn injury, 1971 to 1991. Burn center admissions are presented as portion of total burn admissions. Plotted points are 3-year averages. Burn center admission estimates before 1976 are projections based on number of burn center beds then in operation. (Sources: NHDS and ABA.)

In estimating deaths from electrical injury that can be attributed to burns, we excluded pre-hospital deaths from lightning or electrical injury, the great majority of which result from cardiopulmonary arrest at the scene" and included only those deaths occurring in burn centers. We concluded that about 10 percent of the nation's 800 deaths a year from electrical and lightning injury occur in burn centers, which was calculated as follows. In a region where 5 percent of the nation's burn center patients are treated, electrical injury, which is frequently accompanied by a substantial surface burn resulting from the ignition of clothing, accounted for about 7 percent of burn center admissions (unpublished 1987 to 1992 regional data: Burn Foundation). This total projects to 1200 to 1500 admissions a year nationally. An aggregate 7 percent mortality rate was calculated from a review of 14 studies of high-voltage electrical injuries treated in burn centers, published between 1969 and 1986.[19] Because overall burn treatment outcomes have improved during the past 20 years and the threshold of severity for referral to a burn center has declined, we used a 5 percent mortality rate estimate in deriving our estimate of 80 deaths in burn centers per year associated with both high-and low-voltage (23,000 admissions x 7 percent electrical x 5 percent mortality = 80 deaths) and assumed that no such deaths occurred in general hospitals.

Multiple causes present a particular challenge to coding the cause of deaths of the injured elderly.[20] As burn centers continue to improve in their ability to extend life after severe burn injury, elderly patients are more likely to survive the incident and the acute care hospital stay. Nonetheless, their deaths are likely to be hastened by the impact of severe injury on their physiologic reserves,[21] and "late effect" of burns and other injuries is rarely coded as the cause of death.

Fire Service Reports. The NFPA surveys annually the fire experience of a stratified sample of fire departments, including most large departments, and publishes estimates of civilian and firefighter fire deaths the following year.[22] In 41 states some or all fire departments also contribute data on fire incidents to the USFA-sponsored National Fire Incident Reporting System (NFIRS). USFA relies mainly on NFIRS data for its estimates of fire deaths, which appear in its periodically published reports on the U.S. fire experience.[23] Because the fire death component of the vital statistics count does not differ significantly from fire service survey estimates and because most deaths associated with burns result from fires, NFPA and USFA analyses remain the best sources of detailed information on fatal injury scenarios for the majority of deaths in which burns were a factor.[24-25]

Other Data Sources. The recent estimate of 600 fire-related vehicle crash deaths per year is based on unpublished NFPA data for 1986 to 1992. Several sources confirm a downward trend of about 40 percent in such deaths over the preceding two decades.[26-28]

Hospitalized Burns

From 1991 to 1993, an annual average of 51,000 hospital discharges were recorded for burn injury, an estimated 45 percent of them by the nation's 137 burn centers. Admissions estimates and data sources for the hospitals with and without burn centers are discussed separately. Because of their partial dependence on each other, trends in admissions to the two hospital groups are reviewed together.

Burn Center Admissions

Estimates. There were an estimated 23,000 total burn center admissions in 1992 and an estimated 1200 in hospital deaths among these admissions.

Data Sources. The ABA maintains a burn facility directory based on a regular survey of physician members known to be active in burn care.[29] About 80 percent of the surveyed physicians typically provide counts or rounded estimates of admissions to their burn service. To estimate total burn center admissions, we used the burn center universe of 137 facilities identified in an independent 1992 survey,[30] combined admissions counts and estimates where reported by physicians at these facilities, and assumed that non-responding facilities admitted a similar number of patients per burn unit bed. Allowing for occasional readmissions during the acute care stage, the admissions estimate may be 1 percent to 2 percent higher than the number of injuries it represents.[31]

The estimate of 1200 deaths in burn centers was projected from the 5.1 percent burn center mortality rate in the first compilation of data from the new ABA burn patient registry, to which 22 burn centers contributed data on admissions during 1991 through 1993.[32] The registry is now being merged with the trauma registry of the American College of Surgeons, and the ABA/TRACS registry is likely to become a major source of information on burn epidemiology and trends in burn treatment outcomes. The new registry supersedes the National Burn Information Exchange, which collected data on 110,000 burn injuries hospitalized between 1969 and 1987 in 60 participating burn centers.[33]

NFPA and burn center data show that populations experiencing fire injuries and requiring burn center treatment overlap only moderately. For example, among firefighters only 7000 of the 100,000 injuries reported in 1993 were classified as burns. The rest were attributed to causes such as lacerations, strains, smoke or gas inhalation, and thermal stress.[34] In the absence of a burn injury, a serious fire injury will usually be treated at the closest appropriate general hospital. Conversely, most burns treated in burn centers do not result from fires, and burn centers also admit patients with medical problems such as toxic epidermal necrolysis syndrome,[35] a disorder involving severe skin loss.

Total Burn Hospitalizations

Estimates. The National Hospital Discharge Survey (NHDS) estimated 54,000 hospital discharges with a principal diagnosis of burn injury in 1993. Estimates for the previous 2 years were 46,000 in 1992 and 52,000 in 1991,[1] resulting in a 3-year average of 51,000.

Because most persons with severe burn injuries who survive long enough to reach a hospital alive are transferred to burn centers, deaths from burns in general hospitals are rare. The general hospital burn mortality rate of 1.5 percent in 1991 Pennsylvania data projects to only 200 such deaths nationally per year. Most deaths occur quickly in patients considered unlikely to survive a transfer to a burn center.

Subtracting 1400 combined burn center and general hospital burn deaths from 5500 total fire and burn deaths leaves an estimated 4100 other deaths from fire and burns. Most such other deaths occur at the scene or en route to a hospital. Some may have occurred in hospitals, from inhalation injury, or from other fire-related trauma.

The NHDS estimated in 1991 another 8000 acute hospital discharges in which burn injury was coded as a secondary diagnosis. Most of these patients were treated in non-burn center hospitals, where they have normally made up about one fourth of all admissions for which a burn diagnosis was recorded. Because it is unknown whether the burn injury alone would have been serious enough to have caused these admissions, we have not included them in total burn discharge estimates.

Data Sources. NHDS samples from which acute care discharge estimates are currently drawn include about 250,000 discharges (about 1 percent of the total) from 440 short-term hospitals.[36] The 95 percent confidence interval for NHDS estimates of acute burn discharges from 1991 to 1993 is approximately plus or minus 10,000.

These samples contain too few burns (around 400) for estimates by age or region to have statistical significance. In contrast, state-level hospital databases represent a promising source of data for such analyses. Some 30 states now have published a variety of reports, although data on a subset as specific as burn injury may be accessible only by commissioning a special report from the state data agency.

Trends (in burn admissions to general and specialized facilities). A comparison of NHDS statistics to data collected by the ABA reveals a sharp decline in burn admissions to hospitals without burn centers, which is in contrast with a smaller but steady increase in burn center admissions (Figure 4.2).

In 1970 the NHDS estimated 90,000 hospital discharges in the United States with a principal diagnosis of burn injury. After fluctuating generally between 85,000 and 95,000 until the mid 1980s, the NHDS estimate began to decline at an accelerating rate, failing to just 46,000 in 1992. From 1971 to 1991, the rate of hospital discharges with a principal diagnosis of burn injury dropped almost 50 percent, from 45 to 23 per 100,000. Hospital discharges with a secondary diagnosis of burn injury also fell. Conversely, burn center admissions have increased from roughly 15,000 to 23,000 since the ABA began to survey burn center directors in 1976.

The subtraction of burn center admissions from total burn admissions reveals a decline from 70,000 to 30,000 since 1976 in burn admissions to hospitals without burn centers. This represents more than a simple shift to burn centers, since after 15 years there were five fewer general hospital burn admissions for every added burn center admission. Other factors include a shift in treatment from inpatient to outpatient settings, independent of severity, and improvements in triage that have nearly eliminated general hospital admissions of patients ultimately transferred to a burn center. Even after allowing for these changes in practice, it appears that both the average severity and overall number of burn injuries have declined significantly.

The current dominance of burn center hospitals as the treatment site for burn injuries is greater than admissions totals alone might suggest. The 23,000 burn admissions estimated for 137 burn center hospitals in 1992 represented an average of 168 such admissions per hospital. The nation's other 30,000-odd burn admissions were divided among 5300 other hospitals, an average of only six per hospital. The average length of stay of burn center patients in 1991 Pennsylvania hospitalization data was close to twice that of general hospital burn patients (12 days to 7 days), and because of greater severity of illness, burn center per diem charges were much higher.

Thus burn centers accounted for some two thirds of all hospital days for burn patients and an even greater proportion of all hospital charges incurred by burn patients. In addition to enabling knowledge dispersion among burn treatment specialists to benefit a greater proportion of burn patients, this concentration of burn treatment resources in burn centers increases the value of epidemiologic and treatment cost data to the planning and evaluation of burn prevention programs and safety measures.

Recent regional data suggest that despite the growing concentration of patients with burn injuries in specialized centers, burn center admissions may have begun to decline. For example, annual admissions to the Burn Foundation's regional consortium of four burn centers peaked at 656 in 1991 and had dropped slightly to 642 by the end of 1994. Average length of stay nationally in burn centers has also declined, from about 16 to 13 days since 1980. The combined impact of falling admissions and shorter length of stay is likely to accelerate the closure of smaller burn units or their merger with other services.[37]

By the end of 1995, we expect that national, burn center admissions will reflect a slight decline since 1992. Further projections of burn center admissions remain conjectural, because they depend on future trends in burn incidence and in admissions, referral, and length of stay patterns, as affected by clinical progress and by the major transition that the overall health care system is currently undergoing.

Table 4.4. Estimates of total burn incidence and treated burn injuries (1957 to 1993)

Survey period	Annual incidence estimate*	Percent treated*	Total treated	U.S. population (in millions)	Treatment rate (per 1000)
1957-1961	1,973,000	87.1	1,719,000	175	9.8
1965-1967	2,233,000	86.5	1,932,000	190	10.2
1980-1981	2,130,000	75.8	1,615,000	225	7.2
* *					
1985-1987	1,753,000	92.1	1,614,000	235	6.9
1991-1993	1,129,000	95.0	1,073,000	255	4.2

(*Source: Series 10 Publications of the National Health Interview Survey, originally the National Health Survey*)

*Because NHIS adopted a more restrictive definition of reportable injury when revising its survey method in 1982, total injury point estimates before and after that date do not represent a true time series.

Total Burn Patients Treated and Total Burn Incidence

Estimates. All total treatment and incidence estimates drawn from national surveys have large standard errors because of the relatively small number of burns in their samples. For this chapter we blended point estimates from four federal surveys to derive an estimate of 1.25 million total burn injuries in 1992.

Trends. The National Health Interview Survey (NHIS) is the only federal survey to have published a series of total burn injury and treatment estimates during the period covered in this chapter. The NHIS is also the only survey that embraces all treatment sites and total incidence, based on data collected in household interviews. Estimates reported in two early NHIS injury publications suggest a stable rate of medically attended burn injuries in the late 1950s and 1960s (around 10/1000 population).[38,39] The rate derived from the next estimate published by the NHIS for 1980 to 1981 had dropped to 7.2/1000.[40] Rates derived from more recent NHIS studies were 6.8/1000 in 1985 to 1987[41] and only 4.2/1000 in 1991 to 1993 (Table 4.4).[42] A graph displaying these rates as a time trend is not included, because the potentially large variance resulting from sampling error renders trend lines misleading.

The potential impact of sampling error is reflected in the decline of 38 percent between the point estimates for burn injury in NHIS reports based on 1985 to 1987 and 1991 to 1993 data (from 1.753 to 1.129 million injuries). The unlikely possibility of such a large drop in incidence in 6 years provides a useful caution against over-reliance on the point estimate for burns in any single national survey. The authors accordingly derived a blended 1992 burn incidence estimate by combining NHIS statistics with estimates from three other federal surveys. This blended estimate of 1.25 million burn injuries, whose derivation will be described, also brings the estimated decline in rates of total burn injury during the past 20 years roughly in line with the 50 percent declines in rates for fire and burn death and hospitalized burn injury.

The need to track trends in specific statistics can also conflict with the need to revise continuous surveys. After NHIS tightened its definition of a reportable injury in 1982, as part of the update that follows every decennial census, previous and subsequent estimates of total injuries could no longer be used in a time series.

For historical interest, we have nonetheless displayed in Table 4.4 all published NHIS estimates for total burn injuries as well as for those requiring medical attention, whose definition has not changed.[41] The first estimate of burn injuries per year published by NHIS was based on household survey responses from July 1957 to June 1961.[42] This estimate, 1.973 million, is the apparent original source of the "two million burns per year" statistic frequently, used in the burn literature ever since.

Data Sources. In deriving the estimate of 1.25 total million burn injuries in 1992, we combined NHIS point estimates with recent outpatient treatment estimates from the National Hospital Ambulatory Medical Care Survey (NHAMCS), which began data collection in 1992, the National Ambulatory Medical Care Survey (NAMCS), which has collected data from physicians' offices since 1973, and the 1987 National Medical Expenditure Survey (NMES).

Since 1956 the NHIS has continuously collected in household interviews a wide variety of data on the health status and health service experience of the U.S. population. In recent years NHIS has interviewed an average of 45,000 households, with approximately 120,000 members. An NHIS interview includes both standard and special supplemental questions. In one standard question respondents are asked whether any household member has received an injury, within the previous 2 weeks and whether medical treatment was provided for that injury.

For 1992, NHAMCS calculated a point estimate of 679,000 hospital emergency department visits for burn injury. For those with E codes, an estimated 473,000 were identified in E924 (hot substances, etc.) and 127,000 in the E890-99 series (fire-and flame-related accidents).[43] The presence of repeat visits in emergency department data is reflected in a 1987 NMES estimate of 1.22 emergency department visits for each injury.[44] In 1992 NHAMCS also estimated an additional 121,000 hospital outpatient department visits for burn injury, 56 percent of which represented follow-up visits.

NAMCS estimated 1,073,000 physician office visits for burn treatment in 1991. The survey estimated that 72 percent of the burn visits were either new patients or new problems, but like NHAMCS, did not determine whether patients new to the treatment site had previously been treated elsewhere for the presenting problem.

From these several distinct surveys we derived a 1992 estimate of roughly 1.2 million treated burn injuries, half of which were treated in hospital emergency and other outpatient departments and half by private physician offices. The additional estimated 50,000 unattended burns result from the total definition of burn injury used by NHIS.

(NHIS defines an injury as an event that either necessitated medical attention or caused activity restriction for at least one-half day. For 1991 to 1993, 95.0 percent of all burn injuries were estimated to have received medical attention.)

Given the accelerating transition of health care from inpatient to outpatient settings, major improvements in outpatient care statistics are likely in the near future. Systems managing all care for specific populations are devoting increased attention to distinguishing patients from patient visits and analyzing the reasons for such visits. At the federal level the Prospective Payment Advisory Commission has recommended that the Health Care Finance Administration extend Medicare's prospective payment system to outpatient care. Improvement in diagnosis and cause-specific outpatient statistics is also anticipated at the state level.

Hospital emergency department data have already proved valuable in the surveillance of product-related burn injury. The U.S. Consumer Product Safety Commission derives annual estimates of injuries related to specific products from data on emergency department encounters in a sample of 90 hospitals that currently participate in its National Electronic Injury Surveillance System (NEISS).[45]

State and Local Burn Injury Profiles

With the expansion of inpatient and outpatient data collection and the spread of E code mandates at the state level, there are increasing opportunities to monitor state and local trends in burn incidence and medical care use for the great majority of burn injuries without relying on projections from national sample statistics.

Local and regional subsets of data on inpatient and outpatient burn admissions, combined with population data, may provide a baseline for studies of the effectiveness of educational, social service, and legislative interventions aimed at the prevention of burn injury, although the complexities of real-world conditions make it difficult to evaluate the effectiveness of specific interventions.[46-49]

Although the NEISS system has proved valuable in product-related injury surveillance at the national level, most injury surveillance activity in the United States, as with public health services in general, is authorized and carried out at the state and local level.[50,51] Interest in linking burn injury cause data to prevention strategies, sometimes combined with the desire, to identify potential arsonists through medical reports, has led in at least 21 states to the passage of legislation mandating the reporting of some or all burn injuries to a unit of state government.[52]

The results of these state laws range from minimally monitored data collection efforts to programs with a structured surveillance component. For example, in Oklahoma, detailed reports on hospitalized burn injuries, followed up by state health department personnel to achieve completeness, provide the basis for frequent "injury update" publications dedicated to burns that present detailed anecdotes, discuss burn injury patterns, and recommend prevention strategies.[53] Such active surveillance is expensive, even when limited to hospital admissions, and is unlikely to be established as a routine local or state health department activity throughout the nation.[54]

Summary and Recommendations

Burn incidence and medical care use estimates for the United States from 1971 through 1991 reveal that rates for more serious burn injuries (indicated by death or hospitalization) have declined dramatically, by 50 percent. National sample statistics suggest a similar decline in less severe injuries during the same period. These trends coincide with the development of a national network of burn centers, wide dissemination of fire and burn prevention devices and programs, and broader societal changes whose effect in reducing burn incidence has been positive if not directly intended.

The availability of data making it possible to monitor these trends has improved substantially during this period, reflecting the growth of health-related data systems and the increasing specificity of the code sets used in them. State health care data systems in particular have been expanding in the 1990s.

To enhance the availability of information on trends in burn epidemiology, including medical care use, we urge the continued strengthening of national health surveys and state-level health care data systems, an expansion of such systems, including E coding, to additional states and to outpatient and emergency department records, and the prompt implementation of ICD-10 in the United States. A cooperative effort is also needed at all levels to develop appropriate data sets and establish systems to collect information on long-term outcomes of burn injury.

The publication of E-coded statistics drawn from hospital discharge and emergency department data will improve the overall understanding of burn epidemiology, especially regarding the generally unexplored relationship between cause and severity level. As previously noted, although 125 deaths occurred in 1991 from contact with hot liquids, substances, and objects, such contacts accounted for close to

500,000 emergency department visits. In contrast, fires started by dropped cigarettes are responsible for eight times as many deaths (about 1000/year) but only about 3000 injuries to civilians (non-firefighters).[55]

We encourage individual investigators to take advantage of newly available state and national data to examine burn incidence and epidemiology at all levels of severity. We also suggest that the community most concerned with the prevention and treatment of burn injuries assume the responsibility for compiling and publishing on a regular basis an updated profile of burn injury incidence and medical care use, with a brief guide to data sources.

At the national level the assumption of such a function would be consistent with the mission of the ABA, which embraces the treatment, research, rehabilitation, and prevention of burn injury, with a particular focus on severe injury. Such a profile could be published in the *Journal of Burn Care and Rehabilitation*, the official publication of the ABA, and made available to the public in fact sheet form.

State-level profiles could be developed through cooperation between a state's health data agency and its burn centers or their support organizations, in states where data are now collected on all hospital discharges. This is especially desirable in states where E codes are now mandated.

In an era of rapidly changing patterns of injury incidence and health care responses, the regular preparation and publication of such profiles are important to burn care management and to planning and evaluating burn prevention initiatives.[56,57]

References

1. US Department of Health and Human Services. Reducing the health consequences of smoking: 25 years of progress: a report of the surgeon general. Rockville, Maryland: Department of Health and Human Services, 1989; publication 89-8411.

2. National Institute on Alcohol Abuse and Alcoholism. Eighth special report to the U.S. Congress on alcohol and health. Epidemiology of alcohol use and alcohol-related consequences. Washington, D.C.: National Institute on Alcohol Abuse and Alcoholism, 1993.

3. Neuborne E. Busy people want meals on demand. *USA Today*, October 4, 1994.

4. Israel RA, Rosenberg HM, Curtin LR Analytical potential for multiple cause-of-death data. *Am J Epidemiol* 1986; 124,2:161-79.

5. Morris JA, MacKenzie Ej, Edelstein SL. The effect of preexisting conditions on mortality in trauma patients. *JAMA* 1990;263,14:1942-6.

6A. McGinnis JM, Foege WH. Actual causes of death in the United States. *JAMA* 1993;270,18:2207-12 [Letter].

6B. *JAMA* 1994;271,9:659-61. Comments on JAMA 1993;270, 18:2207-12.

7. Baker SP. Injury classification and the International Classification of Diseases codes. *Accid Anal Prev* 1982;14:199-201.

8. Langley JD. Description and classification of childhood burns. *Burns* 1984;10:231-5.

9. Sniezek JE, Finklea JF, Graitcer PL. Injury coding and hospital discharge data. *JAMA* 1989;262,16:2270-2.

10. Garrison HG, Runyan CW, Tintinalli JE, et al. Emergency department surveillance: an examination of issues and a proposal for a national strategy. *Ann Emerg Med* 1994;24,5:84956.

11. International Statistical Classification of Diseases and Related Health Problems, 10th Revision, World Health Organization, Geneva, Switzerland, 1992.

12. National Center for Health Statistics, *Vital Statistics of the U.S.*, 1991 (unpublished).

13. National Center for Health Statistics, *Vital Statistics of the U.S.*, 1971-1991.

14. Harwood B, Hall JR. What kills in fires: smoke inhalation or burns? *NFPA Journal* 1989;83,3:29-34.

15. Hall JR, Harwood B. Smoke or burns: which is deadlier? *NFPA Journal* 1995;89,1:38-43.

16. Berl WG, Halpin BM. Human fatalities from unwanted fires. *Fire J* 1979;79,9:105-23.

17. Friede A, Reid JA, Ory Hw. *CDC Wonder*: a comprehensive on-line public health information system of the Centers for Disease Control and Prevention. *Am J Public Health* 1993;83,9:1289-94.

18. Wright Rk, Davis JH. The investigation of electrical deaths: a report of 220 fatalities. *J Forensic Sci* 1980;25,3:514-21.

19. Remensnyder JP. Acute electrical injuries. In: Martyn JAJ, Acute management of the burned patient. Philadelphia: WB Saunders, 1990:66-85.

20. Fife D. Injuries and deaths among elderly persons. *Am J Epidemiol* 1987;126:936-41.

21. Clark W, Fromm B. Burn mortality: experience at a regional burn center, literature review. *Acta Chir Scand* 1987; 537(suppl):1-127.

22. Hall JR, Harwood B. The national estimates approach to U.S.: Fire statistics. *Fire Tech* 1989;25:99-113.

23. Federal Emergency Management Agency, U.S. Fire Administration, National Fire Data Center. Fire in the United States, 1983-1990, 8th ed. Emmitsburg, Maryland 1993, *publication FA-140.*

24. See esp. Conley Cj, Fahy RF. Who dies in fires in the United States? *NFPA Journal* 1994;88,3:99-106.

25. Mierley, MC, Baker SP. Fatal house fires in an urban population. *JAMA* 1983;249,11:1464-8.

26. Partyka SC. Fires and burns in towed light passenger vehicle crashes. Washington, D.C.: National Highway Traffic Safety Administration, 1992.

27. Israel RA, Rosenberg HM, Curtin LR. Analytical potential for multiple cause-of-death data. *Am J Epidemiol* 1986;124: 1942-6.

28. Cooley, P. Fire in motor vehicle accidents. Highway Safety Research Institute, Ann Arbor, Michigan, 1974.

29. Burn Care Resources in North America: annual or biennial directories, 1976-1994. Current directory available from the office of the incumbent Secretary of the American Burn Association.

30. Dimick AR, Brigham PA, Sheehy EM. The Development of Burn Centers in North America. *J Burn Care Rehabil* 1993; 14,2(suppl):284-99.

31. Smith GS, Langlois JA, Buechner JS. Methodological issues in using hospital discharge data to determine the incidence of hospitalized injuries. *Am J Epidemiol* 1991;134: 1146-58.

32. Saffle JR, Davis B, Williams P, et al. Recent outcomes in the treatment of burn injury in the United States: a report from the American Burn Association patient registry. J Burn Care Rehabil 1995;16:219-32.

33. Feller I, Jones CA. The National Burn Information Exchange: the use of a national burn injury registry to evaluate and address the burn problem. *Surg Clin North Am* 1987;67:167-89.

34. Karter MJ, LeBlanc PR. U.S. firefighter injuries in 1993. *NFPA Journal* 1994;88,6:57-66.

35. Jordan MH, Lewis MS, Jeng JG, Rees JM. Treatment of toxic epidermal necrolysis by burn units: another market or another threat? J Burn Care Rehabil 1991;12:579-81.

36. National Center for Health Statistics. National Health Care Survey (brochure), Hyattsville, Maryland, 1993.

37. Fortune JB, Luniewski JK, Rodney KE, Feustel Pj, Millett JM. Reorganization of a burn unit in response to under-utilization: a critical assessment. J Burn Care Rehabil 1992;13:348-55.

38. National Center for Health Statistics, Vital and Health Statistics data from the National Health Survey: types of injuries, incidence and associated disability, United States, July 1957-June 1961. Series 10, Number 8, Washington, D.C., 1964.

39. ____. Types of injuries, incidence and associated disability, United States, July 1965-June 1967. Series 10, Number 57, Washington, DC, 1969.

40. ____. Types of injuries and impairments due to injuries, United States, 1980-1981. Series 10, Number 159,Washington, DC, 1985.

41. ____. Types of injuries by selected characteristics, United States, 1985-1987. Series 10, Number 195, Hyattsville, Maryland, 1990.

42. ____. Types of injuries by selected characteristics: United States, 1991-93. Publication pending in NCHS Series 10, Hyattsville, Maryland, 1996.

43. Burt CW. Injury-related visits to hospital emergency depart-ments: United States, 1992. Advance data from Vital and Health Statistics; Hyattsville, Maryland: National Center for Health Statistics. 1995; No. 261.

44. Cited in Miller T, et al. Societal cost of cigarette fires, final re-port, Fire Safe Cigarette Act of 1990, U.S. Consumer Product Safety Commission, 1990, Vol 6: A-8.

45. U.S. Consumer Product Safety Commission, Division of Haz-ard and Injury Data Systems. The National Electronic Injury, Surveillance System: a description of its role in the U.S. Con-sumer Product Safety Commission, March 1990.

46. McLoughlin E, Vince Cj, Lee AM, Crawford JD. Project burn prevention: outcome and implications. *Am J Public Health* 1982;72,3:241-7.

47. MacKay AM, Rothman Kj. The incidence and severity of burn injuries following project burn prevention. *Am J Public Health* 1982;72,3:248-52.

48. Peck MD, Maley MP. Population requirements for statistical analysis of efficacy of burn prevention programs. J Burn Care Rehabil 1991;12:282-4.

49. Christoffel T, Teret SP. Protecting the public: legal issues in injury prevention. New York: Oxford University Press, 1993.

50. Graitcer PL. The development of state and local injury sur-veillance systems. *J Safety Res* 1987;18:181-98.

51. Wharton M, Vogt RL. State and local issues in surveillance. In: Teutsch SM, Churchill R.E. Principles and practice of pub-lic health surveillance. Oxford: Oxford University Press, 1994.

52. Hammond J. The status of statewide burn prevention legisla-tion. J Burn Carre Rehabil 1993;14:473-5.

53. Pagonis J. Gasoline-related burn injuries, Oklahoma, 1988-92. Injury update, Injury Prevention Service, Oklahoma State Department of Health, August 4, 1994.

54. Rossignol AM, Locke JA. An assessment of the completeness of the Massachusetts Burn Registry. Pub Health Rpts 1983; 98,5:492-6.

55. Miller A. The U.S. smoking-material fire problem. National Fire Protection Association, Fire Analysis and Research Division, October 1993.

56. Feck G, Baptiste MS, Tate CL. Burn injuries: epidemiology and prevention. *Accid Anal Prev* 1979;11: 129-36.

57. Haddon W. Advances in the epidemiology of injuries as a basis for public policy. *Public Health Rep* 1980;95:411-21.

*— by Peter A. Brigham, MSW, and Elizabeth McLoughlin, ScD
Philadelphia, Pennsylvania, and San Francisco, California*

Chapter 5

Socioeconomic Factors and the Geographic Distribution of Burn Care Units

Abstract

Age, occupation, and economic circumstances influence both the incidence of burn injury and the risk of burn death. Flame injury is the most common type of burn for which patients are admitted to burn centers, but scald injuries account for 30 percent of all burns necessitating admission to the hospital. Approximately 300 burn patients per million population require in-hospital care each year because of extent of burn or presence of a complicating factor. Forty-two per million population per year within that group require care at a burn center, where the personnel, equipment, and facilities necessary to address the multi-system effects of severe burn injury are available. Transfer of burn patients must be coordinated between originating and receiving physicians and is best done as soon as resuscitation has restored hemodynamic and pulmonary stability. The resources required to deliver this complex system of burn care are expensive. Current prospective payment methods result in large reimbursement deficits, and the national trend favoring such payment mechanisms threatens the future of burn centers.

Epidemiology

Incidence

The precise occurrence rate of burn injury in the United States is unknown because, except in a few states, burn injury is not a reportable

©April/June 1990 *Problems in General Surgery*, Vol. 7, No. 2. Lippincott Co. Reprinted with permission.

disease. It is commonly estimated that more than two million people sustain burns each year in the United States. Annually there are 6,000 burn-and fire-related deaths, and an additional 500 deaths being attributed to arson or "suspicious circumstances[1,12] (Table 5.1).

Burn Hazards

The risk of burn death and burn injury and the frequencies of causative agents are influenced by age, occupation, and economic circumstances. Death by fire and the risk of burn injury are greatest among the economically disadvantaged, apparently as a consequence of residence in older buildings, use of portable, open-flame-type heating equipment, faulty heating or electrical systems, crowded living conditions, and absence of smoke detectors. House fire death rates among black people and native North Americans are more than twice those of white people, presumably a reflection of the hazards associated with residence in low-income census areas.[3] House fires account for 75 percent of all fire and burn deaths, death rates being highest among young children, who have difficulty escaping because of dependency, and the elderly, who have difficulty escaping because of preexisting disease and decreased agility.[2] House fires are more common on weekends, and fatal house fires are most commonly caused by cigarettes.[2,4] More than half of adults who die in house fires have a high blood alcohol concentration.[5] House fires cause only approximately 4 percent of burn admissions, but the fatality rate among patients hospitalized for burns from conflagrations is higher than for patients with burns from other causes, 12 percent vs 3 percent, presumably because of associated inhalation injury.[2]

Clothing ignition is the second leading cause of burn admissions for most ages.[2] In children such burns are most often caused by inappropriate use of matches and lighters.[6] The burn injury rate resulting from the ignition of clothing is highest in low-income census tracts, there being a relation between burn rates and income for burns resulting from ignition of clothing by appliances and equipment.[7] A recent study in Denmark demonstrated that nursing home patients were most frequently burned when unattended as a consequence of fires ignited by cigarettes.[8] The fatality rate among patients with burns resulting from the ignition of clothing is exceeded only by that of patients with burns incurred in house fires.[2] Clothing-related burns caused by synthetic fabrics that melt and adhere to the skin are commonly deeper than burns caused by other agents and often present in a gravity-directed run-off pattern.

Approximately 112,000 patients with scald burns are seen in hospital emergency rooms annually.[9] Although flame injury is the predominant type of burn for which patients are admitted to burn centers, approximately 30 percent of all burns necessitating admission of a patient to the hospital are caused by scalds from hot liquids.[2,10] The case fatality for scald injuries is low, but scalds are a major cause of morbidity and associated costs, particularly among children younger than 5 years and among the elderly.[11] One survey found that 45 percent of all patients in New York State admitted for scalds were children younger than 5 years.[12] Spillage of hot beverages, particularly coffee, is the preponderant cause of scalds among young children. The most common cause of scalds, and of all hospital admissions for burns in the population as a whole, is hot water, including tap water in bathtubs and showers.[2] A recent survey in Denmark revealed that the kitchen is the working place with the highest risk of burns, most commonly as a result of contact with hot liquids.[13]

One epidemiologic study found that in the 15-to 24-year age group the largest number of burn admissions were related to automobiles. Motor vehicle crashes accounted for more than one-fourth of such burns, and steam from automobile radiators was another frequent cause of burn injury.[2] A 1985 review[14] revealed that among patients burned in motor vehicle accidents, 36 percent had other injuries (most of which were fractures), 36.3 percent had inhalation injury, and 24.7 percent died.

Table 5.1. Burn Injury in the United States

Total burns (estimated)	2,000,000+/yr
Burn and Fire Deaths	6,500/yr
Burn patients treated in emergency departments	500,000/yr
Hospital admissions for acute burn injury(300/million population)	74,000/yr
Burn center admissions Major burns (42/million population) Lesser burns with complicating co-factor (40/million population)	20,000/yr

Workers in the chemical industry are the single group at greatest risk for chemical burns. Workers involved in the manufacture of phosphate-based fertilizers are at increased risk for burns because they work with strong acids and those who are involved in the manufacture of soap are at increased risk for burns because they work with strong alkali. People who work with etching processes and in petroleum refineries are at greatest risk for injury due to hydrofluoric acid.[15]

Electric current causes 1,100 deaths annually, one-third of which occur in the home and one-fourth of which occur on industrial sites or farms.[2] Young children are at greatest risk of electrical injury from household current as a consequence of inserting uninsulated objects into electrical receptacles or biting or sucking on electric cords and sockets.[1] Burns resulting from low-voltage direct current can be produced by contact with automobile battery terminals and by defective or misused medical electronic equipment, such as electro-surgical devices.[16] Such injuries may be full thickness in character but are typically of limited extent. High-voltage electrical injury is more frequent in white than in black people, presumably because of employment patterns. Electricians, particularly those working for utility companies; construction workers working with cranes; farm workers moving irrigation pipes; oil field workers; truck drivers; and people installing antennae are at greatest risk of high voltage electrical injury.[17-19] The summertime peak incidence of electrical injury is related to the seasonal intensity of farm irrigation, construction work, and work on outdoor electrical equipment.

Each year 150 to 300 people in the United States are killed by lightning.[20] Approximately one-fifth of lightning deaths occur on farms. Lightning death rates are highest in the Southern and Mountain states. The death rate resulting from lightning injury is highest in the 10-to 19-year age group. As in the case of high-voltage electrical injury, lightning injury is most common during the summer. People in open fields, recreational golfers, fishermen, and campers are at greatest risk for lightning injury.[2]

Fireworks are another seasonal cause of burn injury. The United States Consumer Products Safety Commission estimated that 11,400 people injured by fireworks in 1981 required treatment in hospital emergency rooms.[21] Of those patients, 8.8 percent required in-hospital care and approximately 60 percent of the injuries were burns.[22] On the basis of such studies, it can be estimated that 1.86 to 5.82 fireworks-related burn injuries per 100,000 persons occur in the United States during the 4th of July holiday.[23] During the 15-year period 1960 through 1974, 3,628 burn patients were admitted to the United States

Army Institute of Surgical Research burn center, of which 4, or 0.1 percent, had been burned by fireworks.

Roofers and paving workers are at greatest risk for burn injury caused by hot tar. Burns from hot bitumen constitute 16 percent of all accidents involving roofers and sheet metal workers, 17 percent of those injuries being of sufficient severity to cause "lost time from work." In 1979, in California alone 366 roofers and slaters sustained burn injuries.[24"] Welding is another occupation associated with an increased risk for burn injury, most commonly because of flash burns and explosions, the incidence of which can be reduced if containers are flushed with nitrogen before welding.

Child abuse is a special form of burn injury that is most commonly inflicted by parents but can also be perpetrated by siblings and child care personnel. Factors predisposing to child abuse include teen-aged parents, mental deficits in either the child or the abuser, unwed motherhood, a single-parent household, and low socioeconomic status, although child abuse occurs in all economic strata. Most victims of child abuse are younger than 2 years and have signs of poor hygiene, psychologic deprivation, and nutritional impairment.[25] Contact burns, caused by cigarettes approximately one-third of the time and often not necessitating admission to a hospital, are the most common form of child abuse thermal injury.[26] Burn injuries caused by placing a small child in a microwave oven are typically full-thickness in depth, sharply demarcated, and present on the body parts nearest the microwave-generating element.[27] Child abuse burns requiring in-hospital care are usually scald injuries, often with associated soft tissue trauma, fractures, and head injury. The characteristic distribution of the scald burn (i.e., feet, posterior legs, buttocks, and hands) should alert one to the possibility of child abuse and prompt a thorough evaluation of the circumstances surrounding the injury and the home situation. The importance of such evaluation is emphasized by the fact that if child abuse goes unidentified and the child is returned to the home, there is a high risk of death resulting from repeated injury.[28]

Two studies[29,30] have called attention to burn injuries as a consequence of spousal abuse in which the face or genitalia are intentionally splashed with chemicals or hot liquids and those caused by either abuse or neglect of elderly, disabled, or handicapped adults.

Burn Size

Burn injury elicits the stereotypic biphasic multi-system response that follows any injury.[31] Because the magnitude and duration of organ dysfunction are proportional to the extent of the burn, health care needs increase as the extent of the burn increases. Most burn patients have injuries of such limited extent that they do not require in-hospital care. Even in the population of patients admitted to burn centers, 75 percent have burn injuries that involve less than 22 percent of the total body surface.[10,32] This preponderance of minor burns is surprisingly constant, even in situations and populations in which the risk of burn injury is increased, such as mass casualty disasters and military armed conflict.[33]

Regional epidemiologic studies in Florida and central New York state as well as national surveys in Denmark and Uganda[34-37] found that annually approximately 300 burn patients per million population require in-hospital care because of the extent of their burns or a complicating factor, such as an associated injury. Most of these patients are adequately cared for in a general hospital by personnel experienced in burn care. Within this group of burn patients there is an additional subset of patients with major burn injuries (42 per million population per year) and patients with lesser burns and a complicating co-morbid factor (40 per million population per year) (Table 5.1).

The American Burn Association criteria for major burn injuries are given in Table 5.2. Patients with major burn injuries are best cared for in a specialized burn center.

Table 5.2. Major Burn Injuries

1. Burns >10 percent BSA in patients <10 or >50 years
2. Burns >20 percent BSA in other age groups
3. Burns involving face, hands, feet, genitalia, perineum, or major joints
4. Full-thickness burns >5 percent BSA at any age
5. Electrical and lightning burns
6. Chemical burns
7. Inhalation injury
8. Concomitant mechanical trauma
9. Lesser burns with significant preexisting medical disorders

BSA: body surface area.

Because the extent of a burn is commonly overestimated by persons with limited experience in burn care, it is inevitable that patients with less than major burns will be hospitalized and even transferred to burn centers. Such over-referral must be expected and accepted to ensure that all patients with major burns requiring burn center care are indeed transferred to such facilities.

Burn Care Needs

The intensity of nursing care, the need for medical specialist care, and the volume of laboratory support are greatest in patients with burns of 50 percent or more of the total body surface. The nurse-intensive nature of critical burn care is indicated by the data generated in a nursing workload study conducted at the United States Army Institute of Surgical Research burn center during the period January to December 1988.[38] The average daily direct nursing care hours required by the patients in that burn center's intensive care unit (ICU) were 28.3. The need to staff a burn ICU at a level exceeding one nursing service member per patient per day to provide the nursing care required by an extensively burned patient is one of the factors that has promoted the regionalization of burn care facilities.

The multi-system effects of extensive burn injury that result in myriad complications requiring at least consultative, if not direct involvement, of medical specialists are responsible, at least in part, for the frequent siting of burn centers at academic institutions. The medical specialists most frequently involved in the care of patients at burn centers are ophthalmologists, plastic surgeons, orthopedic surgeons, anesthesiologists, cardiologists, radiologists, psychiatrists, and pathologists.

The wide variety and volume of support services required by severely burned patients have also contributed to the development of dedicated tertiary burn centers. Respiratory therapy is required not only during resuscitation, but also during the treatment of post-resuscitation pulmonary insufficiency. A planned program of progressive physical therapy and anti-deformity splinting initiated on admission necessitates involvement of physical therapists and occupational therapists throughout the entire hospital course. Dietetic services are used from the time resuscitation is complete until far into convalescence. Social services are involved in family support throughout hospitalization and in preparing patients for reentry into society. Educational services are used in the convalescent period to minimize injury-related educational lag in burned children.

The laboratory support required by a burn patient varies across time after injury and depends on the extent of the burn, the presence of associated injury such as inhalation injury, and the occurrence of complications. Clinical laboratory support is most intense during the resuscitation period and during the treatment of complications, such as pulmonary insufficiency, fluid and electrolyte disturbances, and metabolic derangements. In addition to epidemiologic surveillance, microbiology support is required for diagnosis and therapeutic monitoring of infections.[39,40] Pathology support is required for accurate assessment of the microbial status of the burn wound as an integral part of the wound biopsy monitoring program.[41]

Burn Care Facilities

In confirmation of the previously noted tendency to over-referral, approximately 90,000 burn patients, who require an average of 12 days care, are admitted to hospitals in the United States annually.[2] Within that group of burn patients, approximately 20,000 meet the

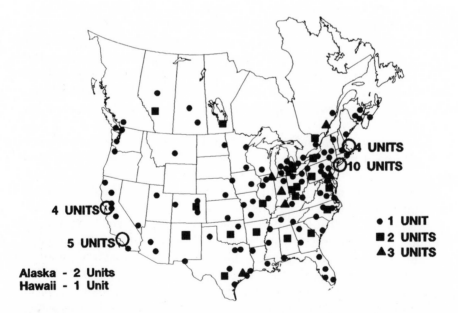

Figure 5.1. *Distribution of burn care centers in the United States and Canada.*

criteria of having major burn injuries and are cared for in burn centers. The American Burn Association burn care resources document lists 182 hospitals with self-designated burn care facilities. One hundred forty-six hospitals have burn centers containing 1,790 dedicated burn care beds, and 36 claim specialized burn care programs but no specific burn unit or center. In 1985 approximately 21,000 acutely burned patients were admitted to those burn care facilities. In Canada there are 25 hospitals with self-designated burn centers containing 158 dedicated burn care beds and two additional hospitals with specialized burn care programs but no dedicated burn care beds.[42] Examination of Fig. 5.1 confirms the regionalization of tertiary burn care facilities in the United States and Canada and also documents that the distribution of those facilities parallels population density. Most burn centers in the United States are located on the Atlantic and Pacific seaboards and in the upper Midwest and Texas, whereas in Canada the burn centers are located in urban areas in the lower latitudes of the provinces.

Transfer Procedures

The regionalization of burn care is made possible by and, in fact, depends on a system of timely transfer of patients with major burn injuries to burn centers. Establishment of transfer agreements ensures access to such a system. Patient safety and continuity of care are ensured by physician-to-physician coordination of the transfer procedure. The receiving physician at a burn center should review with the referring physician each of the items listed on a checklist, such as that displayed in Figure 20.3, to determine the adequacy of resuscitation, personnel, equipment, and supplies needed to effect transfer; the optimal timing and mode of transfer (ground ambulance vs aircraft); and any necessary modifications of treatment before movement.

With rare exceptions, aeromedical transfer is not required for a burn patient if ground ambulance transfer time is one hour or less. When transfer of a patient by ground ambulance would require more time but the patient is still within 150 miles of the burn center, a helicopter is commonly used for transfer. It is particularly important that a burn patient who is to be transferred by helicopter be well stabilized in terms of hemodynamic and ventilatory function before movement. The poor lighting, limited space, vibration, and high noise levels in a helicopter make monitoring difficult and also severely restrict one's ability to carry out emergency therapeutic interventions such

61

as airway intubation or insertion of vascular access lines. When transfer distance exceeds 150 miles, a fixed-wing aircraft is used. The transfer aircraft must be of sufficient size to accommodate a litter and permit continued fluid infusion and continuous ventilatory support, if such are required. The patient area should be of sufficient size to accommodate all equipment and supplies necessary to continue resuscitation and address complications of the injury and therapy, should such arise, during the aeromedical transfer procedure.[43]

Ideally, a physician should be in attendance during the transfer of a patient with a major burn injury. If this is not possible, experienced non-physician burn unit personnel should be used and all details of patient care and transfer closely coordinated with the receiving physician. The burn flight team used by the United States Army Institute of Surgical Research burn center consists of a surgeon, a licensed practical nurse, and a registered nurse. This group is augmented by a respiratory therapist when assistance in ventilatory management is required during intercontinental transfer procedures.[43]

The burn team is transported to the referring hospital, where evaluation and pre-flight stabilization of the patient are carried out

Table 5.3. Pre-transfer Preparation and Stabilization of Burn Patients (148 Patients in 124 Flights)

		Number of Patients
Modification of fluid therapy		42
Cannula and catheter placement or modification		87
Nasogastric tube:	33	
Intravenous cannula:	29	
Urethral catheter:	13	
Endotracheal tube:	8	
Thoracostomy tube:	2	
Tracheostomy tube:	2	
Alteration of pulmonary management		20
Institution of mechanical ventilation:	16	
Administration of oxygen:	4	
Placement of escharotomy incisions		6
Application of wound dressings		38

before movement. A review of management problems encountered in 124 flights, in which 148 burn patients were transferred, revealed that cannula insertion or replacement was the most common intervention required before transfer (87 patients).[44] Placement of a nasogastric tube to reduce the risk of emesis resulting from altitude-related expansion of gas within the gastrointestinal tract was required in 33 patients. Placement of an intravenous cannula was required in 29, placement of a Foley catheter in 13, insertion of an endotracheal tube in eight, and placement of a thoracostomy tube and tracheostomy in two patients each. Alteration of fluid therapy to correct shock or oliguria was necessary in 42 patients before transfer, and alteration of ventilatory support was required in 20: the institution of mechanical ventilation in 16 and the administration of oxygen in four. There were six patients in whom escharotomy of encircling limb burns was required to maintain perfusion of unburned tissue (Table 5. 3). Because pre-flight stabilization is best performed in the referring hospital, flight line delivery and acceptance of a patient with a major burn injury should be discouraged.

In-flight treatment needs and management problems recapitulate pre-flight stabilization problems. A major change in fluid therapy was the most common in-flight intervention and was required in 38 of the previously mentioned 148 burn patients. In-flight ventilatory adjustment was required in seven patients, and 14 required administration of intravenous medications exclusive of analgesics. The frequency of these pre-flight and in-flight treatment needs indicates the importance of the flight team personnel having available all necessary equipment and supplies throughout the transfer procedure.

The aeromedical transfer of burn patients is best carried out as soon as resuscitation therapy has stabilized hemodynamic and pulmonary function, as indexed by adequacy of tissue blood flow and tissue oxygenation. Later transfer of burn patients may be compromised by post-resuscitation complications. Pneumonia, congestive heart failure, cardiac arrhythmias, hyperpyrexia above 39.4°C, and active gastrointestinal hemorrhage are all contraindications to patient transfer that must be addressed and controlled before transfer.[43] Pneumocephalus is an additional contraindication necessitating delay in transfer.

Transfer personnel must be able to recognize the pathophysiologic changes characteristic of burn injury and the common complications of burn therapy and be capable of modifying therapy as necessary both before and during transfer. The continuity and quality of care are optimum when transfer is effected by properly equipped experienced burn care personnel. During the period January 1977 through October 1987, 898 burn patient aeromedical transfers were carried out by the burn flight teams of the United States Army Institute of Surgical Research. Eight hundred seventy-seven flights were conducted within the continental United States to transfer 1,061 patients without a death. Twenty-one intercontinental missions were conducted to transfer 73 burn patients with only two in-flight deaths. One occurred when mechanical ventilation became inadequate in a patient with respiratory insufficiency resulting from severe inhalation injury, and the other occurred when fluid needs were grossly underestimated in a patient attended by non-burn center personnel.

Assessment of Outcome

The endpoints of burn care are survival, functional recovery, and cosmetic result. The latter two endpoints take precedence in the care of patients with burns of limited extent, and survival is the predominant concern and therapeutic guide in patients with major burns. Survival data also serve as indices of the quality of care and provide a means of evaluating treatments and comparing results with those of other institutions.

Raw survival data not only are meaningless but also are potentially misleading because mortality in burn patients is proportional to the extent of burn and strongly influenced by age. The sigmoid dose-response relation between extent of burn and mortality necessitates mathematical transformation by either probit or logit technique to define a linear relation between the two variables, generate a reliable error term, and facilitate statistical comparisons.[45, 46] The effect of age on burn mortality is often dealt with by age-group stratification: 0 to 14 years, 15 to 49 years, and older than 50 years are commonly used groupings. Alternatively, outcome analysis can incorporate a continuous curvilinear function of age.[47]

Assessment of burn patient outcome should be limited to patients received at the individual burn treatment facility within the first 10 days of the injury and treated until discharge or death. The death rate among burn patients is relatively high in the first 10 post-burn days and significantly lower thereafter, and it is clearly unwarranted to tabulate as a survivor a moribund patient who is transferred and dies elsewhere. Because the co-morbid effects of concomitant mechanical injury, particularly head injury, are difficult to quantify, patients with associated injury should be excluded from assays of burn-specific mortality.

Recent studies have documented the mortality-enhancing effects of inhalation injury and infection, particularly pneumonia.[48, 50] The effects of those disease processes on mortality among burn patients, dependent on both age and extent of burn, are independent and additive. When comparing outcomes, it is essential that the populations being compared be comparable in terms of presence of inhalation injury and infection and that those co-morbid factors be comparably distributed in relation to age and burn size within the populations. The distribution of burn size within any population of burn patients being assessed must also be considered because a probit curve of the mortality for a population in which small burns predominate may be upwardly biased. A separate outcome analysis should be performed on the subset of patients within that population with burns of more than 40 percent of the body surface to eliminate such an error.

The LA_{50}, the extent of burn associated with death in half of the patients with burns of that extent, is the statistic commonly used for outcome assessment. Comparison of current LA_{50}s with those of 40 years ago confirms the improvement in burn patient survival that has occurred among the young adult and older adult age groups over the last four decades. In the mid-1940s the LA_{50}s (by probit analysis) was 43 percent for young adults and 23 percent for older adults as compared with 60.8 percent and 39.2 percent, respectively, at the United States Army Institute of Surgical Research during the years 1979 to

Table 5.4. Burn Center Staffing Requirements

Director
Associate director
Fellow
Residents: 2 for every 15 patients
Nurses: 1 for every 2 ICU patients
Clinical nurse instructor
Occupational therapist: 1 for every 7 patients
Social worker: full time assignment to burn center
Nutritionist
Respiratory therapist: 24 hours per day, 7 days per week.

(Modified from standards of Burn Advisory Committee, New York City Emergency Medical Services, 1988.)

1983.[51] A similar improvement in survival rates has been reported at pediatric burn centers, i.e., an LA_{50} of 51 percent in the 1940s compared with the 93 percent rate recently reported in 1986 by one such center.[52] This increase in survival rate represents the aggregate effect of nonspecific improvements in the care of critically ill patients over four decades, the benefits of specialized care and research at regional burn centers, and the effective transfer system that ensures that patients with major burns are referred to burn centers in a timely manner.

Economics of Burn Care

Burn centers were the first successful implementation of the specialty referral center concept. The first burn center was established at the United States Army Surgical Research Unit and opened in 1950. Since that time, this concept has been expanded to create trauma centers, limb replantation centers, and spinal cord injury centers. Although the specialty referral center is the most efficient method to deliver expert medical care for these specific acute medical problems, the expense to the institutions supporting these centers is enormous.

Service standards for specialized burn facilities have been established by a number of accreditation agencies at the local, state and national levels. Individual standards require unit organization and integration with other units in the supporting institution, delineated

Table 5.5. Distribution of Routine Service Costs of a University Burn Center, New York Hospital, 1988

Expense	Percentage
Personnel	43
Medical supplies	17
General administration	14
Unit administration	5
House staff	4
Central services	3
Laundry	3
Other	15

responsibilities of the staff according to special patient-care needs, education, policies and procedures for patient care, and guidelines for facility design and equipment.[53, 54] Required personnel reflect the true interdisciplinary composition of a full-service burn center, the major emphasis being on continuous individualized burn care (Table 5.4). In addition, physician consultative services from all major clinical departments must be readily available at all times.

Severe burn injury is a chronic disease of which hospitalization for acute burn care is only the initial phase. Absolutely implicit in the decision to establish a burn center is the obligation to provide burned patients with the long-term care required before the burn and all of its sequelae have healed and the patient has reentered society productively. Outpatient follow-up care is often long term and may span 4 or 5 years for children with severe burns. Major treatment programs for outpatients include control of burn scar hypertrophy and contractures, treatment of post-injury stress disorders, provision of social worker and home health support, and patient and family education (both in burn care and burn prevention). Without this long-term care, the benefits of acute treatment are often lost.

Costs of Burn Center Care

The costs of burn center care have proved to be relatively elusive to define. One problem has been the diversity of recognized burn treatment facilities, which range from four-bed units to centers with more than 40 beds. It is likely that burn facilities begin to approach economic efficiency at the size of an eight-to ten-bed unit, given the multidisciplinary personnel needed for burn care. Smaller facilities often experience great difficulty in routinely keeping these expensive beds filled and the dedicated staff intact.

The New York Hospital Burn Center is an example of an urban burn care facility servicing the population predominantly of the greater New York City metropolitan area. It consists of a 24-bed ICU floor and a 22-bed step-down area. Census ranges from 35 to 75 patients, with a mean inpatient load of approximately 50 patients. The ICU is configured so that the patients requiring complex monitoring and nursing care are located in half of the ICU, whereas those who are recovering gradually move toward the other half as their conditions improve. Although the latter beds are less densely equipped, all are configured to provide full ICU-level support. The step-down floor is also staffed as described in Table 5.4 and is engineered so that it can act as a primary burn ICU in the event of a mass casualty incident.

Table 5.6. Ancillary Service Utilization of a University Burn Center, New York Hospital, 1988 (Average Cost Per Case [$])

DRG	Lab	Radiology	Blood	Special	OR/RR	Pharmacy	Misc.	Total
456	765	451	207	394	349	432	66	2,664
457	1,610	746	661	369	50	696	0	4,133
458	4,439	2,262	1,339	2,284	1,923	3,463	317	16,027
459	1,974	972	846	534	401	1,204	46	5,976
460	1,071	524	136	314	36	495	11	2,587
472	4,997	2,327	2,249	2,175	1,935	3,175	617	17,474
474	16,290	8,097	2,013	4,988	1,341	14,776	922	49,056

DRG: diagnosis-related group; OR: operating room; RR: recovery room.

Table 5.7. Burn Center Payer Class Distribution (New York Hospital, January 1989 through July 1989, 650 Admissions)

	ICU percent	Step-down-unit percent
Medicare	12.4	13.5
Medicaid	39.3	35.6
Blue Cross	13.3	14.6
Commercial	22.8	27.4
Self-pay	12.2	8.9

ICU: intensive care unit.

In this way, bed occupancy can be maintained while resources and staff are distributed in the most efficient manner. Activity of nursing care is extremely high for massively burned patients and may require one nurse assigned to each of these critically ill patients. Sovie et al[55] found that the proportion of patient days requiring category 3 and 4 nursing intensity (on a four-part nursing intensity scale) was more than 93 percent for extensively burned patients. Both of the categories entail one-on-one staffing assignments.

As is evident, salaries and benefits for clinical personnel are the largest proportion of the operating cost in the burn center (Table 5.5). The smaller unspecified costs include medical records, dietary support, house keeping, legal affairs, and operation and maintenance of the physical plant. In 1988, service costs averaged $1,194 per day per patient in the New York Hospital burn center. Ancillary costs depended on the classification of the patient's injuries (Table 5.6). In general, the more extensive the thermal and associated injuries, the more costly they were. Tables 5.5 and 5.6 do not reflect equipment and other capital costs or depreciation of the physical plant.

Reimbursement

The adequacy of reimbursement in the long term determines whether or not a burn center can survive. The demographic profile of a population of burn patients usually reflects a significant bias toward the less economically advantaged (Table 5.7). In states without regulatory control of hospital reimbursement, significant cost shifting likely plays a role in funding for underinsured or non-insured patients. Commercial carriers usually pay all charges, whereas Blue Cross and Medicare often have restrictions or limits on paying hospital bills. In some states Medicaid pays very little, and self-pay patients usually are indigent. Table 5.7 illustrates the tendency for severely burned patients in the ICU to be the major financial risks to hospitals with burn centers. Until recent years, cost shifting has been the traditional method for paying for under-reimbursed burn care. During the last decade, prospective payment plans have emerged as the alternative and increasingly dominant method for hospital reimbursement. Under these models, cost shifting is rarely feasible, and the financial success or failure of a hospital and its burn center critically depends on the fixed reimbursement rate covering the costs of patient care.

Reimbursement based on the patient's diagnosis is the major prospective payment system used by funding agencies. Diagnosis-related groups (DRGS) were developed in the 1970s initially as a tool for utilization

Table 5.8. DRGs Associated With Thermal Injury

Cutaneous Burns

456—Burn patient transferred to another acute care facility
457—Extensive burns without OR procedures
458—Non-extensive burn with skin grafts
459—Non-extensive burns with wound debridgement and other OR procedures
460—Non-extensive burns without OR procedures
472—Extensive burns with OR procedures

Inhalation Injury

101—Other respiratory system diagnoses
474—Respiratory system diagnoses with tracheostomy
475—Respiratory system diagnoses with ventilatory support
736—Tracheostomy other than for mouth, larynx, or pharynx disorder.

DRGS: diagnosis-related groups; OR: operating room.

Table 5.9. Weight Factors and Reimbursement Rates of Burn-Related DRGs

DRG	Relative Weight	Expected LOS(Days)	Reimbursement Rate($)
456	5.5044	8	24,061
457	5.3930	17	23,574
456	6.5200	24	28,502
459	3.0963	10	13,535
460	1.3967	8	6,105
472	20.3751	36	89,064
101	1.3539	10	5,918
474	123838	45	54,132
475	5,0545	14	22,094
736	16.8390	48	73,610

LOS: length of stay; DRG: diagnosis-related group; CMI: case mix index.
New York State Guidelines, 1988, except for DRG 474, which was calculated from HCFA relative weight.

review. Hospitalized patients were classified according to patterns of care received, lengths of stay, and use of services. The original 383 DRGs recognized only the presence or absence of a secondary diagnosis and did not recognize the variable severity of an illness within broad disease categories. Additional DRGs have been added during the last decade, and the current number exceeds 700.

Each DRG is assigned a case mix index (CMI), which is a weighted average service intensity multiplier that theoretically reflects relative resource consumption associated with each DRG. The higher the index, the more seriously ill the patient is, and the greater are the hospital revenues. Each DRG is characterized by an expected length of stay (LOS) based on statistical evaluation of that disease complex in the past. Long stay outliers occur when actual LOS exceeds the expected LOS of the patient's DRG by 20 days or 1.94 standard deviations, whichever is less. Cost outliers are derived in the same manner based on the reimbursement rate for each DRG.

There are six burn categories ranging from DRG 456 to the new DRG 472, which was added in October 1986 (Table 5.8). In addition, four additional DRGs are frequently used for patients with inhalation injury, with or without cutaneous burns. The burn DRGs are based only on extent of burn injury and the occurrence of a surgical procedure. A non-extensive burn can be as large as 49 percent total body surface area (TBSA) if it is all second degree, and an extensive burn can be as small as 20 percent TBSA if it is all third degree. Debridement that uses surgical excision qualifies for inclusion into DRG 459, whereas hydrotherapy or enzymatic debridement for wound care is not classified as an operative procedure. Furthermore, a number of procedures performed in appropriately equipped and staffed burn centers qualify as operating room procedures. These procedures include tracheostomy, escharotomy, and fasciotomy. Together, the combinations of burn extent and operative status result in 279 ICD-9-CM codes (International Classification of Disease, version 9, Clinical Manual).

Each DRG is associated with a fixed reimbursement rate, and certain strategies to secure optimal reimbursement are evident (Table 5.9). Since October 1988 new codes require medical coders to distinguish between excisional debridement (ICD-9 code 86.22) and non-excisional debridement (86.28). If excisional debridement is performed, it must be documented in the patient's medical record; there is a significant difference in the reimbursement rates for DRG 459 and DRG 460 (Table 5.9). If a patient has both a thermal burn and severe inhalation injury, coding the primary diagnosis as inhalation injury or as a cutaneous burn may have a considerable impact on reimbursement. Thus, it is important to document inhalation injury on admission by bronchoscopic examination or xenon ventilation-perfusion lung scan.

The effect of the initial five burn DRGs (456-460) was evaluated in 275 severely burned patients admitted to the New York Hospital Burn Center in 1983.[51] Charges were documented by the billing department. In addition, the costs of burn care for each of these 275 patients were collected by prospectively following each patient's clinical course during hospitalization. These costs included direct costs, indirect costs, overhead, and ancillary services. Direct costs included all clinical personnel and materials for the care of patients on the burn unit. Indirect costs included labor and supply components of the service departments contributing to burn patient care. The step-down cost allocation method was used to determine the overhead and housekeeping components of the burn unit. Ancillary service costs were obtained by documenting each patient study or treatment and calculating costs using the cost-to-charge ratio for each event.

The step-down cost allocation method, however, reflects accounting costs and not true economic costs. Except for that of ancillary services, all other costs were measured directly either from purchase orders or from hours worked and pay rates.

Daily costs in 1983 averaged $1,216 per patient, whereas hospital daily charges were only $830. Assuming that DRG reimbursement was received for every patient (and this certainly was not the situation because of the large number of worker's compensation and indigent patients), the average payer rate would have been $573 per patient per day, or a real loss of $643 per patient per day. A major cause of per-patient loss (in addition to that for indigent patients) was the proportion of the total hospitalization that was attributed to LOS outliers in Medicare and Medicaid patients (73 percent and 49 percent, respectively).

The ability of the five burn DRGs to explain the variation in resource consumption was further examined in the 400 evaluable burned patients admitted in 1983, including the 275 patients described earlier.[57] The cost data, not charges, were evaluated by a simple analysis of variance to assay degree of variation within each DRG and by a reduced form model relating resource consumption to clinical and nonclinical factors. The burn DRGs explained only 17 percent of the variation of resource consumption, which is lower than other DRGs or competing classification methods.

Uncaptured components of patient severity, especially inhalation injury and larger body surface area burns, explain much of the residual variation within each DRG. Age is positively related to resource consumption (P <.05). For patients between the ages of 20 and 65 years, a 10 percent increase in age was associated with a 4 percent increase in resource consumption. The observable differences in patient severity within each burn DRG allow hospitals without specialized burn facilities to select and transfer nonprofitable patients to regional specialty units, greatly increasing that center's financial risk.

Since this analysis, numerous changes have been made in the DRG method that have benefited burn centers. In 1986, DRG 472 was added, allowing greater reimbursement for massive burns undergoing surgical procedures. In 1987, DRGs 474 and 475 were added. Those two DRGs allow higher reimbursement rates for patients with severe inhalation injury, who incur greater patient care costs than those with cutaneous burns. In addition, the *Budget Reconciliation Act Of 1987* increased outlier payments for burn DRGs from 60 percent to 90 percent.[58] Finally, in 1988 DRG 736 was added, but it applies only to non-Medicare patients; in an all-payer state system, DRG 474 is the equivalent DRG for Medicare patients.

Table 5.10. Case Mix Index by Payer Status

	Number of Patients	CMI	Actual LOS	Expected LOS
ICU patients				
Medicare	46	3.09	29.5	10.3
Medicaid	145	3.73	13.5	10.8
Blue Cross	49	5.29	13.9	14.1
Commercial	84	2.47	9.4	8.3
Self-Pay	45	5.91	2.9	14.4
Step-down unit patients				
Medicare	38	2.65	24.1	11.1
Medicaid	100	3.62	22.3	10.6
Blue Cross	41	3.22	14.5	10.1
Commercial	77	3.28	11.6	10.43
Self-Pay	25	4.78	16.8	12.9

LOS: length of stay in days; ICU: intensive care unit.
New York Hospital, January 1989 through July 1989.

In 1988, New York State introduced the All Payor DRG Program. With this new law, all hospital reimbursement agencies are required to use established fixed payment schedules (Table 5.9). Medicare patients continue to be funded under guidelines set by the federal government, whereas all others follow New York State guidelines. The fixed rate of the latter system is moderately higher than that for Medicare, but LOS outlier payments are greatly reduced. Indigent care continues to remain unfunded.

These new reimbursement guidelines have considerable impact on burn center reimbursement. The elderly and indigent are responsible for disproportionately high excessive LOS and severity of illness indices (Table 5.10). The indigent (self-pay) CMI is four times the mean CMI for the hospital overall. Even when a severely burned patient is covered by a third-party payer, patient care costs far outstrip the DRG fixed-rate reimbursement. The mean LOS for DRG 472 was 70 days in the New York Hospital Burn Center in 1988. Using the mean LOS for that DRG and its burn center daily rate plus ancillary costs from Tables 5.6 and 5.9 (mean LOS X daily rate + ancillary services), the average hospital cost for DRG 474 was $118,309; by comparison, actual reimbursement was only $54,132, a considerable loss for the hospital.

Diagnosis-related group outlier policy is flawed because it assumes that the costs of treating patients decrease near the end of a hospital stay. In reality, severely burned patients require expensive care until the end of hospitalization. Severe illnesses remain uncaptured in the current DRG structure. Age and inhalation injury greatly influence burn management and are major determinants of survival.[57, 59] The high costs of the ICU environment, especially if a patient requires mechanical ventilatory assistance, almost uniformly cause great financial losses for the hospital.[60, 61]

Burn centers continue to be a major source of financial loss for hospitals that support them.[62] The effects of the new DRG 472 are not yet evident, but its addition to the DRG method reduces the magnitude of hospital deficits but likely does not eliminate them. New technologies in wound care have proved cost effective.[63] However, financial solvency will require major changes in current prospective methods before burn center care, with all its advantages for improved patient care and survival, becomes financially neutral. At this time, a reorganization of the present DRG system is being considered, which would redefine and expand the number of DRGs to 1,200 with classification that would recognize the severity of a patient's condition and complications.[58] Until such a system is accomplished, burn centers will continue to close.

References

1. Pruitt BA jr, Goodwin CW. Thermal injuries. In: Davis JH, Drucker WR, Foster RS jr, Gamelli RL, Gann DS, Pruitt BA jr, Sheldon GF, eds. *Clinical surgery*. St. Louis: CV Mosby, 1987; 2823.

2. Baker SP, O'Neill B, Karpf RS. *The injury fact book*. Lexington, MA: Lexington Books, 1984; 139.

3. Callegari PR, Alton JDM, Shankowsky HA, et al. Burn injuries in native Canadians: a ten year experience. *Burns* 1989; 15:15.

4. Birky MM, Halpin BM, Kaplan YH, et al. Fire fatality study. *Fire and Materials* 1979; 4:211.

5. Mierley MC, Baker SP. Fatal house fires in an urban population. *JAMA* 1983; 249:1466.

6. Consumer Product Safety Commission. Bureau of Epidemiology annual report of flammable fabric data, FY 1975. Washington, D.C.: U.S. Consumer Product Safety Commission, 1975.

7. Barancik JI, Shapiro MA. Pittsburgh burn study. Pittsburgh and Allegheny County, Pennsylvania, June 1, 1970-April 15, 1971. Washington, D.C.: U.S. Consumer Product Safety Commission, May 1976.

8. Trier H, Spaabaek J. The nursing home patient, a burn-prone person: an epidemiological study. *Burns* 1987; 13:484.

9. Graitcer PL, Sniezek JE. Hospitalizations due to tap water scalds 1978-1985. *MMWR* 1988; 37:35.

10. Clark WR, Fromm BS. Burn mortality experienced at a regional burn unit. Literature review. *Acta Chir Scand* 1987; (Suppl 537):26-29.

11. Bradshaw C, Hawkins J, Leach M, et al. A study of childhood scalds. *Burns* 1988; 14:21.

12. Baptiste MS, Feck G. Preventing tap water burns. *Am J Public Health* 1980; 70:72 7.

13. Lyngdorf P. Occupational burn injuries. *Burns* 1987; 13:294.

14. Purdue GF, Hunt JL, Layton TR, et al. Burns in motor vehicle accidents. *j Trauma* 1985; 25:216.

15. Mozingo DW, Smith AA, McManus WF, et al. Chemical burns. *j Trauma* 1988; 28:642.

16. Leeming MN, Ray C jr, Holand WS. Low-voltage direct-current burns. *JAMA* 1970, 214:1681.

17. Perrotta DM, Brender J, Suarez L, et al. Occupational electrocution-Texas 1981-1985. *MMWR* 1987; 36:725.

18. Milham S. Irrigation-pipe-associated electrocution deaths: Washington. *MMWR* 1983; 32:169.

19. Lescher Tj, Pruitt BA Jr. Antennas, electricity, and amputations, presented at the American Burn Association annual meeting, Birmingham, AL, March 31,1978.

20. Electrical burns. In: Advanced burn life support course manual. Lincoln, NE: Nebraska Burn Institute, 1987.

21. Kobayashi JM. Fireworks-related injuries--Washington. *MMWR* 1983; 32:285.

22. Kale D, Harwood B. Fireworks injuries 1981, Washington, D.C., U.S. Consumer Product Safety Commission.

23. McFarland LV, Harris JR, Kobayashi JM, et al. Risk factors for fireworks-related injury in Washington State. *JAMA* 1984; 251:325 1.

24. Pruitt BA Jr, Edlich RF. Treatment of bitumen burns [Letter]. *JAMA* 1982; 247:1565.

25. O'Neill JA, Meacham WF, Griffin PP, et al. Patterns of injury in the battered child syndrome. *J Trauma* 1973; 13:332.

26. Showers J, Garrison KM. Burn abuse: a four-year study. *J Trauma* 1988; 28:1581.

27. Surrell JA, Alexander RC, Cohle SD, et al. Effects of microwave radiation on living tissues. *j Trauma* 1987; 27:935.

28. Purdue GF, Hunt JL, Prescott PR. Child abuse by burning: an index of suspicion. *J Trauma* 1988; 28: 221.

29. Krob Mj, Johnson A, Jordan MH. Burned and battered adults. *Journal of Burn Care Rehabilitation* 1986; 7:529.

30. Bowden ML, Grant ST, Vogel B, et al. The elderly, disabled and handicapped adult burned through abuse and neglect. *Burns* 1988; 14:447.

31. Pruitt BA Jr. The universal trauma model, 1984 Scutter Oration. *Bulletin of the American College of Surgeons* 1985; 70(10):2.

32. Mason AD jr, Pruitt BA Jr. Epidemiology of burn injury. Presented at 5th International Congress on Burn Injuries, Stockholm, Sweden, June 19, 1978.

33. Shafir R. Burn injury and care in the recent Lebanese conflict. Presented at 6th International Congress on Burns, San Francisco, CA, September 3, 1982.

34. Linn BS, Stephenson SE jr, Smith J. Evaluation of burn care in Florida. *N Engl J Med* 1977; 296:311.

35. Clark WR, Lerner D. Regional burn survey: two years of hospitalized burns in central New York. *J Trauma* 1978; 18:524.

36. Thomsen M, Sorenson B. The total number of burn injuries in a Scandinavian population. *Scand J Plast Reconstr Surg* 1967; 1:84.

37. Lee JO, Craven JL, Smith PF. A study of burn injuries in Uganda. *Surg Gynecol Obstet* 1972; 135: 600.

38. Molter NC. Workload management system for nursing: application to the burn unit. Presented at American Burn Association meeting, New Orleans, LA, March 30, 1989, paper #45.

39. McManus AT, Mason AD jr, McManus WF, et al. Twenty-five year review of Pseudomonas aeruginosa bacteremia in a burn center. *Eur J Clin Microbiol* 1985; 4:219.

40. Shirani KZ, McManus AT, Vaughan GM, et al. Effects of environment on infection in burn patients. *Arch Surg* 1986; 221:31.

41. Pruitt BA Jr. Opportunistic infections in burn patients: diagnosis and treatment. In: Root RK, Trunkey DD, Sande MA, eds. New surgical and medical approaches in infectious diseases. New York: Churchill Livingstone, 1987, pp. 245-261.

42. Burn care resources in North America 1986-1987. American Burn Association, Office of the Secretary, Shriners Burns Institute, Cincinnati, Ohio.

43. Pruitt BA Jr, Fitzgerald BE. Pre-hospital care: a military perspective. *Mayo Clin Proc,* 1980; 223.

44. Treat RC, Sirinek KR, Pruitt BA Jr.. Air evacuation of thermally injured patients: principles of treatment and results. *j Trauma* 1980; 20:275.

45. Pruitt BA Jr, Tumbusch WT, Mason AD jr, et al. Mortality in 1100 consecutive burns treated at a burns unit. *Ann Surg* 1964; 159:396.

46. Curreri PW, Luterman A, Braun DW jr, et al. Burn injury: analysis of survival and hospitalization time for 937 patients. *Ann Surg* 1980; 192:472.

47. Mason AD Jr, Westfall P, Pruitt BA Jr. Age adjustment in analysis of burn mortality (submitted for publication).

48. Shirani KZ, Pruitt BA Jr, Mason AD Jr. The influence of inhalation injury and pneumonia on burn mortality. *Ann Surg* 1987; 205:82.

49. Mason AD jr, McManus AT, Pruitt BA Jr. Association of burn mortality and bacteremia: a twenty five year review. *Arch Surg* 1986; 121:1027.

50. Zawacki BE, Azen SP, Imbus SH, et al. Multifactorial probe and analysis of mortality in burned patients. *Ann Surg* 1979; 189:1.

51. Bull JP, Squire JR. A study of mortality in a burns unit: standards for the evaluation of alternative methods of treatment. *Ann Surg* 1949; 130:160.

52. Hemdon DN, LeMaster J, Beard S, et al. The quality of life after major thermal injury in children: an analysis of 12 survivors with >80 percent total body, 70 percent third-degree burns. *J Trauma* 1986; 26:609.

53. American Burn Association. Specific optimal criteria for hospital resources for care of patients with thermal injury, 1976.

54. American Burn Association. Appendix B. Guidelines for service standards and severity classifications in the treatment of thermal injury, 1983.

55. Sovie MD, Tarcinale MA, Vanputte AW, Studen AE. Amalgam of nursing acuity, DRGS, and costs. *Nursing Management* 1985; 16:311.

56. Osmanski J. Reimbursement implications and costs of the burn DRGs at the New York Hospital [Dissertation]. New York: Columbia University, 1985.

57. Thorpe KE, Kim JO, Goodwin CW. Variation in resource consumption within burn DRGS. Proceedings of the American Burn Association 1986; 18: 116.

58. Rees JM, Dimick Aj. Increase in the outlier payment for burn DRGS. *Journal of Burn Care and Rehabilitation* 1989; 10:355.

59. Feller 1, Tholen D, Comell RG. Improvements in burn care, 1965 to 1979. *JAMA* 1980; 244:2074.

60. Bekes C, Fleming S, Scott WE. Reimbursement for intensive care services under diagnosis-related groups. *Crit Care Med* 1988; 16:478.

61. Douglas PS, Bone RC, Rosen RL. DRG payment for long term ventilator patients: revisited. *Chest* 1988; 93:629.

62. Chakerian MU, Paiz A, Demarest GB. Burn DRGS: effect of recent changes and implications for the future. Proceedings of the American Association for the Surgery of Trauma, 1989; 31.

63. Smith Dj Jr, Robson MC, Meltzer T, Smith AA, McHugh TP, Heggers JP. DRG-driven change in burn wound management: a success story. *Plast Reconstr Surg* 1988; 82:710.

— by Basil A. Pruitt, Jr., Md,
Arthur D. Mason, Jr., Md, and
Cleon W. Goodwin, Md.

Chapter 6

Smoke or Burns: Which Is Deadlier?

This update of a 1989 report reconfirms that the share of fire deaths caused by smoke inhalation exceeds those caused by burns.

In 1989, we analyzed the respective roles smoke inhalation and burns play in causing deaths in fires in the United States.[1] The subject was already well-traveled at that time, but our approach was new. Its core was a statistical analysis of fire deaths as documented in the national database on death certificates. We used data from 1979, the year in which coding was introduced to distinguish smoke inhalation from burns as the principal cause of fire deaths, through 1985.

The intensity of the national debate over the nature of the toxic hazard component of fire, which underlies the interest in burns vs smoke inhalation, has lessened somewhat in the intervening years, but it has not disappeared. Armed with five more years of data, we can see that the trends we identified in the earlier study, which were based on only seven years of data, still hold. And we find that the share of U.S. fire deaths due to smoke inhalation continues to climb, even as the total number of fire deaths—and the number of smoke inhalation fire deaths, in particular—continues to decline.

Background and Previous Analyses

The classic study of smoke inhalation vs burns—and of many other topics related to fatal fires—was conducted by Berl and Halpin in

©NFPA January/February 1995. Reprinted with permission.

Table 6.1. Fire and Flame Deaths According to Death Certificates, 1979—1990

Year	Total	Home Structure Fire	Other Structure Fire	Clothing Fire	Highly Flammable Material Ignition	Controlled Fire	Outside Fire	Unclassed Fire	Unknown-type Fire
1979	5,998	4,718	208	290	115	53	74	226	314
1980	5,822	4,509	292	311	105	66	66	185	288
1981	5,697	4,516	194	305	95	86	87	173	241
1982	5,210	4,200	171	260	91	66	68	143	211
1983	5,039	4,010	126	270	83	66	63	140	281
1984	5,022	4,035	150	224	80	63	91	146	233
1985	4,952	3,973	186	235	69	63	52	119	255
1986	4,835	3,971	141	179	56	46	63	122	257
1987	4,710	3,909	103	200	55	49	71	95	228
1988	4,965	4,088	118	205	75	54	74	106	245
1989	4,723	3,856	152	222	61	54	82	118	178
1990	4,181	3,510	97	161	54	51	71	99	138
Percent Change	-30 percent	-26 percent	-53 percent	-44 percent	-53 percent	-4 percent	-4 percent	-56 percent	-56 percent

1978.[2] After analyzing fire deaths that occurred in Maryland from 1972 through 1977, they found that roughly half of the victims studied had carboxyhemoglobin levels of at least 50 percent, which is enough to cause death. Another one-fourth of the victims had carboxyhemoglobin levels of 30 to 50 percent, which, when combined with other conditions, such as elevated cyanide levels or preexisting health conditions, would have caused death. Based on these figures, they estimated that smoke inhalation accounts for three-fourths of all fire deaths.

Note that this approach was tantamount to assuming that carbon monoxide poisoning was the most likely cause of death and that any other cause would be considered only after the possibility of carbon monoxide poisoning had proven insufficient to explain the death. Such an approach could overstate the relative importance of smoke inhalation, in general, and of carbon monoxide, in particular.

There are two valid and comprehensive national fire fatality tracking methods that use annually updated data and are coded so as to permit analysis of the respective roles of smoke inhalation and burns. One is derived from the combination of two fire incident reporting systems based on fire department reports, as compiled by the U.S. Fire Administration and the NFPA. The other is the national death certificate database, which is collected by the National Center for Health Statistics from state and local authorities.

The fire incident database reflects the assessments of fire officers, which are typically made at the scene of a fire. In this database, most residential fire deaths—nearly three-fourths in a typical year—are coded as having been caused by an unknown combination of burns and smoke inhalation. Of those attributed to only one or the other cause of death, our original analysis of the data collected from 1981 through 1985 showed that smoke inhalation alone was cited four times as often as burns alone. Analysis of the data collected from 1985 through 1989 shows that the ratio has declined to three and a half to one. Clearly, the large proportion of cases attributed to an undifferentiated combination of causes indicates a great deal of uncertainty about the respective roles of these two effects in most fire deaths.

The death certificate database is a complete census of all deaths and reflects medical assessments, which should be more precise and accurate than fire officer assessments, even though many, if not most, death certificate attributions do not have the benefit of a full autopsy. While the fire incident database probably overstates the share of fire deaths caused jointly by smoke inhalation and burns, the death certificate database probably understates such deaths by not providing any code for them. A coroner or medical examiner is forced to attribute fire deaths in structures to either burns or smoke inhalation or to some other specific injury. He or she cannot attribute them to a combination of causes.

Notwithstanding these limitations, the death certificate database supports some significant conclusions.

Patterns and Trends in Fire Deaths

Table 6.1 summarizes U.S. fire deaths, based on those death certificates on which the coding clearly indicates that fire was the cause of death. These exclude most arson deaths, which are categorized as homicides or suicides, and deaths in fires following vehicle accidents. This identification is done by referring to the National Center for Health Statistics' three-digit "E-codes," which classify deaths that are not due to natural causes.[3]

Table 6.2. Primary Cause of Fire and Flame Deaths in Structure Fires, 1979-1990

Year	Total Structure Fires	Smoke Inhalation	Burns	Unknown	Other
1979	4,926	3,136	1,499	93	198
1980	4,801	3,164	1,347	84	206
1981	4,710	3,163	1,320	95	132
1982	4,371	3,082	1,070	103	116
1983	4,136	2,909	1,026	77	124
1984	4,185	2,962	1,037	79	107
1985	4,159	3,003	958	70	128
1986	4,112	3,016	944	71	81
1987	4,012	3,021	834	66	91
1988	4,206	3,180	875	47	95
1989	4,008	3,055	809	51	93
1990	3,607	2,755	730	72	50
Percent Change	-27 percent	12 percent	5.1 percent	-23 percent	-75 percent

84

There are seven categories of fire deaths in Table 6.1. These are structure fires, which are termed "conflagrations" in the E-codes and exclude fires involving primarily ignition of clothing or highly flammable hazardous materials; clothing ignitions that do not, lead to a full structure fire; ignitions of highly flammable hazardous materials that do not lead to a full structure fire; controlled fires; "conflagrations" outside a building or structure; other specific fires; and fires of unknown type. Note that terms such as "conflagration" are not used in this table the way they are used by the fire community.

Estimating Smoke Inhalation and Burn Deaths

Since 1979, a fourth of the E-Code has, in some cases, differentiated smoke inhalation from burns as the major injury causing death in structure fires, which typically constitute four-fifths of the fire deaths classified by E-codes. Table 6.2 shows the breakdown for the years between 1979 and 1990, inclusive.

For the other five categories of cause of fire deaths—excluding unknown-cause cases for the moment—a special analysis was done for our original study using nature-of-injury data collected by the U.S. Consumer Product Safety Commission between 1975 and 1978, inclusive.

This analysis found that 95 percent of deaths involving clothing ignitions were caused by burns, while 4 percent were due to smoke inhalation and 1 percent to some other injury. Ninety percent of deaths involving the ignition of highly flammable materials were the result of burns, while 9 percent were caused by smoke inhalation and 1 percent by some other injury. Seventy-six percent of deaths involving controlled or outside fires were caused by burns, while 23 percent were due to smoke inhalation and 1 percent to some other injury. And 62 percent of deaths involving unclassified fires were caused by burns, while 37 percent were the result of smoke inhalation and 1 percent of some other injury. In all cases, these deaths are dominated by burns, unlike the deaths that occurred in structures, which are dominated by smoke inhalation.

Table 6.3 provides estimated totals and percentages for all fire deaths due to burns, smoke inhalation, and other causes for 1979 through 1990. This table was developed in three steps. First, Table 6.2 was used for structure fires, and the deaths for which the nature of the injury were unknown were proportionally allocated over the others. Second, the percentages from the special 1975-1978 analysis were used to split the numbers shown in Table 6.1 for all other known

Table 6.3. Burn vs. Smoke Inhalation Shares of Fire and Flame Deaths, 1979—1990

Year	Total	Smoke Inhalation	Burns	Other
1979	5,998	3,515 (58.6 percent)	2,262 (37.7 percent)	221 (3.7 percent)
1980	5,822	3,515 (60.4 percent)	2,079 (35.7 percent)	228 (3.9 percent)
1981	5,697	3,501 (61.4 percent)	2,048 (35.9 percent)	148 (2.6 percent)
1982	5,210	3,396 (65.2 percent)	1,683 (32.3 percent)	130 (2.5 percent)
1983	5,039	3,245 (64.4 percent)	1,654 (32.8 percent)	140 (2.8 percent)
1984	5,022	3,277 (65.2 percent)	1,625 (32.4 percent)	121 (2.4 percent)
1985	4,952	3,311 (66.9 percent)	1,498 (30.3 percent)	143 (2.9 percent)
1986	4,835	3,328 (68.8 percent)	1,415 (29.3 percent)	92 (1.9 percent)
1987	4,710	3,307 (70.2 percent)	1,301 (27.6 percent)	102 (2.2 percent)
1988	4,965	3,480 (70.1 percent)	1,378 (27.8 percent)	106 (2.1 percent)
1989	4,723	3,308 (70.0 percent)	1,311 (27.8 percent)	103 (2.2 percent)
1990	4,181	2,986 (71.4 percent)	1,138 (27.2 percent)	57 (1.4 percent)
Percent Change	-30 percent	-15 percent	-50 percent	-74 percent

causes of fire deaths into burns, smoke inhalation and other. Finally, the fire deaths of unknown cause from the last column of Table 6.1 were proportionally allocated over the previously calculated totals for smoke inhalation, burns and other fire deaths.

Table 6.3 shows that smoke inhalation accounts for the majority of accidental fire deaths in structures and that, as of 1990, the share of deaths due to smoke inhalation has reached roughly seven-tenths of the total, compared to one-fourth for burns. The share of deaths caused by smoke inhalation has risen fairly steadily over these twelve years by just over 1 percent point a year. This means that, if this trend continued into the years for which we do not yet have data, the smoke inhalation share would have reached three-fourths sometime around 1993 or 1994.

Given this trend in the burns and smoke inhalation shares of fire of fire deaths, it is not surprising that the trend in the *number* of fire deaths due to burns vs those to smoke inhalation have been quite different. From 1979 to 1990, total fire deaths fell by 30 percent, or 1,817 deaths. However, the number of fire deaths attributed smoke inhalation fell by only 15, or 529 deaths, while the number attributed to burns fell by 50 percent or 1,124 deaths. Injuries other than burns and smoke inhalation fell by 74 percent, but that represents only 164 deaths.

Trends before 1979 cannot be analyzed as precisely, but the analysis did show that structure fire deaths are mostly due to smoke inhalation and all other known classes of fire deaths are mostly due to burns. Table 6.4 looks at the trends for structure and non-structure fire deaths from 1970 through 1990 as a way of indirectly gauging the longer trend in fire deaths due to burns compared to those due to smoke inhalation.

The validity of this approach can be gauged by comparing the trends Table 6.4 shows for 1979 through 1990 to the trends Table 6.3 shows for those same years. The decline in total fire deaths was 30 percent in Table 6.3, very close to the 29 percent decline in total fire deaths excluding unknown causes in Table 6.4. The decline in smoke inhalation fire deaths was 15 percent in Table 6.3, somewhat less than the 27 percent decline in mostly smoke inhalation fire deaths in Table 6.4. And the decline in burn fire deaths was 50 percent in Table 6.3, somewhat more than the 42 percent decline in mostly burn fire deaths in Table 6.4. The very large percentage decline in fire deaths due to injuries other than burns and smoke inhalation is buried in the mostly burns and mostly smoke inhalation figures and is based on a relatively small number of such deaths.

87

Table 6.4. Deaths Due to Fire and Flames, 1970-1990

Year	TotalDeaths Excluding Unknown Cause	Deaths In Structure Fires Mostly Smoke Inhalation)	Deaths Not In Structure Fires (Mostly burns)
1970	6,188	4,450	1,738
1971	6,115	4,553	1,562
1972	6,182	4,806	1,376
1973	5,914	4,555	1,359
1974	5,701	4,515	1,186
1975	5,640	4,568	1,072
1976	5,972	4,901	1,071
1977	5,970	4,967	1,003
1978	5,822	4,926	896
1979	5,684	4,926	758
1980	5,534	4,801	733
1981	5,456	4,710	746
1982	4,999	4,371	628
1983	4,758	4,136	622
1984	4,789	4,185	604
1985	4,697	4,159	538
1986	4,578	4,112	466
1987	4,482	4,012	470
1988	4,720	4,206	514
1989	4,545	4,008	537
1990	4,043	3,607	436
Percent Change 1970-1979	-8 percent	+11 percent	-56 percent
Percent Change 1979-1990	-29 percent	-27 percent	-42 percent
Percent Change 1970-1990	-35 percent	-19 percent	-75 percent

Thus, this indirect, approximate approach to earlier years is pretty sound. Table 6.4 shows that, by this measure, the differing trends for burns and smoke inhalation as the primary cause of fire deaths were under way for many years before 1979. In fact, the difference in trends appears to have been more pronounced before 1979, when structure fire deaths—mostly due to smoke inhalation—actually increased for several years.

Other Patterns of Interest

Given the fire incident database's separation of fire fatalities into smoke inhalation only, burns only, and smoke inhalation combined with burns, it is possible to analyze each group by other coded data elements. In particular, we can gain some insight into what "smoke inhalation" means—what kinds and quantities of gases produced under what conditions—by analyzing fire deaths in terms of the size of fatal fires and the location of the victims.

A recently published analysis summarized a variety of evidence on the nature of the toxic fire hazard problem and found that fires that spread beyond the room of origin and killed victims in other rooms dominated among fire deaths caused by smoke inhalation.[4] Two-thirds of fire victims coded as killed by smoke inhalation only died in this way, as did more than half the victims killed by burns and smoke inhalation.

Fire spread beyond the room of origin is the best indicator in the national fire incident databases that flash over occurred, and other evidence cited in this article supports this interpretation of these statistical findings. The findings strongly suggest that most victims of smoke inhalation are located some distance from a fire's point of origin and are killed when the gases produced during flash over are driven by the heat-pump effect of a room fire that has flashed over.

What Does All this Mean?

First, it is important to note that fire deaths due to burns and fire deaths due to smoke inhalation have both been declining. So whatever else is true, the level of safety is improving.

It may also be useful to note that, from 1979 to 1990, when total fire deaths measured by death certificates were declining by 30 percent—fire deaths caused by burns by 50 percent, and fire deaths caused by smoke inhalation by 15 percent—total fire deaths measured by the NFPA survey were declining by 31 percent, total reported *fires* were declining by 29 percent, and reported structure fires, where most fire deaths occur, were declining by 40 percent.

To put it another way, the chances of actually experiencing a reported structure fire have been declining rapidly, but the chances of dying if you have a reported structure fire have been rising.

A number of factors could be at work to produce these differing trends. Some fire safety changes, such as the wide-spread adoption of home smoke detectors, can make what might have been fatal fires less likely to be fatal, because people are alerted early enough to escape safely. And what might have been small reported fires are less likely to be reported, because people now discover them earlier and thus control them without any help from the fire department. If the effect on reporting fires is greater than the effect on the lethality of fires, even if both effects are large, there could be a failing trend in reported fires and fire deaths and a rising trend in the rate of deaths per fire. There is some evidence to suggest that this is happening.

Why has there been such a difference in the trends in burn and smoke inhalation deaths? Smoke detectors probably are not part of the answer. From the earlier analysis, we know that the typical smoke inhalation fire death occurs farther away from a fire than the typical burn fire death, which should give smoke detectors more time to help people escape and thus avoid dying of smoke inhalation.

There are other possibilities. First, changes in the composition of furnishings, finishes, and other materials in buildings may generate smoke more rapidly or produce smoke that is more toxic than was true in past decades, leading more quickly to incapacitation and fatalities if a large fire occurs, even as the probability of having a large fire has declined. This possibility is, and has been, at the center of the special concern with toxic fire hazard.

Second, changes in product design and in the public's knowledge of, and behavior toward, fire hazards may have shifted in ways that affect, the kinds of fires that lead to burn deaths—such as matches dropped on clothing and the handling of flammable liquids—more than the kinds of fires that lead to smoke inhalation deaths. For example, the regulation of children's sleepwear in the mid-1970s produced a tremendous reduction in what had been a significant component of children's fire deaths due to burns.

Third, advances in the treatment of fire victims may have changed what would have been fatality victims into injury victims. Those advances may have benefited burn patients more, producing a larger increase in the percentage of badly burned victims who survive than in the percentage of those suffering from serious smoke inhalation who survive.

Unfortunately, while we know enough to realize that changes such as these have occurred, we cannot measure the degree to which the observed changes are due to any single one of these factors.

Ironically, some of our success in reducing the likelihood of fire ignition may have been achieved through design changes that can cause those fires that *do* occur to be more severe, on average. For example, some materials used in upholstered furniture are more, resistant, to ignition by cigarettes, the principal heat source in fatal upholstered furniture fires. But if they are ignited, these materials can produce more severe fire growth.

Conclusions

Smoke inhalation is the leading cause of fire deaths, exceeding burn deaths by roughly seven to three as of 1990 and probably three to one by now, given that the smoke inhalation share has been steadily increasing by slightly more than 1 percentage point a year, since at, least 1979.

Smoke inhalation is the principal part and a growing part of the fatal fire problem. Fortunately, that problem has been shrinking, so much so that smoke inhalation fire deaths are declining in number even though they are increasing as a share of the total.

It is becoming increasingly clear that any future reduction in the total number of fire deaths will have to come from a reduction in those deaths caused by smoke inhalation, because the rest of the problem cannot shrink much further. That probably will mean some new fire safety strategy.

To put it another way, the strategies that produced past successes may be reaching their limits, requiring fresh approaches that target, the major parts of the problem as it now exists. Strategies to prevent smoke inhalation fire deaths could include product design changes that would make ignition even less likely or make fire growth slower should ignition occur. Additional compartmentation, such as more doors between more rooms in homes, as is common in England, would be another approach.

Of course, any strategy should be evaluated in terms of its impact on the whole fire problem, not just on the part of the problem, however large, that inspired that strategy. But in choosing strategies, it is clearer than ever that smoke inhalation is the principal agent of fire deaths that should concern us.

—by John R. Hall, Jr. and Beatrice Harwood

John R. Hall, Jr. is assistant vice-president of NFPA's Fire Analysis and Research Division. Beatrice Harwood recently retired as an analyst with the U.S. Consumer Product Safety Commission.

1. Beatrice Harwood and John R. Hall, Jr., "What Kills in Fires: Smoke Inhalation or Burns?,"*Fire Journal*, May/June 1989, pp29.

2. Walter G Berl and Byron M Halpin. *Human Fatalities from Unwanted Fires,* APL/JHU FPP TR 37, Baltimore: John Hopkins University, December 1978, Figure 14.

3. International Classification of Diseases, 1975 Revision, 1977. Note that this classification system is standardized and set by an international body. Therefore, it may possible to conduct studies similar to this data from other countries.

4. Richard G. Gann, Vytenis Babrauskas, Richard D. Peacock, and John R Hall, Jr.,"Fire Conditions for Smoke Toxicity Measurement," *Fire and Materials*, Vol 18, No. 3 (May/June 1994), pp. 193-199.

Chapter 7

Work-related Burns: A Six-Year Retrospective Study

Abstract

During the six years from July 1984 to May 1990, 193 patients (30.2 percent of all patients) were admitted to our regional adult burn center, for treatment of work-related burn injuries. The median age of patients was 32.5 years (range 18-64 percent), and 94 percent were males, 59 percent of the patients came from metropolitan Toronto, and 40 percent from rural Ontario. Most of the patients (97.3 percent) were referred to the burn center within 24 hours of their injury. The most common aetiology was electrical injury (29.5 percent), followed by flame (24.4 percent), contact (10.4 percent), flash (9.8 percent), tar and asphalt (9.3 percent), scald (7.8 percent), chemical (5.1 percent), steam (4.7 percent) and grease (1 percent). Within the electrical burn group, about one-half were flash burns, one-quarter were clothing fire injuries, and one-quarter were contact injuries.

These occupational burns tended to be extensive injuries. The median body surface area (BSA) was 16.5 percent, with a median full thickness (FT) component of 5.0 percent. The average length of stay was 20.0 days. Inhalation injury requiring intubation occurred in 14.8 percent of patients. Sepsis—confirmed by positive blood cultures— developed in 14 percent of the patients, at an average time of 8.8 days postburn. Staphylococcus aureus was the most common organism isolated from blood cultures. Pneumonia occurred in 6.3 percent of patients.

©Burns April 1991 Printed in Great Britain. Reprinted with permission.

A total of 207 surgical procedures was performed on 113 of the 193 patients. Eleven patients required amputations—seven of these patients had sustained high voltage electrical injuries. The mortality rate for all 193 patients was 6.7 percent. Non-survivors had a median burn size of 85.0 percent, with a median FT component of 85.0 percent.

The total cost of in-hospital patient care was $2.96 million. The total estimated time lost from work for the 193 patients was 459 work-years. Many of these injuries appeared to be preventable.

Introduction

Each year in the USA, burns account for approximately 90,000 hospital admissions and 600 deaths (the fourth leading cause of injury death). In addition, many more patients are treated on an outpatient basis. A recent study in Ohio (Chattejee et al., 1989) indicated that the annual incidence of emergency department-treated burns was 4.7 per 1000 population. This represented 2.4 percent of all trauma incidence visits.

Published literature on burn epidemiology and statistics has been directed primarily towards domestic burns. There are few studies on work-related injuries. The available studies from the USA indicate that the frequency of such burns ranged from 21 to 30 percent of all

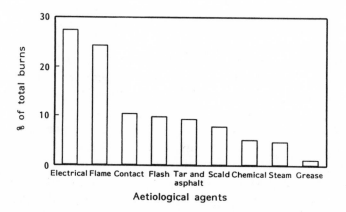

Figure 7.1. Aetiology of 193 work-related burn injuries

94

burn admissions (Iskrant, 1967; Barancik and Shapiro, 1975; MacArthur and Moore, 1975; Clark and Lerner, 1978; Rossignol et al., 1986). In two recent studies of adult patients in the Massachusetts area (Rossignol et al., 1986, 1989), young workers (16-24 years old) sustained burns two to four times more frequently than older patients, men—particularly black-skinned men and young men—sustained injuries much more commonly than their female counterparts, and scald injuries were the most common of burns, accounting for 45 percent of the injuries.

Methods

There are no published studies available on work-related injuries in Canada (Statistics Canada, 1985). The present study was designed to analyze retrospectively all work-related burn patients admitted to the Ross Tilley Burn Center (RTBC) at the Wellesley Hospital, in Toronto, over a 6-year period (from 1984-1990).

When patients are discharged from the RTBC, an extensive database analysis is completed and entered into the center's computer system. This information was subsequently analyzed for this study. In many cases, subsequent chart reviews were also required. In Canada, patients injured in the workplace are financially compensated by the Workplace Safety and Insurance Board (WSIB). To document precisely the time loss from work in this study, the records of the WSIB were reviewed.

The aetiological classification of burn injury has not been standardized in previous studies. In the present study, electrical burns include all thermal injuries resulting from electrical causes, including flash burns, clothing fire, electrical contact, and arcing injuries (Figure 7.1). In both electrical and other categories, flash burns have been separated from other types of flame burns. Flash burns included only explosion types of injuries (Figure 7.1), where the patient's clothing did not catch fire. These burns generally involved the face and hands, and were more superficial than clothing fire injuries (Figure 7.1).

Results

Patient Population

From July 1984 to May 1990 (when the total number of burn admissions was 640), 193 patients (30.2 percent) were admitted for the treatment of work-related burn injuries. The ages of the patients ranged from 18 to 64 years (median 32.5 years). Ninety-four percent

Table 7.1. Aetiology of flame burns

	Patients (no.)
A. Combustible fluid	
Gasoline	10
Xylene	7
Hexane	5
Acetone	3
Diesel fuel	2
Propane	2
Unspecified	2
Alcohol	1
Paint	1
Total	33
B. Intense heat source	
Acetylene torches	5
Molten metal	5
Sparks from machines	3
Open flame	1
Total	14

Table 7.2. Aetiology of the 10 chemical burns

	Patients (no.)
A. Alkali	
Sodium hydroxide	3
Detoxification agent	1
Pulp decomposing agent	1
Unknown	1
B. Acid	
Hydrofluoric acid	2
Sulphuric acid	1
Phenol	1

were males. Fifty-nine percent of the patients were from metropolitan Toronto, and 40 percent were from rural Ontario. Four patients were from other provinces in Canada. The Ross Tilley Burn Center at the Wellesley Hospital serves as the regional adult burn center for metropolitan Toronto and southern Ontario. In this study, 97.3 percent of the patients were referred to the center within 24 hours of their burn injury.

Aetiology

The aetiology of all work-related burn injuries is shown in Figure 7.1.

Electrical Burns. Electrical injury was the most common cause of burn injury and accounted for 27.5 percent (53/193) of all patients. This group can be subclassified into four categories: flash, clothing fire, direct electrical contact, and arcing.

Of the 53 patients with electrical injuries, 26 sustained flash burns, 13 sustained clothing fire injuries, and 14 had contact electrical injuries. There were no arc burns. Of the 26 patients with flash burns, 18 were working with electrical panels or circuits when their injury occurred. The other eight patients were working with electrical relays, wiring or transformers. The 13 clothing fire injuries all resulted when sparks from electrical units ignited the patients' clothing.

Of the 14 contact electrical accidents, five patients sustained low tension less than 1,000 volts) injury, and nine patients sustained high tension (over 1000 volts) injuries. "The high voltage" injuries ranged from 2,400 volts to 115,000 volts. Of these 14 patients, eight unknowingly contacted live components directly. In the other six patients, the vehicles in which they were riding contacted live components.

Flame burns. Flame Burns were the second most common cause of burn injury, and resulted in 24.4 percent (47/193) of the work-related burns. Two main mechanisms were noted—about 40 percent of the patients were injured following the explosion of combustible fluids, and about 60 percent sustained their injury when their clothing was ignited by sparks or flames from intense heat sources (Table 7.1). Gasoline was the most common combustible fluid (10/32 patients), followed by xylene, hexane, acetone, diesel fuel, propane, and alcohol. The nature of the combustible fluid was unspecified in two patients (Table 7.1). Of the 14 patients who sustained clothing fire burns from intense heat sources, acetylene torches and molten metal were the most common aetiological agents, and together caused 10 of the

14 injuries in that group (Table 7.2). The median body surface area (BSA) of the flame burn patients was 15.0 percent (range 2-91 percent).

Thermal contact burns. Direct contact was responsible for 10.4 percent (20/193) of the work-related burns (Figure 7.1). Half of these patients sustained their injuries when their upper extremities were accidentally caught in heated industrial equipment (steam press, dye cast machine and oven door). As expected, burns severity increased with prolonged contact time and temperature elevation. In general, the BSA involved with contact burns tended to be smaller than many other types of burns—median BSA 2.0 percent (range 1-15 percent).

Flash Burns. Flash burns were the fourth most common cause of burns in this series, and resulted in 9.8 percent (19/193) of the injuries (Figure 7.1). Eighteen of these burns were due to explosions. Eleven patients were near compressed fuels (propane or acetylene), which were ignited by adjacent machinery, resulting in an explosion. Other combustible compounds (gasoline, glue and starch) were implicated in five patients. Three other patients sustained injuries following the premature ignition of explosives (ammunition, rocket fuel). Contact with a large industrial furnace produced the only non-explosive flash injury. The median BSA of the flash burn patient was 12.0 percent (range 2-95 percent).

Hot tar asphalt. Hot tar or asphalt was the cause of burn injury in 9.3 percent (18/193) of the patients. In 10 of patients, the heated material spilled directly onto the patient or he fell into it. In three patients, their injury resulted when pipes containing heated tar accidently burst. The median BSA of the group was relatively small— 4.0 percent (range 3–14 percent).

Scald Burns. Scald injury accounted for 7.8 percent (15/193) of the burns (Figure 7.1). Of these 15 patients, eight were accidentally sprayed with heated fluids, four were injured when liquid being poured splashed onto them, and three patients fell into open tanks of heated fluids, when they accidentally lost their footing. The median BSA of the scald burns was 16.0 percent (range 1-90 percent).

Chemical Burns. Chemical agents were responsible for 5.1 cent (10/193) of all occupational burns (Figure 7.1). Five patients sustained alkali burns, four patients had acid burns, and the causative agent was unknown in one patient (Table 7.2). The median BSA of this group of patients was 6.0 percent (range 1-98 percent).

Steam Burns. Steam burns resulted in 4.7 percent (9/193) of the burn injuries. In five patients, these burns were sustained when a steam valve was accidentally opened. In the four other patients, the aetiology was thought to be a faulty valve or pipe system. The median BSA of this group was 25.5 percent (range 10-50 percent).

Grease Burns. Hot grease was responsible for only two burn injuries in this study. Both patients were chefs, one in a fast-food restaurant. These burns were relatively small—1 and 3 percent BSA.

Industrial Sector

The proportion of injuries by employment sector is shown in Table 7.3. The most common sectors involved were manufacturing and construction. Burn injuries were relatively uncommon in the transportation and communication, forestry, agriculture, trade and mining industries.

Table 7.3. Burn incidence by industry sector

Employment sector	percent of patients
Manufacturing	40.4
Construction	38.2
Service	11.8
Transportation and communication	3.7
Forestry	2.2
Agriculture	1.5
Trade	1.5
Mining	0.7

Table 7.4. Anatomical distribution of partial skin thickness (PT) and full skin thickness (FT) Burn injuries

	PT (percent of patients)	FT (percent of patients)
Head and neck	24.2	6.4
Arms	22.6	27.2
Hands	14.5	17.2
Anterior trunk	14.2	12.4
Legs	11.5	16.4
Posterior trunk	8.4	10.0
Genitalia	2.0	2.0
Perineum	1.6	2.4
Feet	1.0	6.0

Table 7.5. Amputations following high voltage electrical injuries

Patient no.	Age (yr)	percent BSA burned	Voltage	Types(s) of amputations
1	35	50	1,000	Left hand
2	28	6	16,000	Left thumb; right below knee
3	31	20	16,000	Left hip disarticulation; right below knee
4	56	3	45,000	Right 4th and 5th toes
5	58	10	16,000	Right 4th and 5th toes, left 4th and 5th metatarsals
6	48	9	16,000	Right below knee
7	21	15	1,000	Right 5th toe; left below knee

Distribution of Burns

The median BSA involved by the burn injury was 16.5 percent, with a range from 1.0 to 98.0 percent. The median full thickness (FT) injury was 5.0 percent, and ranged from 0.5 percent to 98.0 percent. The anatomical distribution of burn injuries is shown in Table 7.5. Partial skin thickness injuries were most common on exposed areas—the head and neck, and arms and hands. Full skin thickness injuries usually resulted from clothing fires, and occurred most frequently on the upper and lower limbs. As expected, burn injuries to the genitalia and perineum were relatively uncommon (Table 7.4).

Surgical Procedures

Of all work-related injuries, 58.6 percent of the patients (113/193) required a total of 207 surgical procedures. Fifteen patients with circumferential or high voltage electrical burns needed 18 sessions of escharotomy and/or fasciotomy, shortly after their admission to the burn center. Of the patients with full skin thickness or deep partial skin thickness burn injuries, 105 underwent a total of 169 debridement and skin grafting procedures.

Eleven patients required total of 16 amputations. Seven of these patients had extensive underlying tissue necrosis from high-voltage electrical injuries. Their amputation levels are shown in Table 7.5. Three patients underwent laparotomy—one for internal injuries, one for acalculus cholecystitis, and one to insert a Greenfield vascular filter, because of a deep vein thrombosis.

Complications

A significant inhalation injury, requiring intubation, occurred in 14.8 percent (29/193) of the patients. The extent of these injuries was confirmed by fibre-optic bronchoscopy. These patients were intubated for an average of 12.2 days. Sepsis—confirmed by the presence of a positive blood culture—developed in 14 percent (27/193) of the patients. The average time of onset of positive blood culture was 8.8 days. The most common organism isolated from blood cultures was *Staphylococcus aureus* (10 patients), followed by *Pseudomonas aeruginosa* (five patients), and *Enterobacteria* (four patients). Two patients had positive blood cultures for methicillin-resistant *Staphylococcus aureus* during a brief outbreak of this organism in the Burn Center.

101

Pneumonia, verified by positive X-rays and/or fibre-optic broncho-scopy, was diagnosed in 6.3 percent (12/193) of the patients. Of this group, approximately one-third had bilateral consolidations. The average time of onset of pneumonia was 9.5 days postburn.

Mortality

The mortality rate in this series was 6.7 percent. The mean age of those patients who died was 39.3 years (range 23-61 years). Their average BSA was 77.78 percent, with 72.1 percent being full skin thickness. The leading cause of death was sepsis with multi-system failure.

Hospital Stay and Treatment Costs

The 193 patients with work-related injuries required a total of 3,844 days in hospital. Their average length of stay was 20.0 days. The total health care cost for this group of patients was $2.96 million.

Work-years Lost

In this series, 89.6 percent (169/193) of the patients were able to return to their previous employment. Their average loss of time from work was 85.0 days. This resulted in a combined loss of 55.1 work-years.

Thirteen patients died, while four others were permanently totally disabled. This resulted in an additional total estimated time loss of 339 years and 58 years respectively. Two patients required extensive job-retraining resulting in a further loss of 6.5 work-years. The total estimated time loss for all 193 patients in this study was 459 work-years.

Discussion

The present study confirms that the work place is a major cause of burn injuries admitted to a burn center. From 1984 to 1990, 30.2 percent (193/640) of all patients admitted to the burn center sustained their injuries at work. Of these 193 patients, 94.3 percent were males, and 64.2 percent were under the age of 35 years. Our burn center serves as a regional adult burn center. This concept appears to be recognized, as 97.3 percent of the burn injuries were referred to our unit within 24 hours of the injury.

The most common causes of work-related burns in this study were electrical (27.5 percent), and flame burns (24.4 percent). Scald burns accounted for only 7.8 percent of the injuries (Figure 7.1). These findings are quite different from other studies of work-related injuries, which have indicated that scald burns were the most common type of work injuries (Rossignol et al., 1986; Inancsi and Guidotti, 1987; Lyngdorf, 1987). Many scald burn injuries at work may be expected to involve smaller burn areas, and may well have been treated at local community hospitals, rather than in our regional adult burn center. In this study, the median BSA was 16.5 percent, which is considerably higher than other studies. Inancsi and Gitidotti (1987) had reported an average BSA of 9.20 percent, and Lyngdorf (1987) had shown an average BSA of 0.66 percent. The higher BSA in our study may well indicate the tertiary referral nature of our burn center.

In this study, work-related injuries tended to be significant burns. The median area of the full skin thickness component was 5.0 percent. Surgical procedures were required in 58.6 percent of all patients. Inhalation injury occurred in 14.8 percent of patients, sepsis in 14.0 percent, and pneumonia in 6.3 percent of all patients. The amputation rate was high in patients who sustained high voltage electrical injuries. The mortality rate in this study was 6.7 percent. These patients who succumbed to their burns tended to have larger burns— their median BSA was 85.0 percent, with a median full skin thickness component of 85.0 percent.

The cost of health care has escalated significantly during the past several years. In this study, the 193 patients with work-related burn injuries required a total of 3,844 days in hospital. The total cost of in-hospital health care for this group was $2.96 million. The cost of work-related burn injuries to society is enormous. In this study, the total estimated time loss from work in the 193 patients, was 459 work-years.

The majority of work-related burns are preventable. Several important occupational hazards were revealed in the present study. Combustible fluids and electrical panels, in particular, accounted for approximately one-third of all work-related burns. It is hoped that a concerted effort could be made, on behalf of both employers and employees, to heighten the awareness of these particular sources of danger. Because of the high incidence of flame burns, further consideration should also be given to the use of flame-resistant clothing, for certain work situations. The devastating nature of high-voltage burn injuries merits special consideration (Table 7.5).

Acknowledgements

The authors are indebted to the burn team, for their unique commitment to the total care of the burn patient. Special thanks are extended to Mr Eric Doucette, Nursing Unit Administrator, for providing a cost analysis of the Burn Center, and to the Department of Medical Records at the Wellesley Hospital. This study was supported in part by MRC grant no. MS-1127.

References

Barancik J. I. and Shapiro M. A. (1975) Pittsburgh Burn Study—Report No. PB 250-737. Springfield VA: National Technical Information Service.

Chatterjee B. F., Barancik, J. I. and Fratianne R. B. (1986) Northeastern Ohio trauma study: V. Burn injury. *J. Trauma* 26, 844.

Clark W. R. Jr and Lemer D. (1978) Regional Burn survey: two years of hospitalized burned patients in central New York *J. Trauma* 18, 524.

Inancsci W. and Guidotti T. L (1987) Occupation-related burns: five-year experience of an urban burn center. *J. Occup. Med.* 29, 730.

Iskrant A-P. (1967) Statistics and epidemiology of burns. Bull. N.Y. *Acad. Med* 45,636.

Lyngdorf P. (1987) Occupational burn injuries. *Burns* 13, 294.

MacArthur J. D. and Moore F. D. (1975) Epidemiology of burns—the burn prone patient. *JAMA* 231, 259.

Rossignol A. M., Locke J. A., Boyle C. M. et al. (1986) Epidemology of the work-related burn injuries in Massachusetts requiring hospitalization. *J. Trauma* 26. 1097.

Rossignol A. M., Locke J. A. and Burke J. F. (1989) Employment status and the frequency and causes of burn injuries in New England. *J. Occup. Med.* 31, 751.

Statistics Canada (1985-1988) Work injuries, Cat. No. 72-208 Supply & Services Canada, Ottawa.

—by D.Ng, D. Anastakis, L. G. Douglas and W. J. Peters Ross Tilley Burn Center, Wellesley Hospital and Division of Plastic Surgery, University of Toronto, Toronto, Canada

Part Two

Types and Degrees of Burns

Chapter 8

Thermal Burns

About two million burn injuries each year require medical attention or restriction of activity. The 90,000 patients admitted to hospitals each year with burns require over a million days of hospital care, or an average of 12 days per admission.

Burns are usually caused by thermal energy. They may also result from exposure to certain chemicals, electricity, ultraviolet radiation and ionizing radiation. This article focuses on thermal energy burns which occur when heat reaches the body in amounts or at rates that exceed the body's ability to dissipate the heat.

The distribution of non-fatal burn causes follows:

Contact with hot objects	24 percent
Scalds and burning grease	21 percent
Explosions (including ovens/furnaces)	10 percent
Fabric ignition only	12 percent
Welding and soldering	4 percent
Trying to extinguish fire in home	11 percent
Electrical short circuits	1 percent
Gasoline related	11 percent
Motor vehicles	10 percent
Other	6 percent

About one in every twenty burns that are treated is serious enough to result in hospitalization. With non-fatal fires, women are involved three times more often than men.

Initially, most burns are minor problems. But without aggressive first aid, these injuries can progress to serious conditions. Early assessment and care of the burn patient is critical in minimizing long-term disability and disfigurement.

Clothing should be quickly and carefully removed. Don't pull a stuck fabric; cut around where it adheres to the skin. The burn can be touched without causing further injury; however, the area shouldn't be handled since bacterial contamination can result. Don't apply petroleum jelly, grease, lard, mineral oil, butter, milk or any burn ointment. They seal in the heat, may have to be removed, and offer no real pain relief.

For most minor burns, a continuous flow of cool tap water stops pain. Cool water works most effectively when applied immediately after the injury, but even up to 45 minutes after the burn cooling can help. The burned area should be immersed in cool water while keeping the tap on to maintain the temperature. If the site of the injury renders this awkward, cool compresses refreshed frequently under cool water will suffice. The patient with a major burn—one involving more than 10 percent of the body surface, or the rough equivalent of the surface of one arm—should be transported immediately to the nearest emergency facility.

Exceptions to using cool water irrigation involve burns caused by burning tar and extensive burns. Burning tar cools quickly when ice or freezing water is applied. The cooled, brittle tar can be brushed or flaked off the wound. The most effective method of removing tar is to dissolve it slowly in an agent such as Neosporin ointment.

While transporting a burned patient to an emergency facility, apply insulated ice packs or ice wrapped in several layers of toweling. It takes from thirty minutes to three hours to stop the pain, depending on the depth and extent of the wound. Cooling is no longer necessary if pain does not recur when the compresses are removed from the burn for a 5-minute period. Cover the burned arm with a dry, sterile dressing or clean sheet.

When the patient is a child, always consider the possibility of child abuse. Deliberately inflicted burns often resemble those of accidental origin. Suspect a deliberate burn when:

- The parent shows either unusual wariness or lack of concern.
- The injury is primarily in the genital/buttocks region.

- There is a long delay before the patient is provided any type of emergency care.

- The child has been involved repeatedly in "accidents." There may be several injuries in various stages of healing.

- There are discrepancies between the explanation of the burn and the nature and type of the injury.

Assess the extent and depth of the burn. The amount of the skin surface involved can be calculated quickly by using the "rule of nines." Each of the following areas represents 9 percent of the body surface in an adult: the head and neck, each arm, the chest, the abdomen, the upper back, the lower back and buttocks, the front of each lower limb, and the back of each lower limb. The genital region is 1 percent. The fact that the patient's hand is about 1 percent of the total body surface is very useful in estimating the size of small or oddly shaped burns.

In children, the head is larger in relationship to the body and should be counted as 18 percent, and the legs are smaller (14 percent); otherwise, the basic rule of nine may be used.

In the severely burned, estimating the percentage of the unburned area can sometimes be more accurate than estimating burned areas. It is better to overestimate the extent of a burn than to underestimate.

Continue evaluating the burn by determining its depth or degree. Even the experienced may have difficulty. It is especially difficult to determine depth of a burn very early after injury. A burn area that is reddened—but not blistered—is a superficial (first-degree) burn. It will he painful. Distinguishing a partial thickness (second-degree) from a full thickness (third-degree) burn can be difficult. Rarely is an entire burn of one degree or another, but rather a combination of first-, second- and third-degree burns. Generally, if several intact blisters are present and are very painful, the burn is probably a partial thickness (second-degree) burn. Soot, until it is washed off, can cause confusion in determining the degree of a burn. If the injury is insensitive to pinprick, has a parchment-like (leathery) appearance, and shows clotted blood vessels, suspect a full thickness (third-degree) burn. Though the nerve endings of the skin may be destroyed and therefore no pain may be felt, the margins of such a burn will not have its nerve endings destroyed and may be extremely painful. The skin often has a burned smell, the odor of burning flesh.

After assessing the extent and depth of injury, determine if the patient requires medical treatment. Burn severity is usually considered either minor, moderate or critical.

Patients with suspected inhalation injuries as suggested by burns that occurred when the patient was in an enclosed space require medical attention. A patient with chronic medical problems, such as cardiac disease or diabetes, should receive medical care.

Also, patients with significant burn involvement of the face, hands, feet or genital area should be seen by a medical authority.

Minor burns can be treated at home. Severe burn care should follow a physician's directions. However, many of these cases may be cared for afterward at home, if the following are kept in mind:

- Wash your hands thoroughly with soap and water.

- Spread the ointment (silver sulfadiazine) on the bandage.

- Wash and remove the dressings:

- Remove the old dressings by cutting off the outer layer and then rolling off the rest. Do not pull the dressing off if it is sticking to the wound; soak it off in a basin or tub.

- Soak the burn for 10 to 15 minutes in a mild detergent solution. Gently wash over the burned area with a soft washcloth to remove any old blood, cream, loose skin, or dry, yellow matter.

- Rinse the wound with clear water. Pat the area dry with a freshly laundered soft towel.

- Cover the wound with one layer of dressing treated with ointment (silver sulfadiazine) and wrap snugly with six to seven layers of dry bandage.

Physician appointments should he kept regardless of how well the patient may feel. If there is any sign of infection such as fever (102 degrees or higher), yellow pus, a foul smell, increase in pain and redness or red streaking, consult with a physician.

As the burn heals, the skin and joints nearby can become stiff. To loosen them you should exercise the joints and muscles around the burn as soon as healing begins.

Burn prevention practices, especially in the home, are of the utmost importance in reducing the incidence of burns.

Here is a safety checklist:

- Do not smoke in bed.

- Keep matches out of reach of children.

- Keep fireplaces well-screened or covered.

- Keep portable heaters in good repair.

- Regularly check your furnace and hot water heater.

- Set the hot water heater no higher than 130 degrees Fahrenheit.

- Always test the temperature of a baby's bath with the wrist or elbow to make sure it is comfortable to the touch (90 to 100 degrees Fahrenheit).

- Store cleaning fluids and paints in a cool, well-ventilated area where children cannot get them.

- Keep rubbish out of basement and attic.

- Cover unused electric outlets with plastic covers.

- Do not overload electric outlets.

- Insulate and ground electric cords

- Use only UL-approved appliances

- Do not obstruct ventilation of TV set.

- Use heating pads according to directions.

- Do not reach across an open burner while cooking.

- Keep hot liquids out of the reach of children. Do not allow pot handles to protrude over the edge of the stove.

- Do not refuel a hot lawn mover, snowblower or other small gasoline engine.

- Do not refuel a hot or lighted kerosene stove.

- Install smoke detectors, especially outside bedroom doors.

- Practice a fire escape plan.

All people have been burned at some time in their lives. Because of its prevalence, all first responders should be prepared to provide emergency care for burn injury.

—by Alton L. Thygerson

Chapter 9

Grease Burns of the Hand

Abstract

Grease burns to the hand represent a serious and preventable hazard. These injuries account for over 10 percent of all major burns seen in the emergency department. These burns occur when the cook attempts to move a pan with burning cooking oil and inadvertently spills the oil on the hand holding the pan. These burns are usually full thickness because of either the high temperatures of the flaming oils or the subsequent ignition of clothing. This article describes a patient who received severe partial and full thickness burns to the dominant hand following a grease burn in the domestic setting. Prevention through improved consumer education and warning labels for cooking oils should reduce the incidence of these serious injuries.

In case fat should ever catch fire, have a metal lid handy to drop over the kettle (*Joy of Cooking*, 1975).[1]

Introduction: Preventable Injuries

Hot cooking oil or grease burns represent a serious and preventable hazard. Second only to hot water as a cause of scald injury, these burns represent 10.4 percent of all major burns and 8.2 percent of all minor burns seen in the emergency department[2]. These grease burns occur most commonly in the domestic setting when an attempt is made

©May/June 1996 *The Journal of Emergency Medicine*, Vol 14, Elsevier Science Inc. Reprinted with permission.

to move a container in which cooking oil has ignited, and it is inadvertently spilled on the hand holding the container[3]. These burns are usually full thickness because of either the high temperatures of the flaming oils or the subsequent ignition of clothing. The severity of these injuries must be recognized in the emergency department since early and aggressive surgical therapy is of special importance for injuries to the hand because of its unique functional importance and long-term cosmetic concerns[3]. Prevention through unproved consumer education and warning labels for cooking oils should reduce the incidence of these serious injuries. This article describes a patient who received severe partial and full thickness burns to the dominant hand following a grease burn. If the patient had understood the hazards of hot grease, she might have been better prepared for the fire and avoided the functional and cosmetic sequelae of severe burns to the hand.

Case Report

The patient is a 23 year-old female who suffered a deep partial thickness and full thickness grease burn on the dorsal surface of her dominant right hand. The accident occurred at home while heating corn oil in a pan. When the grease ignited after reaching its flash point, she quickly moved the pan, inadvertently spilling it on her hand. Five days after the accident, the patient came to the emergency department, where she presented with leathery, insensate skin on the dorsum of her hand. The skin color was pale white, with no capillary refill. Hair was visibly absent. The skin was anesthetic to contact with a sterile applicator stick. Because the burn was judged to be full thickness, plastic surgery consultation was obtained. After tetanus prophylaxis was administered, the patient was admitted to the burn center. The following day, she was taken to surgery for tangential excision of the burn wound until there was a bleeding, viable wound bed. After hemostasis was achieved, a split-thickness skin graft (0.012 in) was harvested from her left thigh and applied to the excised bed. The graft healed without infection. To prevent the development of hypertrophic scar formation, the patient was fitted with an elastic pressure glove garment, which she was to wear each day. Because she was not compliant with this recommendation, she developed a severe, hypertrophic scar.

Discussion

In scald burns, such as those that occur from a hot grease spill, the severity of the injury is related to the rate of heat transfer to the skin[2]. This property is dependent upon the temperature and duration of contact of the agent and the specific heat and conductivity of the local tissues. The initial temperature of an agent at the time of contact is very important. Although water can only be heated to 100°C at atmospheric pressure without vaporizing, grease can attain much greater temperatures. Particularly important is the fact that greases are combustible materials, and instead of vaporizing, they will ignite, posing an even greater danger to the user when the flash point is reached. The duration of contact between the liquid and the skin depends on the viscosity of the liquid as well as the mechanism in which it is applied to the victim's skin. Viscous oils and greases usually cling to the patient's skin, causing extensive local damage. The specific conductivity of the local tissues plays an important role in the rate and degree of thermal injury. Because skin is a relatively poor conductor of heat, it provides a formidable barrier to heat injury. Water content, local oils and secretions, and the cornified keratin layer of the skin all influence tissue conductivity. Moreover, local blood flow produces a profound effect on heat transfer and distribution and enhances the ability of the skin to conduct heat away from the burn site.[2]

The importance of duration of exposure and temperature as factors in the magnitude of burn injury was studied by Moritz and Henriques.[5] They demonstrated irreversible damage to the basal epidermal cells after six hours of contact at a temperature of 44°C. As the temperature increased only 3 degrees to 47°C, they noted significant partial thickness burns in less than 30 min. Further increasing the temperature to 51°C resulted in complete epidermal necrosis after only 4 min. As temperatures increased above 70°C, less than two seconds were needed for complete destruction of the epidermis. Because cooking oils are most commonly heated to temperatures well above these values, and their flash points usually exceed 200°C, it is easy to understand why flaming oils can instantaneously cause full thickness burns.

Our patient had a typical grease burn, which occurred on the dominant hand after grabbing a hot skillet. This experience is consistent with Pegg and Seawright[3], who discuss the hazard of burns received from hot cooking oils. They report 112 cases of hot oil burns, the vast majority of which were received in the domestic setting. Most of the burns occurred when the hot oil ignited, and the patient attempted to move the cooking vessel. Interestingly, the patients in the study had no predisposing factors for burn injury (e.g., alcoholism, drug abuse, anesthetic skin, paralysis). These authors feel that improving consumer education is paramount to the prevention of these burns. In particular, they note that no warning labels were found on any major brands of frozen foods or cooking oils. They suggested the inclusion of precautions on these products, which should mention the risks of ignition and the danger of adding water to hot oil.

Hayes-Lundy et al.[6] report the danger that grease burns present to young adults. They note that grease burns account for 7-8 percent of all serious burn injuries, most frequently resulting from kitchen accidents. In their study, they report the incidence and consequence of grease burns received in restaurant kitchens, which represent 55 percent of all scald burns in this industry. They focus on the large economic burden, which manifests as medical care costs and lost work. Of the patients in their burn center who required surgery, the average cost of care was over $7,000. They also surveyed the state insurance record, which listed 81 reported grease burns over a three year period at an average burn care cost of $660 per patient. Like Pegg and Seawright[3], these authors feel that improved education would dramatically reduce the incidence of these injuries. They discuss specific measures to prevent grease burns, including orientation films, increasing the length of training periods with periodic refresher courses, and specific education on grease handling techniques.

Because grease burns result largely from a lack of consumer education, cooking pans and particularly deep-fryers should provide detailed warning labels, which inform the user of the dangers of cooking with hot grease. Unfortunately, when examining six different brands of skillets and kettles, none were found to have warning labels mentioning the hazards of hot grease. Furthermore, no electric deep-fryer examined had a pamphlet that discussed the possibility of a grease fire. The cook should be aware that vessels used for frying should have a flat bottom, which decreases the likelihood of spilling. In addition, these vessels should have short handles turned away from the edge of the stove, which reduces the chance of accidental spilling. The cooking oils themselves need detailed, easily readable warning labels. Through a survey of cooking oils it was observed that all ten domestic brands had warning labels. Nevertheless, there was a great variation in the readability of the labels. Additionally, no imported oils had warning labels.

The best warning system would be in large, block letters. It needs to be easily read, and the letters should be colored, contrasting with both the general consumer information and the background color of the label. Pertinent points it should address include covering the cooking vessel and turning off the heat when the oil ignites. It should mention the hazard of pouring water on hot grease. Notably absent from all labels surveyed and of special importance were instructions never to move a vessel containing hot grease—particularly one that has ignited. Although some labels mention a recommended frying temperature, it would be practical to also mention the flash point of the oil. Because cooking oils are frequently advertised on television, this medium would provide an excellent opportunity to further illustrate these preventive measures. Visual representation of this safety advice would help to educate consumers about the hazards of grease fires. Because split-second decisions must be made once a fire has started, the cook has little time to formulate a plan. The danger of the situation is attenuated only when the cook is aware of the hazard prior to a grease fire.

When preventive measures are unsuccessful, there is uniform agreement that grease burns usually present with full thickness injury, and surgeons recommend early excision and grafting of these injuries. Parry[4] reviews reconstruction of the burned hand and emphasizes aggressive surgical therapy for these injuries. He reports that the best cosmetic and functional results occur with full-thickness grafts followed by split-thickness and meshed split-thickness grafts. He notes that the availability of an acceptable donor site is an important factor in the determination of the graft type. Leen et al.[7] discuss the efficacy of split-thickness grafting in the case of a hot oil burn of an adolescent female. They discuss the importance of early grafting in the young adult population, for whom immobilization and hospital care are difficult to maintain. They also note the importance of cosmetic result in this population and the undesirable effects of hypertrophic scar, which results from primary healing. Ward[8] reports that hypertrophic scarring can be markedly reduced by the use of continuous pressure over healed burn injury. The use of pressure garments following wound stabilization should be used for 6-18 months. This is the usual period for scar maturation, and it is during this time that the scar will actively contract. In the case reported in this article, poor compliance with the pressure garment likely contributed to the development of a hypertrophic scar.

Conclusion

The mechanism of burn injury described in this article represents the most common scenario seen in grease burns. The patient, who had no particular risk factors for burn injury, was cooking with hot grease in the domestic setting, and she received extensive burns to her dominant hand. Rather than covering the pan with a lid and turning the heat off, she moved the pan, inadvertently spilling hot oil on her hand. This inappropriate management of the grease fire obviously reflects the need for improved consumer education. Because grease burns are usually full thickness, they require excision of the burn wound and the application of skin grafts. Despite thorough debridement of all nonviable tissue along with the placement of split-thickness skin grafts, the patient developed extensive scar hypertrophy, a common sequela of burn injury. Improved warning label systems, which are easily readable and which contrast in color and size with the other information on the label, would help to prevent these injuries.

Acknowledgment—This research was supported by a grant from the Texaco Foundation, White Plains, New York.

References

1. Ronibauer IS, Becker MR. Joy of cooking. New York: Bobbs-Merrill Company; 1975:147.

2. Edlich RF, McCullough JL, Thacker JG, Freidman HI. Scald burn injuries. In Edlich RF, Spyker DA, eds. Current emergency therapy. Rockville, MD: Aspen Systems Corp.: 1985:257-61.

3. Pegg SP, Seawright AA. Burns due to cooking oils—an increasing hazard. *Burns*. 1983;9:362-9.

4. Parry SW. Reconstruction of the burned hand. *Clin Plast Surg*. 1989; 16:577-86.

5. Moritz AR, Henriques FC Jr. Studies of thermal injury: pathology and pathogenesis of cutaneous burns; an experimental study. *Am J Pathol*. 1947;23:915-941.

6. Hayes-Lundy C, Ward RS, Saffle JF, Reddy R, Warden GD, Schnebly WA. Grease burns at fast-food restaurants: adolescents at risk. *J Burn Care Rehabil*. 1991; 12:203-8.

7. Leen ME, Feldman M, Schoenberger S, Chae KC. Split-thickness graft of a pedal oil burn in an adolescent female. *J Am Podiatr Med Assoc*. 1991;81:435-9.

8. Ward RS. Pressure therapy for the control of hypertrophic scar formation after burn injury: a history and review. *J Burn Care Rehabil*. 1991;12:257-62.

—by Timothy J. Bill, BA, David J. Bentrem, BA, David B. Drake, MD, and Richard F. Edlich, MD, PhD. Dept of Plastic Surgery and the DeCamp Burn Center, University of Virginia School of Medicine, Charlottesville, Virginia

Chapter 10

Chemical Burns to the Skin

Abstract

Emergency physicians occasionally encounter patients with chemical injuries. Pathophysiology is related to the chemical characteristics of the offending agent, but treatment follows common, simple principles. Only a few agents require individualized therapy.

The emergency physician must have a general understanding of chemical burns. Fortunately this is relatively easy because most burns can be managed by applying management principles consistent with the basic chemistry learned during premedical education. Only a few chemical burns require specific antidotes.

It has been estimated that 10 percent of the 300,000 chemicals in commercial and industrial use can produce chemical burns. No one knows the exact incidence of significant burns, but one estimate places the number at 60,000 per year. If this number is accurate, the average emergency department will encounter about one chemical burn per month.

General principles to be used in the treatment of chemical burns include the following:

- Immediate treatment is more important than identification of the offending agent.

- Chemical burns may be associated with other injuries. Often the more obvious, injuries may lead the emergency physician to overlook the chemical burn. Of course, the converse may also be true.

- Chemical burns may be more severe if the patient is immuno-compromised or debilitated in other ways.[1,2]

Pathophysiology

The chemical mechanism responsible for producing injury is dependent on the nature of the chemical agent involved. For example, sodium hypochlorite, an oxidizing agent, releases free chlorine, thus coagulating protein. Hydrochloric acid, a reducing agent, rapidly coagulates protein by changing it to the salt of a weak acid. A corrosive, sodium hydroxide, produces liquification necrosis by saponifying and dehydrating cells.[3,4]

While perhaps of some scientific interest, the chemical mechanism of injury is really unimportant to the physician confronted with a patient who requires attention. The emergency physician's decision process can generally be based upon the clinical effects of these chemicals on the patient and on comparison of the clinical effects with thermal injury.

Clinical Manifestations

Burns are classified by a number of factors, including their depth, extent, and location. These factors can be quantified to provide guidelines for the management of the burned patient.

Burn characterization by depth is referred to as degree of burn. First-degree burns are superficial and involve only the epidermis. Clinically this is manifested by reddening of the skin. These burns are moderately painful. Second-degree burns include damage to the entire epidermis with extension into the dermis, resulting in blister formation. These burns are severely painful. Third-degree burns are the most serious types of burns because they are characterized by total destruction of the skin and its appendages (i.e., sweat and sebaceous glands, hair follicles) with formation of a hard eschar. There is generally little or no pain except from adjacent areas of second-degree burn.

The clinical manifestations of the chemical injury may also be described by reference to a burn as a partial or full-thickness injury. Superficial partial-thickness injury involves the epidermis only. The burn is red, moist, and blistered. Tactile and pain sensors are intact.

Deep partial-thickness burns involve the entire epidermis and dermis, leaving only skin appendages intact. The underlying tissue is mottled and appears white and dry. This type of burn requires meticulous care but can be expected to heal without scar formation provided there are no complications during treatment. Full-thickness burns are equivalent to the third-degree classification. Skin is totally destroyed and a hard eschar is present. Spontaneous healing will not occur.

The rule of nines may be used to provide an approximation of body surface for classification of burns and for determination of initial fluid resuscitation. In this classification, first degree burns are not included because they do not affect fluid requirements. Based on the rule of nines, estimates of skin area include the following:

Head and neck	9 per cent
Anterior trunk	18 per cent
Posterior trunk	18 per cent
Upper extremities	9 percent each
Lower extremities	18 percent each
Perineum	1 per cent

The clinical manifestations of chemical burns naturally depend on the organ systems involved.[5,6]

The initial characteristics of a cutaneous injury will be similar to those of a thermal injury, namely, erythema, swelling, and pain. Similar to those of thermal injury, the specific manifestation will depend on the degree and depth of injury. Unlike thermal injury, however, the severity of the burn may initially be underestimated because chemical injury may not become fully manifest for twenty-four to thirty-six hours. Initial injury may appear deceptively mild.[7,8]

Simultaneous with cutaneous injury, there may be damage to other organs. Obviously ingestion of caustic substances may produce some cutaneous manifestations, but the major morbidity will be that related to esophageal burns. The eye is very frequently subjected to chemical injury. Both acids and alkalis penetrate ocular tissue rapidly and may cause permanent injury within thirty seconds.

While beyond the scope of this article, it is necessary to mention that chemical injury to the lungs may result in extreme morbidity and even mortality. Although chemical injury is most commonly seen as the result of fires involving synthetic material that release toxic products of combustion such as hydrochloric acid, acrolein, phosgene, and free radicals, chemical injury may also result from the inhalation of volatile chemicals during their manufacture, transport, and storage.

The manifestations of pulmonary injury include discoloration by soot, coughing, wheezing, and shortness of breath. Like cutaneous injury, chemical injury to the lungs may be delayed, but clinical manifestations are almost always present by six hours. Worsening may occur over a longer time period. The reader interested in learning more about this topic is referred to research by Cohen and Guzzardi.[9]

Treatment

Because of the rapidity with which chemical injury occurs, treatment should begin immediately, preferably at the scene of initial exposure. Contaminated clothing should be removed, and any particulate material should be brushed away without exposing the rescuer to hazardous material. The exposed area should then be copiously lavaged with water for at least fifteen minutes at the scene. Cool water is theoretically preferred because it will reduce any heat of reaction, thereby minimizing concurrent thermal injury. Obviously, treatment should not be delayed if only warm water is available. Oily materials may require light scrubbing for complete removal. Dilution is the key to treatment because neutralization may result in thermal injury secondary to the heat of the chemical reaction.

Upon arrival to the emergency department, the patient is evaluated for other injuries that may have initially been overlooked or that have been of a lower priority. If there is question as to adequacy of lavage, retreatment is initiated with copious amounts of tap water for at least ten minutes. At the York Hospital emergency department, physicians routinely irrigate affected eyes with 1 Liter of Ringer's lactate per eye even if there is history of immediate lavage. The author does not routinely use ph paper to assess the adequacy of lavage, although its use has been recommended by some experts. The author has found the use of the Morgan's lens to improve efficiency and adequacy of eye lavage, if the patient can tolerate the discomfort.[10,11]

Only after these initial steps have been undertaken should the emergency physician consider the use of specific antidotes.

Specific Antidotes

Phenol

The affected area should be lavaged for five minutes to ten minutes. If this is ineffective in relieving the burning, the area should be bathed with polyethylene glycol 300 or 400 and industrial methylated spirits in a 2:1 mixture. Glycerol, or isopropyl alcohol are acceptable alternatives to this mixture. Glycerol can be used safely on mucous membranes.[12,13,14]

Active metals

Chemically active metals such as sodium and potassium may ignite in the presence of air, whereas other less active metals, such as calcium, magnesium, aluminum, and lithium, burn when ignited. These metals should be smothered or extinguished with chemical extinguishers if possible. Oil will prevent further burning of the metal once it has cooled. The affected area should be irrigated with large amounts of normal saline solution, bathed with 1 percent copper sulfate and then 5 percent sodium bicarbonate solution, and then washed again with saline solution.

Metals that burn should be removed if possible before lavage because of the relatively intense exothermic reaction caused in the presence of water. However, copious lavage may minimize the heat of reaction if it is impractical to remove the offending agent.[8]

Hydrofluoric acid

Hydrofluoric acid has traditionally been widely used in industry and certain service industries. Because of its low ph and corresponding strength as an acid, it can readily penetrate both intact and damaged skin. In extensive exposures (large areas of skin exposed for extended time), there is a possibility of fluoride toxicity. Because of its ability to penetrate tissue, the initial manifestations of burns may be absent, and tissue injury may not become manifest for up to six hours. Even asymptomatic individuals with significant exposure should be treated as if they were injured.

If the skin is uninjured, simple lavage is generally adequate followed by application of a bulky dressing impregnated with calcium gluconate, calcium chloride, or magnesium sulfate. If there is cutaneous evidence of injury or if pain is persistent after irrigation, 100 percent calcium gluconate solution may slowly be injected subcutaneously at a dose of about 0.5 ml/kg. This injection may cause compression of tissue and subsequent necrosis if given in nondistensible tissue. Therefore its use is not recommended in fingertips, a common site of fluoride injury.[15-18,19]

Nitrite/Nitrate burns

Chemical injury from nitrite and nitrate liquid and solids has been reported. Individuals exposed to these agents should be evaluated for the potential of methemoglobinemia.

Methemoglobinemia is treated with a 1 percent solution of methylene blue at a dose of 0.1 to 0.2 ml/kg intravenous. Nitrates and nitrites may be absorbed systemically through intact skin and by inhalation.[7,8]

Calcium hydroxide

Calcium hydroxide is the principal chemical agent found in lime. Besides its agricultural uses, lime is found in cement mixtures. Calcium hydroxide is similar to other moderately strong alkalis, since it can cause tissue necrosis and deep chemical burns. Because of its widespread use, unappreciated toxicity, and mild initial manifestations, calcium hydroxide injury may be rather extensive and require debridement. With cement burns, severity of injury is dependent on degree of abrasion, alkalinity, and duration of exposure. If the cement has not yet hardened, additional water added to the mixture may delay the hardening process and reduce chemical injury.[20]

Tar

Tar or asphalt that comes in contact with skin should be allowed to air cool, although water may be used to reduce the degree of thermal injury by dissipating heat. Various authors have recommended both early and delayed removal of tar. The rationales for both appear appropriate. Tar may be removed by applying an emulsifying agent such as Neosporin cream, Vaseline, or ShurClens. These agents should be applied every six hours. In general, mechanical debridement is not recommended because of its propensity to cause both tissue damage and pain. Stripping of tar may also remove hair follicles pigment from the cutaneous tissue.[8]

Hydrocarbons

Emergency physicians are unlikely to see severe burns from medium volatility hydrocarbons such as turpentine or gasoline. Most gasoline available in the United States no longer contains lead. But systemic lead toxicity following ingestion had been reported in the past. Minor irritation is common and should be treated the same as thermal burns of similar depth.[8]

References

1. Deitch FS. The management of burns. *N Engl J Med.* 1990;323:1249-1253.

2. Herbert K, Lawrence JC. Chemical burns. *Burns.* 1989;15:381-384.

3. Mozingo DW, Smith AA, McManus WF, et al. Chemical burns. *J Trauma.* 1988;28:642-647.

4. Davidson EC. The treatment of acid and alkali burns. *Surgery.* 1927;85:481.

5. Demling RH. Fluid replacement in burned patients. *Surg Clin North Am.* 1987;67:15-30.

6. Edlich RF, Rodeheaver GT, Halfacre SE, et al. Systems conceptualization of burn care on a regional basis. *Top Emerg Med.* 1981;3:7-16.

7. Guzzardi LJ. Chemical injuries to skin. In: Rosen P, Baker F, Eds. *Emergency Medicine—Concepts and Clinical Practice.* St. Louis, MO: Mosby; 1983.

8. Haynes BW, Jr. Emergency department management of minor burns. *Top Emerg Med.* 1981;3:35-40.

9. Cohen MA, Guzzardi LJ. Inhalation of products of combustion. *Ann Emerg Med.* 1983;12(10):628-632.

10. Herr RD, White GL, Bernhisel K, et al. Clinical comparison of ocular irrigation fluids following chemical injury. *Am J Emerg Med.* 1991;9:228-231.

11. Morgan SJ. Chemical burns of the eye: causes and management. *Br J Ophthalmol* 1987;71:854-857.

12. Mozingo DW, Smith AA, McManus WF, et at. Chemical burns. *J Trauma.* 1988;28:642-647.

13. Hunter DM, Timerding BL, Leonard RB, et al Effects of isopropyl alcohol, ethanol, and polyethylene glycol/industrial methylated spirits in the treatment of acute phenol burns. *Ann Emerg Med.* 1992;21:11-15.

14. Brown VKH. Decontamination procedures for skin exposed to phenolic substances. *Arch Environ. Health.* 1975;30:1.

15. Caravati EM. Acute hydrofluoric acid exposure *Am J Emerg Med.* 1988;6:143-150.

16. Schultz CH. Hydrofluoric acid burns of the hand. *West J Med.* 1989;151:71.

17. Iversion RE, Laub DR, Madison MD. Hydrofluoric acid burns. *Plast Reconstr Surg.* 1971;48:107.

18. Mayer TG, Gross PL. Fatal systemic fluorosis, due to hydrofluoric acid burns. *Ann Emerg Med.* 14:149-153.

19. Mullet T, Zoeller T, Bingham H, et al. Fatal hydrofluoric acid cutaneous exposure with refractory ventricular fibrillation. *J Burn Care Rehabil.* 1987;8:216-219.

20. Wilson GR, Davidson PM. Full thickness burns from ready-mixed cement. *Burns.* 1985;12:139-144

— by Lawrence Guzzardi, MD

Faculty Physician Emergency Medicine Residency
Department of Emergency Medicine
York Hospital
York, Pennsylvania

Chapter 11

Electrical Burns

Abstract

Electrical injuries are unique with respect to low mortality rates, but very high rates of short-and long-term morbidity, and overall outcome. Controversy still exists regarding the advantages of one-stage debridement versus early serial debridement of necrotic tissue. The purpose of this study was a retrospective evaluation of treatment, morbidity and outcome in a group of patients with electrical injuries. Over a 13-year period 1,992 patients were admitted with acute burns to our burn center. Electrical injuries occurred in 129 (6.5 percent) of these patients. There were thirty-eight high-tension injuries and 91 low-tension injuries. The average age was 33.7 years (five months to 63 years), with burn wounds ranging from 1 percent to 57 percent total body surface area (mean 9.5 percent). Ninety-four (72.9 percent) of these injuries were work related, and most occurred in males (85 percent). A total of 323 surgical procedures were performed on those 129 patients. An average of 0.48 surgical debridements per patient was necessary in the low-tension injury group and only three partial fingers or toe amputations were necessary. In the high-tension group, twenty-seven major limb amputations were performed after 2.3 debridements per patient, resulting in an overall major limb amputation rate of 35 percent. The average length of stay was 22 days, and the cost of hospitalization ranged from $900 to $120,000 (mean

---

©1995 *Burns* Vol. 21, No. 7, Elsevier Science Ltd. Reprinted with permission.

$14,901). Significant long-term neurological deficits persisted in 73 percent of patients at long-term follow-up; (mean 4.5 years). Only 5.3 percent of patients after high-voltage electrical injury were able to return to their premorbid job.

Introduction

The discovery of electricity and the introduction of dynamo machines presented a major industrial advance. It also caused death soon after its discovery. Jex-Blake and Oxon[1] reported that a stage carpenter was killed in 1879 at Lyon, France, by an alternating current of 250 volts. D'Arsonvall[2] discussed the physiological action of high-frequency alternating currents and its possible usefulness in medical treatment. Many electrical injuries have been reported thereafter followed by clinical and experimental investigations on the pathophysiology and causes of death[3-6]. The most striking finding was a high incidence of death after contact with electricity which did not seem to depend upon the magnitude of electrical tension.

Reports include death after exposure to 46 volts or after therapeutic application of so-called sinusoidal currents with tensions as low as 30-50 volts[7]. One of the most effective precautions was expressed by Kennelly[8] in 1927, who recommended keeping one hand in the pocket when visiting an electric plant. Today advanced security precautions help to reduce the incidence of electrical injuries, but the high rate of major limb amputation, between 45 percent and 71 percent, remains essentially unchanged[9-12]. According to Lee[13], mortality ranges from 3 percent to 15 percent and accounts for more than 1,000 deaths per year in the USA. The most common cause of death remains cardiac arrest following acute arrhythmias at the site of the accident. After arrival in the burn center, general morbidity is the major problem, with the mortality rate usually being low.

Electrical injuries are divided into low-tension (<1,000 volts) and high-tension injuries (>1,000 volts)[14]. A low-tension injury can produce death from cardiac arrhythmias. Severe morbidity following high-tension electrical injuries is generally the result of massive necrosis of deeper structures, often necessitating major limb amputations or extensive reconstruction. Several clinical approaches based on different theories regarding the pathophysiology of injury are in current use, but the complete pathophysiological mechanism of electrical injury remains poorly understood.

Early debridement is necessary to prevent wound infection as well as the systemic challenge with myoglobins and toxic waste products[15,16].

128

Different surgical regimens fail to prove the superiority of one regimen over another, since valuable objective measures like rate of return to work are only sparsely reported. The concept of "progressive" wound necrosis has been introduced by Baxter[17], Skoog[18], Bingham[11] and Rouse and Dimick[19] showed beneficial results after debridement of only obviously non-viable tissue, and stated that within two weeks after the injury, there is usually a good wound base for wound closure. Hunt et al.[20], Quinby et al.[21], Luce and Gottlieb[22] and others favor an aggressive surgical approach with early radical debridement and coverage of the wound incorporating the entire reconstructive armamentarium from skin grafts to free flaps[23]. Wang et al.[24] reported the use of early vein grafting to save limbs from amputation. Chick proposed the use of free flaps for wound coverage of radically debrided wounds within 1-10 days after the injury[25]. These different philosophies have led to a controversy over optimal surgical treatment which is still not resolved.

Table 11.1. Involvement of body parts

Involved body parts	Low-tension electrical injury* (no.)	High-tension electrical injury+ (no.)
Head/neck	12	5
Trunk	12	12
Right upper extremity	54	30
Left upper extremity	72	21
Right lower extremity	27	13
Left lower extremity	51	13
Dominant upper extremity	56	31

*n=91.
+n=38.

Table 11.2. Surgical procedures

Treatment	Low-tension electrical injury (no.*)	High-tension electrical injury[+] (no.)
Exploratory laparotomy	0	2
Carpal tunnel release	0	2
Fasciotomy arm incl. carpel tunnel release	0	42
Fasciotomy leg	0	13
Debridement	44	89
Amputation (see Table 11.3)	3	39
Split thickness skin graft (STSG)	38	14
Full thickness skin graft (FTSG)	4	3
Local flop	0	9
Pedicle groin flap	0	9
Pedicle rectus abdominis flap	0	4
Pedicle latissimus dorsi flap	0	2
Free rectus abdominis flap	0	1
Free latissimus dorsi flap	0	3
Free deltopectoral flap	0	1
Free fibula transfer	0	1
Total	89	234
Visits to the operating room	43	89
Visits to the operating room per patient	0.47	2.23
Debridements per patient	0.48	2.34
Amputations per patient	0.03	1.03
Local/distal flaps per patient	0	0.79

*n= 91.
[+]n= 38.

Most patients had more than one procedure per visit to the operating room.

Table 11.3. Amputations

Amputation	Low-tension electrical injury[+] (no.)	High-tension electrical injury[*] (no.)
Thumb, tip	1	0
Thumb, IP joint	0	1
Thumb, MP joint	0	2
Finger, DIP joint	1	1
Finger, PIP joint	0	0
Finger, MP joint	0	2
Below elbow	0	13
Elbow disarticulation	0	1
Above elbow	0	4
Shoulder disarticulation	0	4
Toe	1	4
Foot, distal third	0	1
Below knee	0	2
Above knee	0	3
Ribs (resection)	0	1
Total	3	39
Bilateral major amputations	0	6
Tripod amputation	0	1

[*]n=91.
[+]n= 38.

Clinical Data

The Memorial Medical Center Burn Center admitted 1,992 patients with acute burns between January 1980 and December 1993. One hundred and twenty-nine of these patients (6.5 percent) sustained electrical injuries. The patients ranged in age from 5 months to 63 years, with an average of 33.7 years. All but seven patients were

131

males. The average size of burn wounds was 9.5 percent total body surface area (TBSA), ranging from 1 percent to 57 percent TBSA. Ninety-four (72.9 percent) of the injuries were work related. Involvement of the dominant upper extremity occurred in 56 patients (61.5 percent) in the low-tension group and in 31 patients (81.6 percent) in the high-tension group. The distribution of injuries is shown in Table 11.1. During the time in hospital, the patients' average weight decreased from 81.4 kg to 78.9 kg. The average length of hospital stay was 21.6 days, and the costs of hospitalization ranged from $900 to $120,000, averaging $14,901.

There were 91 (70.5 percent) patients with low-tension electrical injuries, and 46 of those patients required surgery (Table 11.2). Only three minor amputations including one tip of thumb amputation, one finger DIP amputation and one amputation of the fifth toe were performed (Table 11.3). No major limb amputations or major reconstructions were necessary. Cardiac arrhythmias occurred in 31 percent of patients in this group, all started within 24 hours following admission of the patient. The average length of hospital stay was eleven days.

The high-tension injury group comprised 38 patients (29.5 percent). The average number of surgical debridements was 2.3 before final wound closure, and an additional 1.2 procedures per patient were later required to improve the function of the injured site. Compartment syndromes were treated with a total of 55 fasciotomies, forty-two on the upper extremities and 13 on the lower extremities. They resulted

Table 11.4. Complications

Complication	Low-tension electrical injury* (no.)	High-tension electrical injury+ (no.)
Cardiac arrhythmia	37	11
Pulmonary embolism	0	2
Empyema of the elbow	0	1
Heterotopic calcification	1	3
Renal insufficiency/failure	0	0
Death	0	1

*n=91.
+n=38.

in 28 amputations of the upper extremities, and in ten amputations of the lower extremities (Table 11.3). A total of 39 amputations were performed, including six bilateral and one tripod amputation. There were 27 major limb amputations (Table 11.3), and numerous reconstructive procedures including, 15 pedicled flaps and 6 free flaps (Table 11.2). Nine groin flaps, nine local flaps, four pedicled and one free rectus abdominis flap, two pedicled and three free latissimus dorsi flaps, two free deltopectoral flaps, and one free fibula transfer were used to achieve wound closure or lengthening of the amputation stump in these 38 patients. The average length of hospital stay during the acute admission was thirty-eight days. Only 5.3 percent of patients were able to return to their premorbid job.

Complications included two patients with pulmonary emboli, one with empyema of the elbow, two cases of heterotopic calcification, and one death from cardiac arrest prior to admission (Table 11.4). There was no incidence of renal insufficiency or of clostridial infection. Peripheral neurological symptoms of dysaesthesias, cold intolerance, and others persisted in nine patients (10 percent) after low-tension injuries, and in 29 patients (60.5 percent) after high-tension injuries (Table 11.5). Other neurological longterm sequelae in the high-tension group included insensate limbs (four patients), persistent motor palsy (eight patients) and seizures (two patients). The overall mortality rate was 0.8 percent (one patient).

Table 11.5. Long-term sequelae

Neurological problem	Low-tension electrical injury* (no.)	High-tension electrical injury+ (no.)
Persistent dysaesthesias	9	23
Insensate limb	0	4
Persistent motor palsy	0	8
Seizures	0	2

*n=96.
+n=38.

Discussion

Following low-tension electrical injury cardiac arrhythmias presented as the most serious medical problem in our series (41 percent of patients), whereas local wound problems were minor. Surgical treatment included only one debridement before full thickness or split thickness skin graft coverage. No local or distant flaps were necessary. In all patients wound closure was accomplished two to five days after injury. This clinical approach is supported by experimental findings[26] indicating that low-voltage burn wounds did not "progress" more than 48 hours after the injury.

The treatment of high-tension injuries must focus on several problems simultaneously, including maintenance of multiple organ function, elimination of waste products, accompanying injuries related to fall or unconsciousness, and obvious as well as occult soft tissue destruction. The rate of renal failure has been drastically reduced over the last decades due to vigorous fluid supplementation (i.e. 9 ml/kg/percent TBSA)[27]. Furthermore, the overall mortality has been reduced.

Our principles for wound treatment following high-tension electrical injuries included early serial debridement of obviously dead tissue to minimize the risk of infection and subsequent complications. Four patients required acute amputations following admission because life-threatening systemic challenges from myoglobin, potassium and toxic waste products was expected. The remainder of the initial debridements was performed as soon as the patient was stable, usually one or two days post-injury. The debrided wounds were temporarily covered with porcine xenograft or allograft to prevent desiccation. Definitive wound closure was achieved on the second or third visit to the operating room in 87 percent of our patients (day

Table 11.6. Comparison of amputation rates

Injury	Overall amputation (percent) rate	Major limb amputation (percent) rate
Low-tension electrical injury	1.5	0
High voltage electrical injury	49.4	35.1

five after injury). This regimen, in our opinion, preserves the greatest amount of structures and tissues because it reduces desiccation of vital tissues and diminishes the rate of wound infection. Great care was taken to preserve the maximum functional limb length. A free fibula transfer was performed in one case to lengthen the amputation stump to achieve a better functional result. The major limb amputation rate in our series (Table 11.6) was 35 percent, which compares favorably with major limb amputation rates reported in the literature, which are as high as 71 percent[19].

The highest hospital cost ($120,000) was in a patient who sustained deep partial and full skin thickness injuries of 38 percent total body surface area from a high-tension injury. He required seven surgical debridements prior to final wound closure. The high number of surgical procedures was the most expensive factor during the acute hospital stay, but this helped to preserve a maximum of amputation stump length. He and four other patients had preservation of below-elbow stumps instead of proximal amputations of the humerus. Below-elbow prostheses were fitted in all patients, two of whom were able to return to work. The most important economic factor was not the cost of medical treatment and rehabilitation, but the life-long disability of these young handicapped patients. We feel strongly that the whole spectrum of reconstructive surgery, including free fibula transfer, should be applied to preserve or restore maximal stump length in order to provide optimal function. If an amputation cannot be avoided, great care must be taken to provide sufficient stump length and stable soft tissue coverage for adequate prosthetic fitting.

High-tension electrical injuries carry a low mortality but exceedingly high morbidity. Early serial debridement and adequate fluid resuscitation[28] decrease mortality and morbidity, but amputation rates are still high. Artz compared the complexity of the injury pattern to crush injuries[29]. Early fasciotomy did not reduce significantly the amputation rate in our series. We performed 39 amputations in 38 patients with high-tension injuries, and three amputations in 91 patients with low-tension injuries. The mechanisms of muscle necrosis from electrical injury remain incompletely understood. However, several promising approaches have been presented to explain the pathophysiology. Those include thermal damage[30], direct cellular damage by strong electric fields[13], rupture of the cellular membrane by electrical and thermal forces[12,31], biochemical alteration[32], and others. Our own experimental in vivo microcirculatory studies in a rat gracilis muscle have shown severe coagulation necrosis close to the interfaces between electrical wires and muscle tissue after a standardized electrical injury.

The middle portion of the muscle, however, showed increased leucocyte adherence in postcapillary venules and initial arteriolar vasodilatation followed by progressive vasoconstriction during the four hour observation period after the injury[33]. Studies using monoclonal antibodies against CD-18 or ICAM-1 have shown partial reversibility of tissue changes in this experimental electrical injury model[34]. Similar tissue responses have been reported following ischaemia-reperfusion injury[35].

Treatments which have been shown to be beneficial after ischaemia-reperfusion injury might also be applicable after electrical injuries.

References

1. Jex-Blake AJ, Oxon BC. The Goulstonian Lectures on death by electric currents and by lightning. *Br Med J* 1913; 1: 425-430.

2. D'Arsonval MA. Action physiologique des courants alternatifs a grande frequence. *Arch Physiol Norm Pathol* 1983; 5: 401-408.

3. Di Vincenti FC, Moncrief JA, Pruitt BA Jr. Electrical injuries: a review of 65 cases. *J Trauma* 1969; 9: 497-507.

4. Stances A Jr, Larson SJ, Mykleburst J et al. Electrical injuries. *Surg Gynecol Obstet* 1979; 149: 97-108.

5. Hunt JL, Sato RM, Baxter CR. Acute electrical burns; current diagnostic and therapeutic approaches to management. *Arch Surg* 1980; 115: 434-438.

6. Hanumadass ML, Voora SB, Kagan Rj et al. Acute electrical burns: a 10-year clinical experience. *Burns* 1986; 12: 427-431.

7. Meinhold G. Zur Frage der Todesfalle bei sinusoidalem Strom. *Dtsch Med Wochenschr* 1918; 44: 490.

8. Kennelly A. The danger of electric shock from electrical engineering standpoint. *Phys Ther* 1927; 45: 16-23.

9. Solem L, Fischer RP, Strate RG. The natural history of electrical injury. *J Trauma* 1977; 17: 487-492.

10. Nafs FJE, Aromir CF, Carreira S et al. High tension electrical burns. *Eur J Plast Surg* 1993; 16: 84-88.

11. Bingham H. Electrical burns. *Clin Plast Surg* 1986, 13: 75-85.

12. Lee RC, Gaylor DC, Bhatt D, Israel DA. Role of cell membrane rupture in the pathogenesis of electrical trauma. *J Surg Res* 1988; 44: 709-719.

13. Lee RC. The pathophysiology and clinical management of electrical injury. In: Lee RC, Cravalho EG, Burke JF, eds. *Electrical Trauma*. New York: Cambridge University Press, 1993; p 33.

14. Lee RC, Gottlieb LJ, Krizek Tj. Pathophysiology and clinical manifestations of tissue injury in electrical trauma. In: Habal MB, ed. *Advances in Plastic and Reconstructive Surgery,* Vol 8. St Louis. Mosby Year Book, 1993; p 1.

15. Sevitt S. A review of the complications of burns, their origin and importance for illness and death. *J Trauma* 1979; 19: 358-369.

16. Parshley PF, Kilgore J, Pulito JF et al. Aggressive approach to the extremity damaged by electric current. *Am J Surg* 1985; 150: 78-83.

17. Baxter CR. Present concepts in the management of major electrical injuries. *Surg Clin North Am* 1979; 50: 1401-1418.

18. Skoog T. Electrical injuries. *J Trauma* 1970; 10: 816-830.

19. Rouse RG, Dimick AR. The treatment of electrical injury compared to burn injury: a review of pathophysiology and comparison of patient management protocols. *J Trauma* 1978; 18: 43-47.

20. Hunt JL, Mason AD, Masterson TS et al. The pathophysiology of acute electrical injuries. *J Trauma* 1976; 16: 335-340.

21. Quinby WC, Burke JF, Trelstad RL et al. The use of microscopy as a guide to primary excision of high-tension electrical burns. *J Trauma* 1978; 18: 423-431.

22. Luce EA, Gottlieb SE. True high-tension electrical injuries. *Ann Plast Surg* 1984; 12: 321-326.

23. Lister GD, Scheker L. Emergency free flaps to the upper extremity. *J Hand Surg* 1988; 13A: 22-28.

24. Wang X, Roberts BB, Zapata RL et al. Early vascular grafting to prevent upper extremity necrosis after electrical burns. Commentary on indications for surgery. *Burns* 1985; 11: 359-366.

25. Chick LR, Lister GD, Sowder L. Early free flap coverage of electrical and thermal burns. *Plast Reconstr Surg* 1992; 89: 1013-1019.

26. Laberge LC, Ballard PA, Daniel RK. Experimental electrical burns: low voltage. *Ann Plast Surg* 1984; 13: 185-190.

27. Luce EA. The spectrum of electrical injuries. In: Lee RC, Cravalho EG, Burke JF, eds. *Electrical Trauma*. New York: Cambridge University Press, 1993; p-106.

28. Barisoni D, Bertolini D. Kidney function in the extensive burn. *Burns* 1981; 7:361-364.

29. Artz CP. Electrical injury simulates crush injury. *Surg Gynecol Obstet* 1967; 125: 1316-1317.

30. Lee RC, Kolodney MS. Electrical injury mechanisms: dynamics of the thermal response. *Plast Reconstr Surg* 1987; 80:663-671.

31. Benz R, Beckers F, Zimmermann U. Reversible electrical breakdown of lipid bilayer membranes: a charge-pulse relaxation study. *J Memb Biol* 1979; 48:181-204.

32. Robson MC, Hayward PG, Heggers JP. The role of arachidonic acid metabolism in the pathogenesis of electrical trauma. In: Lee RC, Cravalho EG, Burke JF, eds. *Electrical Trauma*. New York: Cambridge University Press, 1993; pp 179-188.

33. Hussmann J, Zamboni WA, Russell RC et al. A model for recording the microcirculatory changes associated with standardized electrical injury of skeletal muscle. *J Surg Res* (in press).

34. Hussmann J, Kucan JO, Russell RC et al. Partial reversibility of tissue changes following high voltage electrical injury after use of MAB against CD-18 or MAB against ICAM-1 in a standardized rat model. *Surg Res* (accepted).

35. Zamboni WA, Roth AC, Russell RC et al. Morphologic analysis of the microcirculation during reperfusion of ischemic skeletal muscle and the effect of hyperbaric oxygen. *Plast Reconstr Surg* 1993; 91: 1110-1123.

—by J. Hussmann, J. 0. Kucan, R. C. Russell, T. Bradley and W. A. Zamboni Southern Illinois University, School of Medicine, Institute for Plastic and Reconstructive Surgery, Springfield, Illinois, USA.

Chapter 12

Lightning Strikes

Lightning kills more people each year in the United States than either tornadoes or hurricanes. Even if a bolt is not fatal, the millions or billions of volts in a single strike can destroy nerves and blood vessels, damage the brain and burn skin.

Michelle Daugherty was puzzled as she scanned the bright, blue sky over a lake in Hot Springs, Ark. She and her teenage nephew, Brian, had spent much of the muggy morning of July 21, 1992, zipping around on personal water craft when she saw a flash out of the corner of her eye.

"We stopped to see what it was. At first, I thought it could have been from a car mirror or a windshield," says Daugherty, 32, who now lives in Phoenix, Ariz. "I didn't think about lightning. Then I heard a faint rumble and thought a storm might be coming. It was weird, there wasn't a cloud in the sky."

The pair immediately gunned the throttles and headed for shore. "That's the last thing I remember," says Daugherty. "I was hit by lightning and went into cardiac arrest." Her nephew—skimming along about fifty feet away—was shocked and felt the searing heat from the bolt but suffered no visible injury.

The lightning struck Daugherty in her left shoulder and exited through her right hand and foot. A flotation device kept her face-up in the water until her nephew and a family cruising nearby maneuvered her into their boat and began mouth-to-mouth resuscitation.

When they reached shore, a bystander began CPR. Paramedics worked on Daugherty for four minutes before they detected a heartbeat. They then rushed her to a hospital, where she spent three days in the intensive care unit.

"I could hardly talk, my motor skills were gone," says Daugherty. "It was like I'd had a stroke. I had to learn to talk again. I shook when I tried to feed myself. I couldn't even squeeze toothpaste out of a tube."

Daugherty is one of the lucky ones. According to the National Oceanic and Atmospheric Administration, lightning was responsible for 2,566 deaths and 6,270 injuries during a 17-year period ending in the mid-1980s. Estimates on the number of lightning-related deaths in the United States each year range from 50 to 300—with 100 often cited in scientific literature as the average.

Among weather-related hazards, only flash floods kill more. Tornadoes rank third and hurricanes fourth.

"Cardiac arrest at the time of the injury is the thing that kills people who get hit by lightning," says Mary Ann Cooper, M.D., a lightning expert and assistant professor of emergency medicine at the University of Illinois at Chicago. Dr. Cooper estimates that about 90 percent of people hit by lightning live to tell about it.

Even if a bolt isn't fatal, the millions or billions of volts in a single strike can destroy nerves and blood vessels, damage the brain, break bones and burn skin—all in under a second. Lightning can literally knock your socks and shoes off as superheated perspiration on the body turns to explosive steam.

While many recover completely without extended medical care, some feel the effects of the jolt for weeks, months or even years, according to Dr. Cooper, who directs the lightning injury research program at UIC.

Precautions

Dr. Cooper advises that it makes good sense to stay indoors if electrical storms are a threat. Unplug your computer, television and VCR during storms. Surge protectors will not save them from the kind of voltages generated by a lightning strike. To decrease your chance of injury from lightning that follows pipes and wires into the home, avoid the telephone and bathroom during lightning storms.

If you are caught outside during a lightning storm, stay low and away from tall trees or metal objects. Carrying an open umbrella can make you a more attractive target for lightning.

Lightning Injuries

The severity and types of lightning injuries vary widely from trivial to fatal. Indeed, lightning seems to be unpredictable in its physical effects, according to Dr. Cooper, who co-authored the chapter on lightning injuries in the medical textbook, "Wilderness Medicine: Management of Wilderness and Environmental Emergencies."

Those suffering minor injuries may say they feel as though they had been hit in the head or been in an explosion. They are often confused, can't remember the incident and may suffer from temporary deafness or blindness. Some may be knocked unconscious; few exhibit burns or paralysis. Dr. Cooper says patients often have at least one eardrum ruptured by the shock wave produced by the lightning. Recovery in these cases is usually gradual but complete.

Moderate injuries from lightning include temporary paralysis, especially of the lower extremities. Lightning strikes often cause interruptions in breathing that may become prolonged and lead to cardiac arrest due to diminished oxygen in the blood.

Seizures also may occur. Burns may become visible within several hours after the strike.

"Chronic pain and weakness tend to last a long time," says Dr. Cooper. "People hit by lightning may be able to work for two or three hours and then become fatigued."

Patients with severe injuries may be in cardiac arrest when found. Brain damage may occur from the lightning strike, the shock waves caused by the lightning, or cardiac arrest. Those with severe injuries usually don't survive because of direct lightning damage and delay in CPR. However, resuscitation should be attempted in all lightning strike cases, even if the victim appears to be dead.

In her research, Dr. Cooper found that 74 percent of sixty-six lightning-injured patients studied had permanent after-effects, many of which were neuropsychological, including amnesia and confusion.

Dr. Cooper found that permanent physical injuries were rare among those studied and included slight paralysis, hearing loss, burn scars and cataracts.

"Lightning patients often have short-term memory problems, are easily distracted and have difficulty completing tasks," says Dr. Cooper. "I've had people who before they were hit had no problem making dinner for fifty people. Now, it takes four hours for them to make dinner for two. They can't seem to keep things straight or organized."

Lightning injuries differ from those shocked by power lines or household current, says Daniel G. Hankins, M.D., a Mayo Clinic emergency department physician who has treated several hundred cases involving lightning-strike and electrical shock since 1975.

"With lightning, what you see is what you get," says Dr. Hankins. "You don't have the deep damage to tissue you see with electrical injuries. For example, in cases where someone touches a power line, there's a lot of damage to structures deeper in the body—what we call the "iceberg effect." A lot of the damage isn't immediately evident in an electrical shock case."

Origins

Lightning results from friction generated by swirling updrafts within towering storm clouds that create layers of oppositely charged particles. Upper portions of the cloud tend to become positively charged, while lower levels tend to carry a negative charge.

When the charges within the cloud become strong enough to overcome the insulating qualities of air, a leader stroke from the cloud to the ground initiates the lightning flash. A return stroke then rises from the ground to the cloud causing a bright flash as huge amounts of energy are discharged. Flashes also occur from cloud to cloud and from buildings or mountains to clouds. Scientists attribute thunder to shock waves stemming from the explosive expansion of air superheated to 14,000 F by lightning, which may pack ten million to two billion volts.

Research in Colorado suggests that lightning strikes create intense, local magnetic fields that may induce dangerous electrical currents in nearby human bodies. In theory, such currents may cause life-threatening disturbances in the heart's rhythm and tissue damage without leaving visible marks, according to Michael Cherington, M.D., and others at the Lightning Data Center in Denver.

Dr. Cherington, a neurologist whose work focuses on lightning cases, says his team's theory would explain the death of someone like a 32-year-old golfer who went into cardiac arrest after lightning struck a nearby tree. There were no burns or other signs on the man's body to suggest he had been hit directly, according to Cherington, lead author of a report on the data center's research published in the June 13, 1998, issue of *The Lancet*.

Chapter 13

Sunburns:
Sunlight, Ultraviolet
Radiation, and the Skin

Introduction

It is ingrained in humans to love light and, indeed, since mankind's first wanderings from the caves, worship of the sun has been a fundamental tenet that many societies hold even to the present.

The properties of the sun that have inspired such reverence include its light (visible radiation) and its warmth (infrared radiation). Additional portions of the solar spectrum that cannot be perceived directly by the senses (ultraviolet) are capable of evoking both physiologic and pathologic events in the skin.

Sunlight is the ultimate source of energy and is vitally important to life as we know it. However, absorption of incident solar energy by components of the skin can cause a variety of pathological sequelae.

Until the 20th century, the sun was the predominant source of human skin exposure to energy within the photobiologic action spectrum. More recently, artificial devices capable of mimicking the emission of some or all of the solar spectrum have been introduced, compounding the opportunities and risks of ultraviolet radiation (UVR) exposure.

Despite the undeniable importance of cutaneous exposure to ultraviolet radiation for vitamin D homeostasis, there is little evidence to indicate that there are additional beneficial effects of such exposure. Indeed, overwhelming evidence exists to support the concept

NIH Consensus Statement, May 1989. May 8-10:71-29.

143

that the skin is damaged in many different ways by its direct exposure to natural or artificial UVR. Some exposure is virtually unavoidable over a lifetime and is dramatically dissimilar in different
populations depending upon climate, geography, occupation, and recreational activities. The consequences of this exposure are also influenced by factors such as the degree of melanin pigmentation. The
effects of UVR can be divided into two general types, acute and
chronic. Acute effects include sunburn, and chronic effects include,
among others, the development of certain forms of skin cancer. In
addition, the skin is a major site of immunologic activity, and UVR is
capable of affecting the immune system via its effects on the skin. The
skin is also susceptible to degenerative changes evoked by chronic
UVR. These changes are a major component of the constellation of
physical changes perceived as skin aging but, which in reality, are due
to chronic photodamage.

It is now possible to measure the effects of solar radiation on the
skin, and epidemiologic studies from around the world have provided
important new knowledge concerning the risks and benefits of exposure to sunlight and UVR.

Expanding knowledge about the hazards of exposure to sunlight
and UVR has been accompanied by improved approaches to
photoprotection, including the development of more effective sunscreen formulations. In addition, there is increasing interest in pharmacologic agents such as the retinoids that may be capable of
inhibiting the development of or possibly even reversing certain
chronic effects of cutaneous sun exposure.

Considerable controversy remains concerning the specific adverse
effects caused by various wavelengths of UVR, the magnitude of the
adverse effects, and potential strategies for their prevention and/or
treatment. A Consensus Development Conference was undertaken in
an effort to define the specific interactions of sunlight, UVR, and the
skin as well as to identify methods for preventing and/or treating the
adverse effects of UVR. Sponsored by the National Institute of Arthritis and Musculoskeletal and Skin Diseases, the Office of Medical Applications of Research, the National Cancer Institute, and the
National Institute of Child Health and Human Development of the
National Institutes of Health, the Food and Drug Administration, and
the Environmental Protection Agency, the conference brought together
physicians, scientists, and other health care professionals, along with
representatives of the public on May 8-10, 1989. Following 1 1/2 days
of presentations and discussions by the invited experts and the audience, members of the consensus panel drawn from the biomedical

144

research community and the public weighed the scientific evidence in formulating a draft statement in response to several questions:

- What are the sources of ultraviolet radiation, and is the extent of human exposure changing over time?

- What are the effects of sunlight on the skin?

- What factors influence susceptibility to ultraviolet radiation?

- Can ultraviolet-induced changes be prevented? If so, how?

- Are sunlight-induced adverse skin alterations treatable and/or reversible? If so, how?

- What are the directions for future research?

In applying the recommendations of this consensus conference, it is important to recognize that special circumstances may exist for each patient. These may include unavoidable exposures to UVR or the inability to use certain of the preventive strategies. There are clearly some areas in which final recommendations cannot yet be made due to insufficient data. In these situations, physicians must use their best clinical judgment in advising patients.

What are the sources of ultraviolet radiation, and is the extent of human exposure changing over time?

There are both natural and artificial sources of UVR. Although there are many artificial sources of this energy, sunlight is the only natural source.

The sun emits a wide variety of electromagnetic radiation, including infrared, visible, ultraviolet A (UVA; 320 to 400 nm), ultraviolet B (UVB; 290 to 320 nm), and ultraviolet C (UVC; 10 to 290 nm). The only UVR wavelengths that reach the Earth's surface are UVA and UVB. UVA radiation is 1,000-fold less effective than UVB in producing skin redness. However, its predominance in the solar energy reaching the Earth's surface (tenfold to one hundredfold more than UVB) permits UVA to play a far more important role in contributing to the harmful effects of sun exposure than previously suspected.

Sunlight is the greatest source of human UVR exposure, affecting virtually everyone. The extent of an individual's exposure, however, varies widely depending on a multiplicity of factors such as clothing, occupation, lifestyle, age, and geographic factors such as altitude and latitude. There is greater UVR exposure with decreasing latitude.

Residing at higher altitude results in a greater UVR exposure such that for every 1,000 feet above sea level, there is a compounded 4 percent increase in UVR exposure. UVR exposure increases with decreased stratospheric ozone. Other factors that influence exposure to UVR include heat, wind, humidity, pollutants, cloud cover, snow, season, and time of day.

Solar flares (sunspots) also alter the amount of UVR reaching the Earth. Solar flares increase ozone concentration in the stratosphere (above 50 km) thereby reducing the amount of surface UVB. This 11-year cycle of solar flares causes as much as a 400-percent variation in UVB at 300 nm reaching the earth. When solar flares are inactive, there is a decrease in the ozone concentration, allowing increased UVB to penetrate to the Earth's surface.

There is also serious concern about depletion of stratospheric ozone by manmade chlorofluorocarbons (CFC). These extraordinarily inert chemicals are used in many commercial products, including aerosols and refrigerants. The U.S. Environmental Protection Agency has been charged with estimating the effects on health associated with changes in stratospheric ozone levels. In a recent risk assessment document, the Agency predicted that without controls on CFC production, there would be a 40 percent depletion of ozone by the year 2075. The Agency further concluded that for every 1 percent decrease in ozone, there will be a compounded 2 percent increase in the more damaging shorter UVB wavelengths reaching the Earth's surface. Such an increase in UVB penetration to the earth is predicted to result in an additional 1 to 3 percent increase per year in nonmelanoma skin cancer (NMSC).

Recent satellite measurements already indicate a worldwide decrease in stratospheric ozone over the last decade. Both satellite- and land-based measurements have revealed a seasonal hole in the ozone layer over the Antarctic secondary to its destruction by CFC's. Although increased surface UVB has been measured in the Antarctic, there has not yet been a measurable change in UVB as a consequence of CFC's in the stratosphere in the United States.

Over the past several decades, the average American's exposure to UVB has increased considerably due to changing lifestyles—more outdoor recreational activities, more emphasis on tanning, scantier clothing, and a population shift to the sunbelt.

The most common sources of artificial UVR exposure are various kinds of lamps that emit this form of energy. These lamps are used primarily for recreational tanning and phototherapy of skin diseases (e.g., psoriasis and cutaneous T-cell lymphoma (mycosis fungoides). UVR lamps can emit UVA, UVB, and/or UVC. Those lamps currently used for recreational tanning emit UVA primarily or exclusively. Some UVA lamps generate greater than 5 times more UVA per unit time than solar UVA radiation reaching the Earth's surface at the Equator. At these doses, "pure UVA" is likely to have adverse biologic effects. However, UVB remains a potential problem with most of these sources. Even 1 percent UVB emission from a UVA source can cause a significant increase in the potential for skin cancer.

The tanning industry is rapidly growing in the United States. Currently, more than 1 million Americans use commercial tanning facilities every day. The biggest categories of users are adolescents and young adults, especially women.

The use of artificial ultraviolet sources for the phototherapy of dermatologic diseases has increased substantially in recent years and has exposed a group of people to markedly increased doses of UVR. Epidemiologic studies of these patients have shown an unequivocal dose-dependent increase in the incidence of NMSC, especially squamous cell carcinoma (SCC).

Another potential but as yet unexplored source of artificial UVR is unshielded fluorescent bulbs used for illumination. An unresolved issue is the amount of UVA emitted by such sources and the long-term effects of this exposure. More research is needed to clarify these problems.

What are the effects of sunlight on the skin?

Marked morphologic changes in all parts of the skin, except perhaps the subcutaneous tissue, are recognized as consequences of exposure to UVR. These changes underlie the clinically observed sagging, wrinkling, leathery texture, and blotchy discoloration of skin typically associated with actinic damage. It is unclear how much exposure and how much time is required to effect these changes, although it is evident that clinically normal appearing skin can show pathologic signs of sun damage upon histologic and ultrastructural examination. It is known that individuals with fair complexions are more susceptible to this damage.

In the epidermis UVR-induced changes include aberrant tissue architecture and alterations in keratinocytes and melanocytes and functional changes in Langerhans cells. Sun-exposed epidermis becomes thickened as much as twofold compared to sun-protected skin and is disorganized, showing evidence of hyperkeratosis, parakeratosis, and acanthosis. Keratinocytes lose their typical alignment and progressive flattening, show inclusions in the nucleus, and accumulate excessive amounts of melanosome complexes above the nucleus (capping). At the ultrastructural level, clumped keratin filaments and alterations in electron density of some basal cells are characteristic. Keratinocytes of the more differentiated epidermal layers (upper spinous, granular, and cornified) show few, if any, cytologic changes.

In spite of evidence for morphologic change, there are no data indicating altered keratinocyte differentiation as a result of sun exposure. Furthermore, it is not known how UVR interactions with light-absorbing molecules within the keratinocytes (e.g., DNA, keratins, lipids) correlate with the changes in morphology. Two other cells of the epidermis are also affected by UVR. The melanocyte, with its melanin pigment-containing melanosomes, is the primary cell involved in photoprotection of the skin. In sun-damaged epidermis, these cells enlarge, increase in number, and migrate to higher levels of the epidermis. UVR also affects Langerhans cells in both animal and human skin by altering their immunologic function. Even low doses of UVB can reduce their antigen-presenting capability, block the normal effector pathway, and evoke an inappropriate response by activating T suppressor networks. It is unclear whether UVR affects Langerhans cells both directly and indirectly through soluble factors released by damaged keratinocytes.

The dermal-epidermal junction loses its rete ridges forming a flattened interface between the epidermis and dermis. This kind of abutment is more susceptible to shearing forces than the normal interlocked system of epidermal rete ridges and dermal papillae. At the ultrastructural level, regions of reduplicated lamina densa are evident. This change is not unique to photodamage but is characteristic of trauma to the epidermis by wounding and/or by disease.

UVR causes unique dermal damage such as alterations in architecture, matrix composition, vascular structure and function, and cellular activities. The connective tissue immediately beneath the epidermis (Grenz Zone) contains large bundles of densely packed, normal-appearing collagen fibrils. Beneath this region, a broad zone of electron-dense elastotic material is evident. There are no data that demonstrate how newly synthesized or degraded, previously existing elastic fibers contribute to this material. Abnormal collagen fibrils can be admixed with the elastotic substance. Other studies show changes in the type III:I collagen ratio and an increase in glycosaminoglycans. Fibroblasts appear to be metabolically active. It is not clear whether this is a transient response to the UVR or whether there is a change in cell phenotype that can be retained *in vitro*. The mechanisms for the altered connective tissue responses are not understood. Dermal vessels become dilated, leaky, and accumulate excessive basement membrane-like material. Inflammatory cells collect around the vessels; mast cells are increased and may show evidence of degranulation and apparent physical associations with fibroblasts. Although the nature of this relationship is unknown, it is a common observation in other disorders in which fibrosis occurs.

Sunburn is UVR-induced erythema of the skin caused by vasodilatation of dermal vessels. This may be mediated through cyclo-oxygenase and lipoxygenase products of arachidonic acid. Generation of the prostaglandins associated with UVB erythema produced within the first 6 to 12 hours can be blocked by topical nonsteroidal anti-inflammatory agents such as indomethacin. These anti-inflammatory agents, however, cannot inhibit the delayed, post 24-hour erythema that is modulated by lipoxygenase products. The time-dependent release of varying mediators during the UV-induced inflammatory process underscores the need for further exploration into selective inhibitors of both the cyclo-oxygenase and lipoxygenase pathways in the prevention and treatment of sunburn erythema.

Also associated with UVR irradiation of human skin is the appearance of dyskeratotic keratinocytes, known as sunburn cells, in the superficial layers of the epidermis. The mechanisms of the development of these cells are still unclear and warrant further exploration.

Tanning is the term applied to the increase in melanin pigmentation following UVR exposure. It is mediated by a combination of immediate pigment darkening (IPD) and delayed pigment darkening (DPD). IPD is caused by UVA and is due to photo-oxidation of preformed melanin. It is not protective against UVB erythema. DPD occurs about 72 hours after UVR exposure and does not afford much protection against UVB erythema and pyrimidine dimer formation. It is accompanied by an increase in the number of DOPA-positive melanocytes, an increase in the number and melanization of melanosomes, and an increase in dendricity of melanocytes. The degree of protection afforded by melanin is unclear. Individuals with dark complexions are still susceptible to UVR-induced photodamage. UVR also increases the transfer of melanosomes from melanocytes to keratinocytes. Following UVR melanosomes diffusely distributed within keratinocytes collect above the nucleus, forming a "cap" over it. DPD occurs with either UVB or UVA. DPD induced by UVB is more protective against UVB erythema than is DPD induced by UVA. Both UVB- and UVA-induced DPD protect equally well against UVB dimer formation.

In addition to certain genetic and metabolic disorders that are precipitated by UVR, there are many photosensitive diseases of unknown cause. These include lupus erythematosus and polymorphous light eruption, which are elicited by certain wavelengths of the UVR spectrum. Photosensitivity disorders may also occur due to the interaction of UVR with many commonly used drugs, as well as chemicals used in industry and consumer products.

UVR modifies local and systemic immune responses, functionally alters Langerhans cells, and activates the T cell suppressor pathway. Soluble factors released from UV-irradiated epidermal cells also may be responsible for this altered immune response. In certain experimental systems, UVR-induced tumors transplanted into genetically identical animals are normally rejected. If these host animals are UV-irradiated before transplantation, the tumor will be accepted. These conclusions are based on animal studies. The role of UVR in the immunobiology of human skin cancer and, particularly, in susceptibility against certain cutaneous infectious diseases is unclear. More studies on the effect of UVR on human neoplastic and infectious disease are warranted.

There is extensive epidemiological evidence supporting the direct role sunlight plays in human skin cancer. Basal cell carcinomas (BCC), the most common skin cancers in Caucasians, are found primarily on sun-exposed areas such as the head and neck where a dose-response relationship exists. Furthermore, patients with skin cancer generally have decreased melanin pigmentation and associated photo-protection; people with light complexion and who sunburn easily have a higher incidence of tumors. There is even stronger evidence for the role of sunlight in causing SCC's. Although both BCC's and SCC's are more prevalent in geographic areas of high sun exposure, there is a much greater increase in SCC with decreasing latitude and increasing sun exposure. A reasonable correlation exists between sunlight exposure and melanoma, but the relationship is not as clear as with NMSC. It should be emphasized that the incidence of NMSC and melanomas has been steadily increasing. Unlike NMSC, melanomas occur most frequently on the upper back in males and lower extremities in females. Melanoma incidence does not follow a pattern of increased risk with cumulative UVR exposure whereas the incidence of NMSC does.

Extensive data also exist concerning UVR-induced skin cancer in experimental animals. In mice and guinea pigs, UVR induces mainly SCC whereas in rats both SCC and BCC are produced by repeated doses of UVR. In general, UVR induces SCC's in mice somewhat more effectively in young animals than in older ones. The cancer response is preceded by photodamage to the epidermal DNA, inflammation,

150

epidermal hyperplasia, and dysplasia. Although there are several animal models in which chemical carcinogens can induce melanomas, the induction of melanomas by UVR has been very difficult if not impossible. Recent studies suggest that the opossum may be a reasonable model for UVR-induced melanomas.

Experiments in animals indicate that UVB is much more effective than UVA in causing NMSC. Nevertheless, UVA can induce DNA damage, erythema, and SCC in both pigmented and albino mice and in guinea pigs. Recent evidence suggests that the longer UVA wavelengths (UVA I:340 to 400 nm) of the UVA spectrum are less damaging than the shorter UVA wavelengths (UVA II:320 to 340 nm), but further research is needed to confirm this distinction.

The exposure of skin to UVB is essential for the endogenous production of vitamin D_3. In areas of the world where there are inadequate levels of nutritionally available vitamin D, UVB is the only source. The relationship of sunshine to vitamin D_3 and the normal growth and development of the skeleton is well known. Exposure of skin to UVR in the region of 290 to 315 nm is essential for the formation of vitamin D_3 in the epidermis.

There is evidence that vitamin D_3 synthesis is inhibited by the use of sunscreens. In the United States, this does not represent a health hazard for the pediatric population that receives adequate vitamin D supplementation in milk. In other countries this may not be the case. Deficiencies in elderly populations may exist.

What factors influence susceptibility to ultraviolet radiation?

Susceptibility to damage by UVR may be influenced by genetic and acquired disorders, genetic traits, age-related factors, and the use of some medications.

Genetic abnormalities can increase the susceptibility to UVR damage. These include disorders manifested *in utero* that may be lifelong or that may appear shortly after birth. Among them are disorders of keratinization and pigmentation. Several inherited disorders in which there is marked susceptibility to UVR in early childhood include xeroderma pigmentosum, Bloom's syndrome, Rothmund-Thomson syndrome, the porphyrias, phenylketonuria, dysplastic nevus syndrome, and the basal cell nevus syndrome.

There are also numerous and diverse acquired diseases that manifest increased light susceptibility. Examples include persistent light reaction, actinic reticuloid, polymorphous light eruption, solar urticaria, hydroa aestivale, hydroa vacciniforme, actinic prurigo, lupus erythematosus, dermatomyositis, Darier's disease, and disseminated superficial actinic parakeratosis.

Significant factors that influence susceptibility to UVR damage include race, ethnicity, eye and hair color, and the tendency toward formation of freckles and nevi. One approach to categorizing humans in terms of susceptibility to UVR is typing according to history of sunburning and tanning. Six skin types have been defined. Type I individuals always burn and never tan; type VI individuals always tan and never burn. The age of an individual may be correlated with factors that influence the susceptibility to UVR. These may include age-related structural differences in the skin, behavioral differences (e.g., adolescent risk taking) and, hypothetically, age-related immunological differences.

Numerous systemic medications may augment UVR susceptibility. Increased UVR damage may occur with the use of oral antibiotics, antihypertensives, psoralens, immunosuppressive agents, nonsteroidal anti-inflammatory drugs, and numerous other agents. In addition, a number of topical medications and industrial chemicals may increase the susceptibility to damage by sunlight. These include topical psoralens, tretinoin, and other photosensitizing and depigmenting agents.

Can ultraviolet-induced changes be prevented? If so, how?

Skin cancers in which UVR exposure plays an important role are the most common form of cancer. In 1978, there were more than 500,000 new cases of skin cancer. This is probably a substantial underestimate for 1989, because the number of office visits for NMSC has increased more than 50 percent in the past decade while the overall increase in office visits has only been 11 percent. Therefore, it is imperative to consider ways to minimize the deleterious effects of UVR.

What measures can be taken to diminish the risk of UVR exposure? There is considerable information that can serve as a basis for developing a policy of "low-risk" behavior.

- First, susceptibility to UVR damage can be reduced through use of *proper clothing* made of tightly woven fabrics with long sleeves, long pants, wide-brimmed hats, etc.

- Second, a significant reduction in certain types of UVR damage can be achieved through the proper use of *physical and chemical sunscreening products*. Maximum photoprotection is afforded by chemical sunscreens with SPF ratings of 15 or higher. Although

152

most sunscreens on the market today are appropriate for UVB protection, combination sunscreens that are effective against UVB and at least part of the UVA spectrum are preferable. Waterproof sunscreens should be selected by swimmers and those who perspire sufficiently to wash off nonwaterproof products. Daily use is recommended during appropriate times throughout the year. Sunscreens should be applied before exposure, with frequent reapplications thereafter.

- Third, one must strive to enhance behavior that *limits sun exposure*. Data exist to suggest that 50 percent of an individual's total lifetime UVR exposure occurs by 18 years of age. Therefore, parental education with subsequent direction of the behavior of children is important during childhood. Modified schedules for outdoor activities at school, camp, daycare centers, or the beach should be considered whenever possible so as to minimize UVR exposure. Time of day and time of year have a major impact on the extent of UVR exposure. For example, on a sunny day in June between 10:00 a.m. and 3:00 p.m., fully 60 percent of the daily UVB radiation reaching the Earth's surface arrives during this period. If exposure during this time could be minimized, a significant reduction in the number of NMSC's would almost certainly occur. Adults and children should limit their exposure during this peak period of UVR.

- Fourth, one must be aware of *photosensitizing medications* and chemicals because it is known that these can exacerbate the effects of UVR exposure.

- Fifth, the adverse *effects of intentional UVR exposure* must be considered. All evidence indicates that UVR-induced suntanning, whether from natural or artificial sources, is harmful to the skin.

There is a critical need to educate the public about all of these factors, consideration of which will show that the low-risk strategies described above are compatible with normal, active lives.

Are sunlight-induced adverse skin alterations treatable and/or reversible? If so, how?

Sunlight-induced adverse skin alterations include NMSC, melanoma, actinic keratoses, as well as textural and pigmentary changes

153

characteristic of chronic photodamage. All of these cancers are treated by standard surgical techniques. Precancerous lesions such as actinic keratoses are treated by topical chemotherapy (e.g., by the use of 5-fluorouracil) and physical methods of superficial skin destruction (e.g., cryosurgery). Various therapies to improve the features of chronic photodamage (scaliness, coarse and fine wrinkling, telangiectasis, and irregular pigmentation) including chemical peels, the topical use of 5-fluorouracil, alpha-hydroxy acids, and all-transretinoic acid have been tried. Although the beneficial cosmetic effects of some of these treatments have received wide publicity, there are insufficient data demonstrating sustained improvement, reversibility of tissue pathology, or the preservation of normal skin function by those agents. There is no information regarding long-term positive, negative, or toxic effects of these agents. Conflicting data exist demonstrating both prevention and potentiation effects of topical retinoids in the development of UVR-induced skin tumors in animals. There are indications that systemic use of beta-carotene and certain retinoids may be beneficial in prevention of sun damage in people with certain disorders. Long-term, large-scale studies of normal individuals in the general population are in progress.

What are the directions for future research?

The following recommendations for future research are not listed according to any particular priority.

- There is a need for updated epidemiologic data concerning NMSC in the United States. Evidence exists to suggest that the incidence of NMSC is increasing, but no new data have been obtained since 1978.

- There is a need for more research to define the action spectra of sunlight and UVR in the pathogenesis of cutaneous melanoma and to develop better animal models for the study of this disease.

- Studies are needed to define more precisely the phenomenon known as "photoaging" of the skin and to compare this with chronologic aging insofar as pathophysiological mechanisms are concerned.

- Studies are needed to better define the immunological effect of UVR exposure and its potential role in the development of skin cancer and cutaneous infections.

- In particular, the biological effects of UVA radiation require further study, particularly with the increased use of UVB sunscreens and UVA tanning equipment, both of which result in increased UVA exposure.

- The importance of UVB radiation in vitamin D homeostasis requires additional study; alternatives to sun exposure should be considered as sources of vitamin D.

- New approaches for behavior modification and education are needed to reduce skin exposure to UVR during childhood and adolescence because it is estimated that as much as 50 percent of an individual's lifetime sun exposure occurs by 18 years of age.

- More effective sunscreens and nontoxic anticarcinogenic agents should be developed as approaches to diminishing the risk of UVR exposure.

- The risk/benefit ratio of widespread, long-term sunscreen use should be monitored.

- There is a need for more research in age-related optical properties of skin and acute and chronic cutaneous responses to UVR.

- There is a need for epidemiologic study of individuals who use sunscreens that block UVB radiation.

- Data are needed that quantitatively assess UVR exposure in normal populations at all ages and under various conditions.

Conclusions and Recommendations

- Human exposure to UVR from natural sunlight and artificial sources is increasing substantially.

- UVR in sunlight is critical for vitamin D synthesis in the skin. However, it produces a variety of pathologic effects, including sunburn, pigmentary change, immunologic alterations, and neoplasia. A constellation of structural alterations of the epidermis, the dermal-epidermal junction, and the dermis is uniquely characteristic of photodamage.

- Factors that influence susceptibility to UVR include genetic abnormalities, skin type, acquired diseases, medication, and chemical exposures in consumer products and industry.

155

- UVR-induced changes can be minimized or prevented by the use of proper clothing, appropriate application of physical and/ or chemical sunscreens, behavior modification, and awareness of photosensitizing medications.

- Sunlight-induced adverse skin alterations can be treated by standard surgical techniques and superficial destructive modalities. There is insufficient evidence concerning the reversibility of adverse effects by topical and systemic agents.

- There should be better education of the public with regard to the hazards of tanning parlors, and there should be greater regulation of tanning facilities to protect the public against inadvertent injury by UVR.

Chapter 14

Chemical Photosensitivity: Another Reason to Be Careful in the Sun

Since childhood, my brother Blair always developed a dark tan without ever sunburning. Now a college soccer coach in Iowa, he is constantly outside practicing in the sun. Recently, Blair suffered a severe sunburn after only forty-five minutes of sun exposure on a cool, partly sunny morning. Consulting his physician, he learned that the commonly prescribed colitis medication Azulfidine (sulfasalazine), which he was using at the time for a colon infection, was the cause of his problems.

Azulfidine is one of the many medications included in the Food and Drug Administration's most recent listing of medications that increase sensitivity to light and can cause a wide variety of health problems known as photosensitivity disorders. In some individuals, these medications can produce adverse effects when the person is exposed to sunlight and other types of ultraviolet (UV) light of an intensity or for a length of time that would not usually give the person problems. Some products are more likely to cause reactions than others. And not everyone who uses the products will be affected.

Photoreactions

Chemicals that produce a photoreaction (reaction with exposure to UV light) are called photoreactive agents or, more commonly, photosensitizers. After exposure to UV radiation either from natural sunlight or

FDA Consumer, May 1996.

an artificial source such as tanning booths or even those "purple-lighted" mosquito zappers, these photosensitizers cause chemical changes that increase a person's sensitivity to light, causing the person to become photosensitized. Medications, food additives, and other products that contain photoreactive agents are called photosensitizing products.

FDA has also reported that photoreactive agents have been found in deodorants, antibacterial soaps, artificial sweeteners, fluorescent brightening agents for cellulose, nylon and wool fibers, naphthalene (mothballs), petroleum products, and in cadmium sulfide, a chemical injected into the skin during tattooing.

Photoreactive agents, such as Azulfidine, can cause both acute and chronic effects. Acute effects, from short-term exposure, include exaggerated sunburn-like skin conditions, eye burn, mild allergic reactions, hives, abnormal reddening of the skin, and eczema-like rashes with itching, swelling, blistering, oozing, and scaling of the skin. Chronic effects from long-term exposure include premature skin aging, stronger allergic reactions, cataracts, blood vessel damage, a weakened immune system, and skin cancer.

Widely used medications containing photoreactive agents include antihistamines, used in cold and allergy medicines; nonsteroidal anti-inflammatory drugs (NSAIDs), used to control pain and inflammation in arthritis; and antibiotics, including the tetracyclines and the sulfonamides, or "sulfa" drugs.

Sometimes this quality can be put to good medical use. For example, two well-known photoreactive chemicals, psoralens and coal-tar dye creams, are used together with UV lamps to treat psoriasis, a chronic skin condition characterized by bright red patches covered with silvery scales.

Pioneering Research

European scientists pioneered photosensitivity disorder research during the 1960s. In 1967, Danish researchers attributed strange skin lesions (any abnormal change on the skin) on women to perfumed soap. In 1967, British researchers discovered that sandalwood oil in sunscreens and facial cosmetics caused photoallergies and later reported that quindoxin, a food additive in animal feed also caused phototoxic erythemal skin patches on British farmers handling the feed.

Shortly thereafter, French scientists demonstrated that bergamot oil in sunscreens caused photosensitivity disorders. German researchers isolated photoreactive agents in colognes, perfumes and oral contraceptives.

In 1972, American scientists linked sunlight-activated aniline compounds (found in drugs, varnishes, perfumes, shoe polish, and vulcanized rubber) to hives and skin conditions such as dermatitis and dandruff.

Scientists were soon publishing laundry lists of photoreactive agents found in these substances as well as those in hair dyes, hair styling creams, and household items such as shoe polish and mothballs. Current research focuses on identifying what photoreactive agents are found in which medicinal products and how to control photosensitivity disorders.

Photosensitizers can cause either photoallergic or phototoxic reactions.

Photoallergies

In photoallergic reactions, which generally occur due to medications applied to the skin, UV light may structurally change the drug, causing the skin to produce antibodies. The result is an allergic reaction. Symptoms can appear within twenty seconds after sun exposure, producing eczema-like skin conditions that can spread to nonexposed parts of the body. But sometimes, photoallergic reactions can be delayed. For example, Yuko Kurumaji reported in the October 1991 issue of *Contact Dermatitis* that photoallergic sensitivity disorders to the topically applied NSAID Suprofen (not approved for use in the United States) took up to three months to develop.

Other regularly used products that can cause photoallergic reactions are cosmetics that contain musk ambrette, sandalwood oil, and bergamot oil; some quinolone antibacterials; and the over-the-counter (OTC) NSAID pain relievers Advil, Nuprin and Motrin (ibuprofen), and Aleve (naproxen sodium).

Phototoxicity

Phototoxic reactions, which do not affect the body's immune system, are more common than photoallergic reactions. These reactions can occur in response to injected, oral or topically applied medications.

In phototoxic reactions, the drug absorbs energy from UV light and releases the energy into the skin, causing skin cell damage or death. The reaction occurs from within a few minutes to up to several hours after UV light exposure. Though sunburn-like symptoms appear only on the parts of the body exposed to UV radiation, resulting skin damage can persist.

159

For example, Henry Lim, M.D., reported in the March 1990 issue of *Archives of Dermatology* that several patients previously exposed to photoallergens continued to have phototoxic skin eruptions up to twenty years after discontinuing medication use, even though they avoided further exposure to the photoallergens.

Frequently prescribed medications that cause phototoxic reactions include tetracycline antibiotics, NSAIDS, and Cordarone (amiodarone), used to control irregular heartbeats.

Because drug-induced photosensitivity disorder symptoms mimic sunburns, rashes and allergic reactions, many cases go unreported. Also, although research has shown that the numbers of photosensitized individuals may be high, most people do not associate the sun's light with the development of their skin eruptions.

Photophobia

Some medications can cause photophobia. Although literally, photophobia is fear of light, photophobic photosensitivity disorder patients avoid light not because they're afraid of it but because their eyes are painfully sensitive to it.

Some medications that induce photophobia include several drugs prescribed for irregular heartbeat, such as Crystodigin (digitoxin) and Duraquin (quinidine), and several drugs for diabetes, such as Tolinase (tolazamide) and Orinase (tolbutamide).

Who Gets a Reaction?

The degree of photosensitivity varies among individuals. Not everyone who uses medications containing photoreactive agents will have a photoreaction. In fact, a person who has a photoreaction after a single exposure to an agent may not react to the same agent after repeated exposures.

On the other hand, people who are allergic to one chemical may develop photosensitivity to another related chemical to which they would normally not be photosensitive. In such cross-reaction, photosensitivity to one chemical increases a person's tendency for photosensitivity to a second. For example, J.L. deCastro reported in the March 1991 issue of *Contact Dermatitis* that 17 patients allergic to the antiseptic thimerosal, used in some contact lens preparations, developed photosensitivity to the NSAID Feldene (piroxicam), yet none of them had any previous photoreaction to Feldene.

Although those with fair skin are more susceptible to photosensitizing, it is not uncommon for dark-skinned individuals to have chronic photodermatitis.

People infected with HIV, the virus that causes AIDS, are more susceptible to photosensitive disorders so they need to exercise special care in UV light exposure. In a study published in the May 1994 *Archives of Dermatology,* Amy Pappert, M.D., reported that if apparently healthy patients exhibit certain photodistributed skin problems of unknown origin, the possibility of HIV infection should be considered.

What is termed a "photo-recall" can take place when a non-photoreactive product prompts the repeat of a previous reaction to a photoreactive agent.

Photoreactive products can also aggravate existing skin problems like eczema, herpes, psoriasis and acne, and can inflame scar tissue. They can also precipitate or worsen autoimmune diseases, such as lupus erythematosus and rheumatoid arthritis, in which the body's immune system mistakenly destroys itself.

A Few Common Photosensitizers

These are just a few of the more commonly used drugs that can cause photosensitivity reactions in some people:

Brand Name	Generic Name	Therapeutic Class
Motrin	ibuprofen	NSAID, antiarthritic
Crystodigin	digitoxin	antiarrhythmic
Sinequan	doxepin	antidepressant
Cordarone	amiodarone	antiarrhythmic
Bactrim	trimethoprim	antibiotic
Diabinese	chlorpropamide	antidiabetic (oral)
Feldene	piroxicam	NSAID, antiarthritic
Vibramycin	doxycycline	antibiotic
Phenergan	promethazine	antihistamine

Do Sunscreens Help?

Does using sunscreens help protect against photosensitivity? The answer is not clear. Sunscreens do lessen the effects of UV radiation, but some contain ingredients that themselves may cause photosensitivity in some people. Also, most sunscreens protect only from short-wave

UV light (UVB), whereas most phototoxic compounds are activated by longer wavelengths of UV light (UVA). Sunscreens containing bergamot oil, sandalwood oil, benzophenones, PABA, cinnamates, salicylates, anthranilates, PSBA, mexenone, and oxybenzone can all cause photosensitivity reactions. Titanium dioxide is the least likely sunscreen to cause photosensitivity disorders.

Before going out in the sun, it's a good idea to check with your doctor to see if any of the medications you're taking is likely to cause problems and decide how to best avoid such reactions. Read the labels of OTC drugs and note if they may be photosensitizing.

If you get symptoms after being out in the sun, you may want to consider what drugs and chemicals you are using and contact your doctor immediately for advice.

—by Craig D. Reid, Ph.D., is a writer in New Haven, Conn.

Chapter 15

Work-related Burns

Diagnosis and Management of Common Industrial Burns

Approximately 5 percent of all occupational injuries are burns.[12] Many work-related burns are minor and can be treated on an outpatient basis; however, multiple studies have confirmed that the workplace is a major site of burns requiring hospital care. Serious occupational burns result in significant risk of temporary or permanent disability or even death.

In 1981 an estimated 150,000 occupational burns were treated in emergency departments in the United States.[12] An annual incidence of 4.7 per one thousand populations was noted in another study.[2] Industrial injuries account for 14 percent to 32 percent of all burns requiring hospital admission and are most commonly related to food preparation, motor vehicle repair, and use of flammable liquids.[6, 7, 9, 11, 13] In most burn center experience, scald injuries are most frequent, followed by burns secondary to flame and contact mechanisms.[7, 9, 13] Although less common, electrical injuries are more likely to lead to permanent disability. At most risk for industrial burns are young males. This results in a significant economic as well as medical impact from these injuries.[13]

Thermal Burns

Workers are at risk for a wide variety of thermal burns including scald, (hot water, grease), contact (liquid metal, hot equipment, tar), and flame (ignited clothing, explosions), depending on their type of employment. Scalds, especially from hot grease, are common and often related to food preparation, particularly among teenagers working at fast-food restaurants.[5] Explosions and use of flammable liquids result in most industrial flame burns, whereas roofers experience most tar burns.

The severity of a burn is related to the depth of burn and the extent of surface area involved. Thermal burns are categorized as first, second, or third degree, depending on the layers of the skin injured. A first degree burn is superficial and involves only the epidermis. The typical appearance of a first degree burn is a pink or light red color with dryness, lack of blistering, and pain on touch. Healing occurs within three to seven days and does not result in scar formation.

Second degree burns involve injury to the dermis of the skin. Second degree burns are further described as either superficial partial thickness involving the upper one third, or deep dermal burns involving the lower two-thirds of the dermis. The former typically appear as bright pink, moist, occasionally blistered, and extremely painful to touch. Such a burn, when pressed by a gloved finger, will blanch and immediately return to its pink color, signifying that the capillary circulation to the dermis is intact. Superficial second degree burns generally heal in two to three weeks.

They do not require skin grafting or result in significant scarring, as long as infection is avoided. Deeper second degree burns vary in appearance but often are a deep red with a dry, granular whitish surface. Spontaneous healing of burns at this depth generally takes greater than three weeks and commonly results in hypertrophic scar formation. When hypertrophic scar formation occurs in cosmetic areas or near joints, motion may be restricted and cosmetic appearance altered, leading to potential functional and psychologic problems.

Third degree burns involve the entire thickness of the skin. These frequently present as white or charred surfaces, waxy and leathery in appearance. The skin loses its pliability and elasticity, and thrombosed superficial blood vessels may be visible. Pain sensation is absent because of destruction of nerve endings in the dermis. Flame injuries, particularly involving combustion of clothing, cause temperatures to reach thousands of degrees and almost uniformly result in full-thickness third degree burns. The depth of a scald injury depends on the temperature of the scalding liquid and the length of time it is in contact with the skin. Scald burns can range from first to third degree.

The first principle of initial care of thermal burns is to remove the source of heat or the offending agent and then apply cool water. In scald injuries, clothes saturated with hot liquid should be removed, whereas any flame needs to be extinguished if possible. Burns of any significant size should be evaluated by a medical professional, particularly if they involve the face, hands, feet, or perineum. Treatment of first degree burns is straightforward and generally includes use of analgesics and application of moisturizing agents that help reduce pain and promote healing. Superficial second degree burns should be covered with barrier-type dressings, for example, petrolatum-impregnated gauze (Xeroform, Sherwood Medical, St. Louis, MO), Op-Site, Smith and Nephew, Inc., Columbia, SC, Biobrane, Dow B. Hickam, Inc., Sugarland, TX, or Duoderm, Conratec, Princeton, NJ. Our preferred dressing for smaller burns is Xeroforin, which, once adherent, can remain on the wound until healing occurs.

Biobrane, a synthetic laminate of nylon, silicone, and collagen, can be particularly useful in larger superficial scald burns. It must be applied early after the initial injury and after complete cleansing of the wound and copious flushing with saline. Advantages of its use include ease of application, decreased pain, and fewer dressing changes. Disadvantages include increased costs and slight risk of infection. If Biobrane is used, the wound is inspected daily until healing begins.

Deep second degree and third degree burns are treated initially with topical antimicrobial agents. The most commonly used topical agent is silver sulfadiazine cream, which has antimicrobial properties and is able to penetrate into burn eschar to help prevent deep burn wound sepsis. Twice daily dressings are generally adequate. Presently, the preferred treatment for deep second degree burns, particularly in cosmetic areas or around joints, is early burn excision with split thickness skin grafting. This usually results in improved cosmesis, better joint function, and earlier return to work. Third degree burns of any significant size are usually best treated by excision and skin grafting. Extensive full thickness burns usually cause a multitude of physiologic changes and pose a significant threat to the patient's life. These burns are best treated in a center specializing in the management of severe burns.

Molten Metal Burns

Molten metal burns, most commonly encountered in foundries, smelting plants, and steel mills, occurs in one of two ways. First, metal may be spilled from containers directly onto workers' clothing and boots. The clothing may be vaporized and the molten metal may penetrate through thick work boots, causing severe burns of the lower leg, ankle, and foot. In addition, burns occur when molten metal is poured into containers containing a minute amount of water. The water quickly vaporizes and "explodes," showering workers nearby with small drop-lets of hot metal, resulting in splatter burns that may affect large body surfaces. These burns are small in diameter but quite deep.

Molten metal generally has temperatures exceeding 1,000°F. With liquid metal of this temperature, the briefest exposure causes seri-ous burns. If the metal stays in contact with the skin for any length of time, fourth degree burns may occur. These burns penetrate below the muscle fascia and can involve muscle, tendon, and bone. Such burns require immediate attention by qualified surgeons with expe-rience in managing major burns.

Prompt removal of molten metal that adheres to clothing, boots, and so forth is then followed by rapid cooling of the affected areas. Splatter burns may require dousing the patient under a shower be-cause of the multiple areas of the body that may be involved. Such burns are generally less than 0.5 inch in diameter and are most of-ten treated by silver sulfadiazine applications twice daily, allowing the damaged tissue to spontaneously slough and healing to occur from the edges of the wound. Larger areas, particularly on the feet and ankles, require prompt surgical attention.

Burns of the lower limbs, including the foot and ankle, that are not fourth degree are often treated with excision and split thickness skin grafting followed by the immediate application of a gauze im-pregnated with zinc oxide, calamine, and gelatin (Dome Paste) boot dressing. This often allows the patient to be treated on an ambula-tory basis with follow-up provided first by the operating surgeon and then by the plant dispensary nurse. Burns that expose tendons, par-ticularly the Achilles tendon, or damage bone and muscle tissue re-quire prompt excision to viable fascia or muscle with immediate application of split thickness skin grafts. In some patients in whom there is destruction of significant amounts of soft tissue or exposed major tendons and bones, a free tissue transfer may be required to avoid amputation. Latissimus dorsi muscle transfers are most com-monly used in these situations.

Electrical Burns

Electrical burns are generally divided into high and low voltage burns.[1] Any electrical burn can cause cardiac arrest, and victims of electrical burns should be assessed promptly for the need for cardio-pulmonary resuscitation. High voltage burns are caused by voltages above 1,000. These voltages have the potential to cause deep tissue destruction, leading to possible amputation of limbs. Low voltage burns are often serious but are less likely to produce extensive deep tissue injuries. Alternating current is more dangerous than direct current. Alternating current by its nature causes tetanic contraction of muscles and frequently exceeds the "let-go" threshold so that patients cannot remove themselves from the current source.

Electrical burns may consist of three forms. Flash burns occur when current is shorted in devices such as junction boxes, producing a very brief, high intensity flash or fireball that causes thermal injury in proportion to the distance the victim is from the flash-point. These burns produce a charring of the superficial layers of skin; however, the destruction of tissue does not penetrate deeply because the source of heat lasts only a fraction of a second. These burns are generally partial thickness and heal spontaneously with appropriate care. Flash burns, however, may ignite clothing and should that occur, the flame burn may do extensive damage as described previously.

The second form of electrical burn is arc burn. With high voltages, current may jump from one high electromotive potential to a lesser potential across an air gap. The propensity for the current to arc depends on the humidity and the potential difference between the contact points. In burns of this type, the skin offers high resistance; however, that resistance is lowered when the skin is moist, particularly with perspiration, which contains salts.[3] When current arcs across an air gap, significant temperatures (in the range of several thousand degrees) are generated. This high temperature can vaporize tissue and frequently causes deep destruction of skin, muscle, bone, nerve, and tendon.[8]

Arc burns also may be associated with electrical conduction, the third form of electrical burn that may occur with high voltage. Current may actually flow through the patient and dissipate into the tissues, then exit from the body wherever a potential difference exists to allow for an arc. The combination of arc burns plus conduction of current leads to deep extensive tissue destruction that requires immediate attention by surgeons experienced in the care of electrical injuries.

In the initial assessment of electrical burns be aware that there may be more extensive deep damage than can be seen on the surface.[1] This means the need for increased fluid replacement, vigorous monitoring of the patient, and early treatment of hemochromogens, which are released from devitalized tissue. The hemochromogens can result in damage to the kidney, which is best averted by maintaining an alkaline urine by administering sodium bicarbonate in the patient's intravenous solution and by maintaining the urine output at approximately twice the usual amount (2 mL/kg/min).[1]

Initial surgical management of high voltage electrical burns involves decompression of compartment syndromes and decompression of nerves. Compartment syndrome develops early in an electrical injury when muscle has been damaged. The muscle compartment needs to be rapidly assessed and surgically decompressed if compartment pressures are found to exceed thirty to thirty-five cm of water. In addition, burns of the hand require immediate decompression of the median nerve by dividing the carpal ligament in the hope of sparing further pressure damage to the nerve. At the initial surgery, muscle that is completely devitalized should be removed before it becomes infected. Because the electrical damage to the endothelium of blood vessels manifests over a period of time, repeat examinations are required to sequentially remove tissue that is nonviable. The progressive loss of circulation may affect medium and larger arteries, It is not uncommon for limbs that seem to be viable soon after injury to be amputated a week or 10 days later. To date, there is no treatment to stop this progression. Once all ischemia has resolved, skin grafting or other forms of reconstructive surgery (which often involves local muscle flaps or free tissue transfers) is indicated.

Chemical Burns

It has been estimated that more than 25,000 different chemicals can cause skin and other tissue damage.[4] Their wide distribution and availability make chemicals a potential source of occupational injury. Indeed, up to 83 percent of chemical burns are work related, frequently occurring in young men.[15] Five to 16 percent of burns that require hospitalization are secondary to chemicals.[6, 11]

The extent of a chemical burn is determined by the concentration, quantity, and type of agent as well as duration of contact and extent of skin penetration. Injury is usually biochemical as opposed to thermal. Chemical burns may initially appear deceptively superficial, making evaluation difficult. However, damage can continue to occur after the initial exposure, resulting in extensive tissue necrosis and potential systemic toxicity.

The first priority in the treatment of chemical burns is to minimize the contact time. All exposed clothing and solid chemical should be removed, followed by immediate and copious lavage of the affected area with water. Use of specific neutralizing agents is rarely indicated and irrigation should not be delayed to wait for their arrival. Burns may then be covered with moist compresses prior to transfer of the patient for medical evaluation.

Alkali Burns

Most chemical burns involve the limbs. The more common agents associated with this type of burn include sodium hydroxide, hydrofluoric acid, sulfuric acid, and cement.

In general, alkali burns are more dangerous than acid burns. Acid burns result in tissue dehydration and protein binding of the acid, which limits the extent of penetration, depending on the concentration of the agent.[6] Alkalis, on the other hand, saponify fat, resulting in easier penetration of cell membranes and wider spreading in the lipid layer of the skin and subcutaneous tissue. The extent of spread can be difficult to appreciate from simply looking at the wound. In addition, alkalis are viscid whereas acids are more like water. Alkalis, therefore, are "sticky" and tend to resist irrigation, requiring mechanical wiping as well as copious flooding with water to prevent deep and extensive burns.

Alkali burns of the eye are especially dangerous.[13] The lipid in the layers of the cornea is readily damaged, leading to opacification and pterygia formation. When irrigating alkali burns of the eye care must be taken to flush all layers of the conjunctiva including the underside of the lids as well as the cornea. This is most effectively accomplished using plastic eye caps with topical anesthesia and often requires continuous irrigation with saline or Ringers' lactate solution for twelve or more hours in order to obtain a neutral pH in the eye fluids. Eye irrigation for alkali exposure must be begun promptly in order to prevent blindness.

Hydrofluoric Acid Burns

Hydrofluoric acid is a strong acid used frequently in etching processes and rust removal that can readily penetrate intact skin.[10] Pain and hyperemia can be delayed up to twenty-four hours after contact, until release of fluoride ions occurs in deeper tissue. Treatment after initial lavage uses topical therapy of calcium gluconate (2.5 percent gel) to allow neutralization of the fluoride ion.[16] If pain persists, subcutaneous injection of a 5 percent calcium gluconate solution can be made directly into the burn. In severe hand and finger burns, we prefer an intraarterial infusion of calcium gluconate via the radial artery, which is continued until pain abates.

Phosphorus Burns

Phosphorus is used in the manufacture of insecticides and fertilizers, and ignites spontaneously on exposure to air. Treatment consists of removal of the phosphorus, submersion and lavage with water, and debridement of residual phosphorus. The latter is aided by topical application of a 1 percent copper sulfate solution, which leads to formation of a black precipitate that allows identification of remaining phosphorus. Subsequent care depends on the depth of the burn.

Cement Burns

Cement is a mixture of several metal oxides (e.g., calcium and aluminum). Alkaline and thermal burns can result from the exothermic process occurring when water is added to the cement.[15a] Anterior leg burns may result when a worker kneels in the cement and symptoms may not become apparent until significant injury has occurred. Treatment consists of initial copious lavage and subsequent standard wound care.

Tar/asphalt Burns

Skin exposure to hot tar and asphalt results in a contact thermal burn.[4a] Although injury occurs with initial contact, removal of the tar using topical mineral oil or petroleum-based ointments (Bacitracin) facilitates subsequent wound management.

Prevention

Certainly the most effective "treatment" for work-related burns is to prevent the burn. Indeed, most occupational burns are preventable. Strategies for prevention include workplace regulation, improvements in equipment design, and worker education, much of which falls under the aegis of the Occupational Safety and Health Administration. The study and implementation of future prevention programs must be ongoing.

Conclusion

The presence of thermal, electrical, and chemical hazards in virtually any worksite places workers at risk for occupational burn injury. An awareness of the common mechanisms and agents that result in industrial burns optimizes treatment. Appropriate and timely initial care, expert evaluation and careful wound management, and use of surgery when indicated are critical in minimizing the disability associated with these injuries.

References

1. Baxter CP, Present concepts in the management of major electrical injury. *Surg Clin North Am* 50:1401, 1970

2. Chattejee, BF, Baranci JL Fratianne RB: Northeastern Ohio Trauma Study: V. Burn injury. J Trauma 26.844, 1986

3. Chilbert M, Maiman D, Scances A Jr, et al: Measure of tissue resistivity in experimental electrical burns. *J Trauma* 25(3):209, 1985

4. Curreri PW, Asch Mj, Pruitt BA Jr. The treatment of chemical burns: Specialized diagnostic and prognostic considerations. *J Trauma* 10:634, 1988

4a. Demling RH, Buerstatte WR, Perea A: Management of hot tar burns. *J Trauma* 20:242, 1980

5. Hayes-Lundy C, Word RS, Saffle JR, et al: Grease burns at fast food restaurants: Adolescents at risk. *J Burn Care Rehabil* 12:203,1991

6. Herbert K, Lawrence JC: Chemical burns. *Burns* 15:381, 1989

7. Inancsi W, Guidotti TL: Occupation-related burns: Five-year experience of an urban burn center. *J Occup Med* 29:730,1987

8. Lee RC, Kolodney MS: Electrical injury mechanisms: Dynamics of the thermal response. *Plast Reconstr Surg* 80:5, 663, 1987

9. Lyngdorf P: Occupational burn injuries. *Burns* 13:294, 1987

10. MacKinnon MA: Hydrofluoric acid burns. *Derm Clin* 6:67,1988

11. Ng D, Anastakis D, Douglas LG, et al: Work-related burns: A 6-year retrospective study. *Burns* 17:151, 1991

12. Occupational Injury Surveillance—United States. *MMWR* 30:578, 1981

13. Rossignol AM, Locke JA, Burke JF: Employment status and the frequency and causes of burn injuries in New England. *J Occup Med* 31:751, 1991

14. Rozenbaum D, Bamchin AM, Dafna Z: Chemical burns of the eye with special reference to alkali burns. *Burns* 17:136, 1991

15. Singer A, Sagi P, Ben Meir P, et al: Chemical burns: Our 10 year experience. *Burns*, 18:250, 1992

15a. Skiendzielewski JJ: Cement burns. *Ann Emerg Med* 9:316, 1980

16. Upfal M, Doyle C: Medical management of hydrofluoric acid exposure. *J Occup Med* 32:726, 1990

—by Christopher P. Brandt, M.D., and Richard B. Fratianne, M.D.

Part Three

Treatment Protocols for Severe Burns

Chapter 16

Initial Burn Care at the Fire Scene

Rescue and the initial care of patients with severe burns can be an intimidating, overwhelming experience. You will undoubtedly encounter your share of these patients during your EMS career, as an estimated two million burn injuries occur each year in the United States, resulting in 200,000, hospitalizations and 8,000-12,000 deaths.[1] Burns occur in every age group and across all socioecononic levels both at home and in the workplace, and in urban, suburban and rural settings.

This chapter will present:

- A brief demographic profile of the burn victim.
- An overview of the mechanisms responsible for burn injuries.
- A discussion of the principles and practices of emergency burn care.

Patterns of Burn Distribution

It's been estimated that 65 percent-75 percent of all burn injuries occur in the home, with house fires responsible for the majority of fire deaths. Careless use of smoking materials, heating-equipment malfunctions and cooking accidents are the leading causes of house fires.[2] Within the home, kitchens and bathrooms are the highest risk areas

©September 1993 Emergency Medical Services. Reprinted with permission. Information in this chapter is aimed primarily at emergency medical personnel but the protocols exercised will interest the burn patient and family.

for burn injury, as potential victims have access to hot liquids and foods, electrical appliances, stoves and space heaters. Scalds from hot liquids are a major cause of nonlethal burns.[3]

When you treat patients with burns that have occurred outside the home, you will no doubt find them in their workplaces, including industrial and agricultural settings; institutions like hotels, schools and health-care facilities; and in transportation-related incidents.[4]

Who Is Burned?

Burn-injury victims may be described in terms of the circumstances of their injuries or their age group. Most burn patients are injured because of their own actions, as when children play with matches or adults use gasoline improperly. Other victims are innocent bystanders or rescue workers burned in the line of duty.

Prior medical conditions such as stroke, epilepsy, decreased sensation due to diabetes or nerve damage may predispose a person to accidental burns. An estimated 4 percent of victim are burned intentionally, as in cases of child abuse or arson.[4] Alcohol use has been identified as a contributing factor in burn injuries because it affects victims' judgment and reaction time. It's also associated with complications in survivors and increased mortality.[5]

The highest-risk age groups for burn injuries are children younger than two years and adults over age sixty.[2] Both groups may have a limited ability to recognize and escape from a fire or burn-inducing incident and their relatively thinner skin predisposes them to more serious injuries. They're also less able to withstand the physiological stress of a burn. Burns are the third leading cause of accidental death in children, and those who are five years old or younger are the most frequent victims of scalds.[6]

Table 16.1. Signs and Symptoms of Inhalation Injury

Shortness of breath
Hoarseness
Stridor
Burns to face, neck, mouth
Singed facial hair
Sooty sputum
Exposure to smoke and/or fire in a confined space

Mortality and complication rates increase dramatically for burn victim older than 50 due to the likelihood of preexisting health problems and their immune system's decreased ability to fight infection.[6]

Burn Physiology

A burn is a traumatic injury to the body's largest organ: the skin. With thermal burns, skin cells are exposed to temperatures that are incompatible with life. Cell death and injury occur as the applied heat exceeds the body's ability to dissipate it. This threshold temperature has been identified as 43°C-45°C.

The amount and depth of skin damage depends on the heat's intensity, duration of contact and skin thickness.[1,4] The skin's specific functions—water conservation, body-temperature control and protection against infection—are hampered when a burn destroys skin integrity.

Mechanisms of Injury

Burn injuries may be classified by causative factors: thermal, chemical or electrical. Inhalation injuries are often seen in conjunction with thermal burns, especially in residential fires.

Thermal Burns

Not all thermal burns are caused by flames. Contact with hot objects, flammable vapor that ignites and causes a flash or explosion, and steam or hot liquid scalds are other common mechanisms of injury.

Just two seconds of exposure to water at 150° can cause a full-thickness or third-degree burn in an adult.[4]

Chemical Burns

A wide range of chemical agents are capable of causing tissue damage and death upon skin contact. As with thermal burns, the amount of tissue damage depends on duration of contact, skin thickness in the area of exposure and the strength of the chemical agent. Chemicals will continue to cause tissue destruction until the chemical agent is removed.[7]

Two types of chemicals—acids and alkalis—are responsible for most chemical burns. Acids generally cause cell damage by coagulation of proteins or desiccating/dehydrating cells. Alkalis dissolve cellular proteins and membranes, producing a liquefaction necrosis and loosening of tissues, which may allow the chemical to diffuse more deeply into the tissues, producing a deeper, more extensive burn.[4]

Electrical Burns

Electrical energy is converted into heat as it encounters varying degrees of resistance along the path of current flow. The injury severity resulting from exposure to electrical current depends on the type of current (direct or alternating), current voltage, the area of the body exposed and the duration of contact.

Alternating current (AC), used in lights and household appliances, may be significantly more dangerous than direct current (DC) at low voltages. It can induce ventricular fibrillation; cause respiratory arrest from involuntary, sustained contraction of the respiratory muscles; or "freeze" the victim to the electrical contact point with powerful muscle spasms that increase the amount of exposure.[8] Direct current at high voltages may also cause fibrillation, but more commonly results in asystole.

Victims of low-voltage electrical injury may have no skin burns at all yet suffer cardiac or respiratory arrest. High-voltage exposure usually results in extensive tissue destruction due to conversion of the electricity to heat and the direct electrochemical effects of the current on living tissue. Once the victim has completed the "circuit," current may penetrate the skin, distribute throughout the body and then collect at exit sites. Burns are seen at entrance and exit sites, as the skin's normally high resistance is overcome by the heat generated. Additionally, heat is generated along the pathway of current flow.

Electricity can also disrupt the movements of charged molecules within the cell, coagulating proteins and causing cell death.[4] Internal damage to nerves, blood vessels and muscle as "preferred" electrical conductors manifests as loss of sensation or movement, hemorrhage or disruption of circulation due to vessel spasm or clot formation and massive tissue destruction similar to that seen with crush injuries.[8] It may be helpful to think of an electrical injury as an iceberg, since a very extensive injury may be present below the surface, despite relatively small entrance-and exit-site burns.

Victims of electrical injuries may also experience minor flame burns if the electricity ignites clothing. Involuntary muscle contractions induced by electrical current can be strong enough to fracture long bones or ribs. Since contact with high-voltage current commonly involves power lines or transformers, victims may suffer falls or be forcefully thrown from the site of contact by powerful muscle spasms.

Inhalation

Inhalation injury and smoke inhalation describe several distinct clinical responses to exposure to incomplete combustion, Asphyxia, carbon monoxide, heat toxic chemicals and particulate matter damage a variety of respiratory structures in different ways, but any combination of these effects may exist in a fire environment.

Fire in an enclosed space may consume all available oxygen, leading to fatal asphyxia in trapped victims.

Carbon monoxide generated by incomplete burning of many fuels displaces oxygen on the hemoglobin molecule and prevents adequate oxygen delivery to tissues.

Inhalation of heated gases can burn the oropharynx, nares and upper airways, causing sloughing of mucous membranes and subsequent swelling, as well as death. Steam has a much higher heat-carrying capacity than air, and inhalation may result in direct thermal damage to lower airways and terminal lung tissue itself.[9]

Toxic chemical products of combustion include water-soluble gases like ammonia and sulphur dioxide, lipid-soluble gases like nitrogen oxides, and cyanide, among others. Toxic gases are absorbed onto soot or particulate matter and deposited in the airways. Tiny particles may travel all the way to terminal airways.[9]

Tissue damage from chemical exposure may be distributed throughout any portion of the respiratory tract including upper airways, larynx, trachea and lower airways, lung tissue or any combination thereof. Increased secretion production and swelling may lead to airway obstruction. Collection of soot and debris may cause small airways and lung air sacs to collapse. Ultimately, the smoke-damaged lung is unable to support adequate gas exchange.

Emergency Measures

The first step in emergency care of the burn victim is to stop the burning process.

How you do this depends on the various mechanisms of injury.

Thermal Burns

Control thermal burns as quickly as possible by removing the heat source.

If clothing has ignited, extinguish flames by having victims roll on the ground, smothering them with a blanket or dousing them with water. If possible, remove smoldering clothing, as it may hold heat near the skin and extend the burn. Cool scald or contact burns by briefly rinsing them with cool—*not* cold—water.

Chemical Burns

Since chemicals continue to "burn' as long as they're in contact with the skin, you must rapidly attempt to remove all residue from the victim.

Thorough dilution with copious amounts of water decreases the chemical concentration and helps physically wash it away. If the chemical is in powder or crystal form, carefully brush it off before irrigating the area. Clothing may hold chemical residue, so remove any contaminated items, keeping in mind the danger of spreading the chemical to uninvolved areas.

Initial water irrigation is recommended for at least thirty minutes. If no water supply is available at the scene, arrange to transport the patient as quickly as possible.

Early and massive dilution of the chemical agent is essential to limiting the injury's depth and magnitude.[4] You can carry out continuous irrigation of the exposed area during assessment, monitoring of vital signs and transport preparation.

Do not attempt to neutralize the chemical, even if you know which agent is involved. The neutralization reaction always generates heat potentially causing additional skin damage.

Chemical splashes to the eyes are particularly serious. Continue eye irrigation until the victim is seen by a physician.

Table 16.2. Physical Assessment of Burn Depth

Superficial or First-Degree	Partial-Thickness or Second-Degree	Full-Thickness or Third-Degree
Red	Red, pink or mottled	White, brown, black or charred
Dry	Weepy, wet, blistered	
Painful	Painful	Dry, leathery
Blanches to touch		Painless or numb

You can set up a bag of normal-saline intravenous solution for eye irrigation by cutting off the bag tip and directing the flow across the eye as the patient lies on his side.

Electrical Burns

Attempts to stop the burning process in cases of electrical injury may pose significant risks to you. You may need to coordinate your efforts with fire fighters so victims can be safely separated from the current source. It may be necessary to wait for authorities to shut off electrical power before you try to rescue anyone.

Ideally, you'll be able to coordinate rescue efforts with other fast-response personnel who are trained to use specially insulated equipment or nonconductive tools. If a victim's clothing is on fire, it may then be extinguished and removed.

Burn wounds can be cooled as described earlier.

Inhalation Injuries

Rescuing patients with inhalation injuries may also place you at risk. Close cooperation with fire fighters is essential to minimize danger and ensure optimum patient care.

Stopping the burning process means extricating victims and moving them to a safe environment, away from smoke and toxic gases.

Table 16.3. American Burn Association Referral Criteria (Partial)

Second- and third-degree burns: >10 percent TBSA in patients younger than ten years and older than fifty

Second- and third-degree burns: >20 percent TBSA in other groups

Third-degree burns: >5 percent TBSA in any age group

Second- and third-degree burns to face, hands, feet, genitals, and major joints

Electrical burns, including lightning injury

Chemical burns

Burn injury with inhalation injury

The ABCs

Once you halt the burning process, your immediate focus must shift away from the burn wound itself. You must now concentrate on the ABCs, as you would do with any trauma victim.

Airway

Securing the airway is of obvious importance in victims with suspected smoke inhalation. Some of the signs and symptoms of inhalation injury are listed in Table 16.1.[9] Evaluation of respiratory status should include level of consciousness, as both hypoxia and carbon-monoxide poisoning can cause confusion, agitation or a depressed level of consciousness.

The major threat to life in the initial stages of inhalation injury is swelling-induced upper airway obstruction. Upper airway edema formation may progress rapidly. Endotracheal intubation is necessary to manage acute obstruction. Esophageal obturator airways will not be helpful because they're not designed to maintain patency of the narrowest portion of the upper airway, the larynx and vocal cords. All victims of suspected inhalation injury should receive oxygen through a well-fitting mask at high flow rates, as well as continuous monitoring of airway status.

Keep in mind that acute obstruction is possible in the absence of exposure to smoke if the victim has an extensive surface burn to the neck. Swelling accompanying a surface burn may be severe enough to compress internal airway structures to the point of obstruction.

Transcutaneous measurement of capillary oxygen saturation is now possible using portable pulse oximetry. This can be a valuable monitoring tool during patient transport, but be aware that it's unreliable in cases of carbon-monoxide poisoning. Hemoglobin saturated with carbon monoxide registers on a pulse oximeter as saturated with oxygen and the machine cannot differentiate between the two. It's therefore dangerous to rely on pulse oximetry for reassurance that the victim is oxygenating well if carbon-monoxide exposure is suspected. Again, highflow oxygen delivered through a mask is recommended until carbon-monoxide levels and arterial blood gases can be determined in the Emergency Department (ED).

Electrical injury may most seriously compromise breathing and circulation by causing cardiac and/or respiratory arrest.

Start standard American Heart Association BLS or ALS measures as soon as possible. Cardiac, monitoring is essential for early detection of rhythm disturbances in all victims of electrical injury. Prolonged resuscitation may be necessary, but efforts can be successful if patients are otherwise healthy.[8]

You must be alert for dysrhythmias, especially supraventricular tachycardia, ventricular fibrillation and PVCS. Treat them according to established protocols or medical-control orders.

Victims of electrical injuries may present with disruption of circulation to the extremities due to damage to major blood vessels along the pathway of current passage. Additionally, patients with circumferential burns to an extremity—for example, a burn completely encircling the forearm—are at risk for decreased perfusion to the portion of the limb distal to the burn The burned tissue is very tough and inelastic. It cannot stretch to accommodate the swelling that inevitably accompanies tissue injury, and it creates a tourniquet effect that cuts off circulation to the extremity. Remove all constricting clothing and jewelry. Assess and document the presence of pulses. Elevate the burned extremities.

Common Associated Injuries

A quick secondary survey should include a search for fractures and blunt trauma, which may be associated with explosions or a fall. Vigorous muscle contraction and/or tetany induced by electrical current can cause long bone, C-spine or rib fractures. Lacerations are common when victims flee from burning buildings by breaking windows. It's important to remember that burn victims are usually alert and lucid in the absence of hypoxia and other injuries. A change in level of consciousness should prompt you to make a quick search for the causative factor.

First responders can often provide valuable information about the injury scene. Details like amount of smoke, labels from chemical containers, evidence of an explosion, electrical voltage and the exact time the injury occurred can make a difference in the care a patient receives at the hospital.

In situations where abuse or intentional infliction of a burn inhury is suspected, provide any potentially relevant information about the scene's physical characteristics, accounts of how the injury occurred and who was present to ED staff upon your arrival. Document these details in your report, as well.

Preparation for Transport

You may be asked to make a preliminary estimate of the depth and extent of a patient's burns. This information is used by medical control to guide fluid resuscitation and plan appropriate triage.

Burn *depth* refers to the specific skin layers and structures that have been damaged or destroyed. Physical assessment characteristics for the three commonly identified burn categories are listed in Table 16.2.

Burn depth is very difficult to estimate accurately in the field, even by experienced personnel. In reality, several days may pass before a deep partial-thickness burn can be differentiated from a full-thickness burn.

A burn is also a dynamic injury. Shock, infection and improper handling can extend a burn, causing it to become deeper or larger.[5]

Extent of the burn is described as a percentage of the patient's total body surface area (TBSA)—an estimate of how large the burn is in relation to the total amount of skin surface area. The Rule of Nines is an easy-to-remember reference, providing approximate TBSA percentages for different areas of the body (see Figure 16.1). Children's bodies are differently proportioned than adults'; their heads and necks are larger, and their limbs are shorter. A person's palm is roughly equal to 1 percent of TBSA.

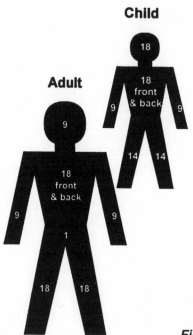

Figure 16.1. *Figure 16.1 Rule of Nines*

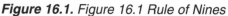

Calculating the extent of the burn is of immediate importance to the victim. Any second-or third-degree burn involving more than 20 percent of the patient's TBSA is considered a major burn. If the victim is younger than ten or older than fifty, a 10 percent-TBSA second-or third-degree burn is considered major.

Expect to transport these patients to a facility with a specialized burn center. Table 16.3 offers a partial list of the American Burn Association's recommended criteria for referring patients to a burn center.[10]

As you prepare the patient for transport, the issue of burn-wound dressings arises. Patients may request ice or cold-water applications to help control pain. At this time, it's important for you to remember the skin's role in body-temperature maintenance. A patient with a major burn is already experiencing a significant body-heat loss through the burn wound; thus, application of wet dressings or ice courts potentially fatal hypothermia. The body's attempt to increase heat production by shivering raises the tissue's oxygen demand to a level the patient with an inhalation injury or preexisting lung disease may be unable to meet.

Cooling by direct application of ice or the evaporative action of wet dressings can cause the network of capillaries and small vessels supplying the skin to constrict. This decreases the flow of oxygen and nutrients to tissues surrounding the burn—tissues that are stressed and damaged, but not yet dead. The result may be an extension of the burn wound.

It's therefore a high priority to keep the victim of a major burn warm and dry. A clean or sterile dry sheet is all that is necessary to dress the burn wound before and during transport. Dry gauze dressings may also be used, if desired. Protecting the burn from exposure to air will help decrease pain. Any cream or salve applied to the burn will have to be washed off in the ED so a physician may evaluate the injury, which ultimately inflicts greater pain on the patient.

A patient with a major burn also, requires fluid resuscitation to maintain his circulating blood volume and prevent shock. Burn victims lose tremendous amounts of fluid by external evaporation through the burn wound and by internal flow of fluid from the circulation into the tissues through "leaky" capillaries. This significant edema formation and depletion of circulating blood volume continue throughout the first 24 hours following the burn, and several formulas have been proposed for optimum fluid replacement. If you're authorized to begin intravenous fluid therapy, medical control will most likely order lactated Ringer's at a rate based on the burn's TBSA percentage and the patient's weight. A sample fluid-replacement formula is outlined in Table 16.4.[5]

If intravenous therapy is ordered, first choice for access is a large-bore catheter in a peripheral vein. Avoid placing catheters through burned skin because they're very difficult to secure (tape won't stick to a burn) and serve as a potential port of entry for bacteria. Catheters placed through burned skin will also have to be changed to another site when the victim reaches the ED or burn center.

Be sure to monitor the patient for shock and airway problems during transport.

Table 16.4. Sample Fluid Resuscitation Formula (Parkland)

Ringer's lactate 4cc/kg/percent TBSA burn

Give half during first eight hours post-injury, remainder over next twenty-six hours.

70-kg. patient with 25 percent TBSA burn

Total fluid requirement(estimate):7,000 cc

Infuse 3,500 cc over eight hours, then 3,500 over next sixteen hours.

Final Thoughts

As an EMS provider, you're an important member of the burn-care team. Appropriate prehospital burn care helps limit tissue damage and prevents extension of the burn. You can also protect your patient from the risks of hypothermia.

Providing accurate information about the patient and the circumstances of his injury to ED staff is vital to triage and treatment decisions. Timely detection of airway compromise and initiation of supportive care may be critical to the patient's survival.

References

1.   Cooper D, Tew KK. The burn injury: Incidence, initial assessment and management *Emerg Care Quarterly* 1(3):1-11, 1985.

2. Silverstein P, Lack B. Fire prevention in the United States.*Surg Clin N Am* 67(1): I14,1987.

3. Dyer C. Roberts D. Thermal trauma. *Nurs Clin N Am* 25(1):85-117,1990.

4. Bostwick JA. *The Art and Science of Burn Care*, pp. 13, 16, 17, 26, 234, 235, 242. Rockville, MD: Aspen, 1987.

5. Demling RH, LaLonde C. *Burn Trauma*, pp. 33, 44-48. New York: Thieme Medical Publishers, 1989.

6. McLoughlin E, Crawford JD. Burns. *Pediatr Clin N Am* 32(1):61-75, 1985.

7. Saydjari R, Abston S, Desai MH et al. Chemical burns. *J Burn Care Rehab* 7(5): 404-408,1986.

8. McCabe CJ, Browne BJ. Electrical and chemical burns. *Emerg Care Quarterly* 1(3):31-40,1985.

9. Orlando R. Smoke inhalation injury. *Emerg Care Quarterly* 1(3):22-30, 1985.

10. American Burn Association. Hospital and prehospital resources for optimal care of patient with burn injury: Guidelines for development and operation of burn centers. *J Burn Care Rehab* 11(2):97-104,1988.

— by Monika J. Guyette, RN, BSN

Monica J Guyette, RIV, BSN, is burn outreach coordinator at the University Of Wisconsin Hospital and Clinics Burn Center in Madison.

Chapter 17

A Simple Guide to Burn Treatment

Burns

Burns or thermal injuries occur when hot liquids (scalds), hot solids (contact burns) or flames (flame burns) destroy some or all of the different layers of cells that form the human skin. For traditional reasons, skin injuries due to ultraviolet radiations or radioactivity, electricity and chemicals, as well as respiratory insults resulting from smoke inhalation, are considered as fire/burn injuries.

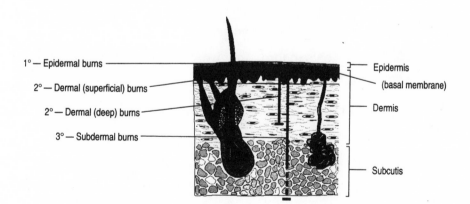

Figure 17.1. *Classification of burns according to depth.*

©1995. Burns Vol. 21, No. 3. Reprinted with permission.

Table 17.1. Classification of burns according to depth

First Degree Burns:

Clinical Signs	painful erythema
Histology	epidermis partially destroyed; basal membrane intact.
Prognosis	heals in a few days

Second Degree Burns (superficial):

Clinical Signs	erythema, blisters, underlying tissue blanches with pressure
Histology	basal membrane partially destroyed
Prognosis	heals in ten-fifteen days

Second Degree Burns (deep):

Clinical Signs	erthyema, blisters, underlying tissue does not blanche with pressure
Histology	basal membrane entirely destroyed; dermis partially destroyed, epidermal cells still present around hair follicles.
Prognosis	heals in three-four weeks, or does not heal; may require grafting.

Third Degree Burns:

Clinical Signs	brown, black or white; no blister, no sensitivity.
Histology	epidermis and dermis totally destroyed; subcutaneous tissue more or less injured.
Prognosis	does not heal except from edges; Requires grafting

Burn Depth

Burn depth depends upon the amount of heat transmitted to the skin. This depends upon two elements: the temperature of the flame, hot liquid or solid and the duration of exposure. (For adults exposed to hot water, a deep burn will result from exposure of two minutes at 50°C (122°F), twenty seconds at 550C (131°F) and five seconds at 60°C (140°F).) Burns are classified according to depth and are identified by three degrees of burn, as shown in *Figure 17.1*.

Burn Severity

Burn severity depends on:

- **Burn depth**—The deeper the burn, the more severe it is. Superficial burns heal spontaneously if correctly treated, while deep burns require grafting.

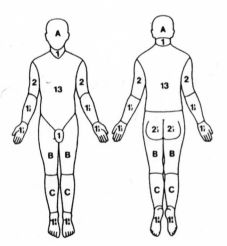

Age in years	0	1	5	10	15	Adult
A – head (back or front)	9$^{1/2}$	8$^{1/2}$	6$^{1/2}$	5$^{1/2}$	4$^{1/2}$	3$^{1/2}$
B – 1 thigh (back or front)	2$^{3/4}$	3$^{1/4}$	4	4$^{1/4}$	4$^{1/2}$	4$^{3/4}$
C – 1 leg (back or front)	2$^{1/2}$	2$^{1/2}$	2$^{3/4}$	3	3$^{1/4}$	3$^{1/2}$

Figure 17.2. *Lund-Browder Chart.*

191

- **Burn surface area**—The larger the damaged area, the more severe the burn is, taking into account burn depth. The ultimate outcome (death, disfigurement) is closely related to burn size. How much of the skin is damaged can be estimated using the Lund-Browder chart (Figure 17.2) which takes age into account.

- **Body region**—A burn on a "functional" area (i.e., face, hands, feet, joints, perineum) is more difficult to treat and more likely to result in disability and/or disfigurement.

- **Smoke inhalation**—This can cause severe respiratory insufficiency resulting from injuries, oedema and obstruction of the laryngo-tracheo-bronchial tree, and from alveolar destruction.

- **Previous health condition**—Previously healthy, well-nourished people are better equipped to survive a severe burn than are those with pre-existing health problems.

Burn Healing

Healing requires:

- absence of infection
- proper oxygen supply
- proper nutritive supply
- protection from further trauma (epidermis is fragile).

First Aid

These recommendations are intended as a guide for "first responders," i.e. informed bystanders, health clinic workers, paramedics and other emergency medical personnel:

1. Remove heat source.

2. Look for associated trauma.

3. Remove non-sticking garments.

4. Cool the burn with cool water (best between 8°C and 23°C; 45°F and 75°F) as soon as possible. Cool water eases the pain, removes the heat and lowers the temperature in the injured tissue. This prevents further injury to the skin, and increases the chances of survival of damaged but still living cells. Cooling

192

can be effective for thirty-sixty minutes after injury, and can be continued until pain no longer returns after cooling stops. Water must be "clean" but sterility is of no concern. NOTE: The patient must be kept warm. In extensive burns, cool for no longer than five minutes, especially in infants.

5. Estimate surface area burned and burn depth.

6. Apply first aid dressing: if hospital or clinic is near, simply wrap up the wound in a clean towel and transport. Otherwise:

    • Clean the burn with a non-alcoholic antiseptic solution or with soap and water.

    • Dress the burn. To prevent the dressing from adhering to the wound and getting soaked by exudates, apply one layer of gauze impregnated with petroleum jelly and cover it with layers of absorbent gauze.

    • Separate fingers and toes with layers of dressing.

    • Leave the face exposed to air.

7. Bring patient to a medical care facility for treatment.

Criteria for Admission to Hospital

This depends upon the country's available medical facilities. If possible admit to hospital:

• Patients with burns over 10 percent body surface.

• Patients with deep burns (deep second degree or third degree) (unless outpatient treatment is possible until grafting).

• If dressing is impossible (i.e., burn of perineum).

• If ambulatory treatment is impossible due to social or health conditions.

• If smoke inhalation is present; suspect smoke inhalation with a flame burn if any of the following elements are present:

    i.   fire occurred in enclosed space
    ii. facial burn
    iii. soot in nostrils or sputum
    iv. stridor.

Ambulatory Care of a Burn Patient

- Give tetanus prophylaxis.

- Clean the burn with a non-alcoholic antiseptic solution or with soap and water.

- Dress the burn wound by applying one layer of gauze impregnated with petroleum jelly and cover it with enough layers of absorbent gauze. The dressing should not adhere to wound nor become soaked by exudates. Keep fingers and toes separate.

- Some parts of the body require special attention:

  i. a hand can move freely and be functional when treated inside a plastic bag filled with silver sulfadiazine (to be changed every twenty-four hours)

  ii. superficial burns of the face can be treated by regular dressings or by air exposure, allowing a crust to form which will peel off as healing progresses.

- *Always* treat the pain of a burn:

  i. give paracetamol or codeine at scheduled intervals to relieve continuous pain

  ii. before dressings, give a potent oral medication: i.e., codeine or morphine (p.o 0.3-0.5 mg/kg); patients will appreciate it and be less anxious; dressings will be easier to perform and therefore be of higher quality.

- Give written instructions to patient or family member to come back before the end of the third day in case of fever, or if the dressing soaks through, is malodorous or is disrupted.

- Admit patient who returns with an infection or who has insufficient healing after twelve days.

Hospital Admission Checklist

- Vital signs:
  i. respiration
  ii. heart rate
  iii. blood pressure
  iv. body temperature.

- Associated trauma:
  - i. head
  - ii. spine
  - iii. chest
  - iv. abdomen
  - v. extremities.

- Diuresis (color).

- Thirst.

- Nausea, vomiting (color).

- Pain (score).

- Burn injury:
  - i. agent and circumstances: how it happened
  - ii. body region(s); circumferential
  - iii. burns
  - iv. surface area burned
  - v. depth
  - vi. inhalation injury.

- Patient information:
  - i. height
  - ii. usual weight
  - iii. past pathology
  - iv. known allergies
  - v. last meal.

- Tests:
  - i. blood (electrolytes, urea, proteins, glucose, Hb, coagulation, cross-matching, CoHb, arterial blood gases)
  - ii. chest X-Ray
  - iii. EKG
  - iv. surface cultures at wound.

Treatment Checklist

- Restore ventilation (corticoids are useless).

- Restore haemodynamics with i.v. infusions if necessary (for shock, use plasma or albumin), according to the chosen formula (Evans, Parkland, Brooke, etc).

- Restore and maintain body temperature.

- Cool the burn (useful only within one hour after injury).

- Treat pain (i.v. morphine, 0.05 mg/kg/hour starting dose).

- Perform escharotomy if necessary (intramuscular compartmental pressure must be below thirty mmHg).

- Clean and dress the burn (only when ventilation, haemodynamics and temperature are normal).

- Elevate burns of the head and of extremities above heart level.

After Admission, Control Vital Signs

- Clinical values:
  i.   systolic blood pressure: >100 mmHg
  ii. heart rate: <120
  iii. diuresis: for adults 0.5 ml/kg/hour; for children 1 ml/kg/hour (no less, no more) (If myoglobinuria, demand two ml/kg/hour; add i.v. bicarbonate to enhance myoglobin elimination).

- Laboratory values:
  i.   haematocrit <50
  ii. blood sodium <150 mEq/l
  iii. serum albumin >20 g/l
  iv. urinary sodium >40 mEq/l.

Fluid Loss and Replacement

After a serious burn, there are substantial fluid leaks throughout the body.

Fluid losses from damaged blood vessels happen immediately, are maximal at two hours postburn, and last 8 to 36 hours. Plasma leakage can cause hypovolaemic shock when the burn surface is greater than 15 percent in adults and 10 percent in children and infants. Water losses from evaporation through the burn will continue to occur, depending upon environmental conditions.

Replace fluids—Two vitally important factors for the treatment of burn hypovolaemic shock are sodium and water (if one of these is not given, the patient will die).

The most frequently used fluid replacement formulae are Evans and Parkland.

Evans: Day 1

If burned surface area (BSA) >50 percent, use 50 percent.
Ringer lactate 1 ml/kg/ percent BSA
Plasma 1 ml/kg/ percent BSA
5 percent dextrose 2000 ml/m^2 body surface

Evans: Day 2

50 percent of first day requirements.

Parkland

Ringer lactate 4 ml/kg/percent BSA for the first 24 hours.

For Children

Use Evans formula, or Ringer's lactate: 5000 ml/m^2 BSA + 2000 ml/m^2 body surface for the first 24 hours. Small children are more sensitive than adults to insufficient or excessive fluid loading; accurate burn surface estimation is mandatory; beware of insensible water losses; use weight for monitoring.

Other Notes

At least 50 percent of the first day's fluid load must be given during the first eight hours.

- If blood pressure and diuresis do not respond adequately to fluid therapy, check renal and cardiac function.

- After 48 hours, return to normal intake; beware of evaporative losses for water ((25 ml + percent BSA) x (body surface in m^2) per hour) and of wound losses for albumin.

Hypermetabolism and Nutrition

After a serious burn, the body enters a hypermetabolic state.
Hypermetabolism is caused by heat losses through the injured skin, fever, tissue mediators coming from the burn, stress hormones and infection. It can appear precociously by day three postburn and will

last as long as skin coverage is not completed. It is correlated with the amount of burned tissue with a maximum of twice the theoretical resting metabolic expenditure for burns of 50 percent or more. Its main characteristic is protein hypercatabolism, which can lead to autocannibalism of the body cell mass and death.

Nutrition Is Essential for Healing and Survival.

- Nutritional needs are correctly approximated by widely used formulas such as:

    Curreri formula for adults: (25 kcal/kg) + (40 kcal/ percent burned surface area)

    Galveston formula for children:

    (1800 kcal/m^2 body surface) + (1300 kcal/ml^2 burned surface area)

- Nutrients will consist mostly of carbohydrates (60-65 percent) and proteins (25 percent), with 10-15 percent liquids.

- Enteral nutrition is preferred since it is technically easier, less dangerous (infection), and more efficient than parenteral nutrition.

- Vitamin and trace elements supply must be increased (especially vitamins A and B, copper and zinc which are essential for healing).

- Control of adequate nutrition relies mostly on body weight and nitrogen balance.

- Heat loss will be limited by raising the ambient temperature to a level of patient "comfort" (usually above 27°C or 80°F).

Infection Control

Infection of the burn wound should be prevented by proper local treatment. Treatment is essentially topical using antiseptic solutions to clean the wound and bacteriostatic creams applied in dressings containing silver sulfadiazine, mafenide acetate, sulfamylon or polyvidoneiodine. Dressings are made with non-adherent material and several layers of absorbent gauze so that the surface of the dressing remains dry. Changes should be performed every 12 to 24 hours.

There are two different ways to treat a burn wound to enhance healing and prevent infection:

- *Open method*—Air exposure gives rise to the formation of a dry crust; the environment must be clean and the patient rather motionless.

- *Closed method*—This is more widely used. The wounds are cleaned every day at bedside or in a hydrotherapy tank with antiseptic solutions, then covered with dressings impregnated with topical agents.

The application of cerium nitrate/silver sulfadiazine or mafenide acetate, which penetrate deeply into the eschar of deep burns, can prevent microbial penetration for long periods.

The diagnosis of contamination or invasive infection will be best performed by the means of biopsies including organism count ($>10^6$/g = infection) and histological examination, rather than by superficial wound culture.

Antibiotics will be used only if there is sepsis or prophylactically before surgery in patients with burns covering more than 15 percent of the body surface.

Intravascular catheters are especially prone to infection and should be changed every 72 hours.

Removal of Burned Tissue and Wound Covering

A burn injury has three zones, as shown in Figure 17.3.

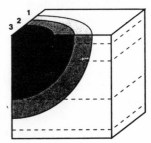

1 a zone of hyperaemia (enhanced circulation)

2 a zone of stasis (impaired circulation)

3 a zone of coagulation (cell-death)

Figure 17.3. Three zones of a burn injury.

The zone of cell death must be removed. Burned tissue easily becomes infected. Dead tissue is an easy prey for exogenous or endogenous infection which can overwhelm a depressed immune-defense system during the first week in severe burns. Infection can be limited to the burn eschar (contamination) or invade viable subeschar tissue (invasive infection), deepening the burn and causing septicaemia.

Decision-making Guidelines for Removal of Burned Tissue

"Easy" Situations:

- *Superficial Burns* will heal spontaneously in 10 to 15 days if no infection occurs.

- *Small but obviously deep burns* can be excised and grafted without delay.

More Complex Situations:

- *Burns of doubtful depth* should be dressed and watched up to day 12, when the decision for further spontaneous healing or excision and grafting will be made.

- For patients with *extensive deep burns*, survival will rank before aesthetics or even functional considerations. Maximum spontaneous healing will be encouraged. Obviously deeply burned tissue will be removed as soon as possible by excision to fascia and replaced by viable coverage (temporary or permanent).

- *Facial Burns, hand Burns and Burns of other functional areas* will have priority for surgical treatment. In case of incomplete occlusion, eyes must be protected by blepharorraphy or grafting of the eyelids.

Removal of Dead Tissue

Removal of dead tissue can be made by several means:

- *Enzymatic debridement* (sutilain ointment or benzoic acid) is still used by a number of physicians. Drawbacks: may be costly and/or painful and/or toxic.

- *Tangential excision* is the "state of the art" technique for burn specialists. Drawbacks: blood loss can be enormous and sudden (0.5-3 ml/cm^2), and much experience is needed for assessment of the viability of the wound bed for grafting.

- *Excision to fascia* — causes less bleeding, and the burn wound is almost always suitable for grafting. Drawbacks: aesthetic results may be disappointing, due to little or no subcutaneous tissue.

Wound Coverage

- *Dermo-epidermal autografts* can be harvested from any body region, although the back, scalp and thighs are preferred. Autografts should be 0.2-0.3 mm thick in adults. Donor sites and graft dressings are not different from fresh burns dressings; they should not be removed before the fifth day.

- *Dermo-epidermal allografts* are harvested from fresh cadavers and kept in skin banks. They can be used as temporary coverage, with rejection in two or three weeks, and give the best preparation for autografting. They can provide permanent coverage in combination with autografts ("sandwich" technique or Jackson's technique or "chinese" technique).

- *Meshed dermo-epidermal grafts* (1.5 x 1, 3 x 1, 6 x 1) allow expansibility, better conformity with the wound bed and drainage of subgraft exudates.

- **Cultured epithelium autografts** grow in two or three weeks and give a permanent coverage; the wound bed must be well prepared and protected after grafting, since cultured epithelium is fragile. This technique is costly but very promising.

- *Dermal-equivalents* combine a collagen matrix and a synthetic film; they provide satisfactory temporary cover. Drawbacks: costly and sensitive to contamination.

Other Important Considerations

- **PAIN**—*Pain must be treated from the start* by potent analgetic drugs:

  i.   For background pain: continuous infusion of morphine (0.05 mg/kg/hour starting dose) with the possibility of rescue

201

doses for breakthrough pain (best administered by means of patient-controlled analgesia devices); or scheduled administration of oral morphine at fixed intervals (2 mg/kg/24 hour, starting dose).

ii. For pain due to therapeutic procedures (i.e., bedside dressing): repeated boluses of i.v. morphine (0.1-0.15 mg/kg, starting dose).

- **Psychological**—*Possible psychological disorders:*

i. These include delirium and maladaptive behaviors during the early period (first month), depression and post-traumatic neurosis later on. Appropriate pain management lessens their incidence.

ii. Drug therapy or individual psychotherapy can help.

iii. Psychological support from the entire burn team is essential. Physiotherapy: must start on day one with positioning and mobilization of joints; compression may be necessary early after grafting.

- **Psychosocial**—*Psychosocial care:*

i. Permit patients to exercise as much control as possible over their own treatment.

ii. Permit family members to participate in caring for patient.

iii. Keep communication clear and open between patient, medical staff and family.

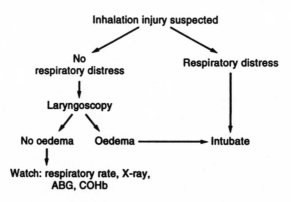

Figure 17.4. *R. H. Demling diagram.*

Care for Special Types of Burns

Smoke Inhalation

Smoke inhalation can cause severe respiratory insufficiency from oedema and obstruction of the laryngo-tracheo-bronchial tree, and from alveolar destruction. These lesions come from the chemicals contained in smoke (and not from heat). Associated carbon monoxide and/or cyanide poisoning is not uncommon.

Smoke inhalation is a special entity:

- Beware of three dangers:

  1. undiagnosed CO poisoning
  2. sudden laryngeal obstruction
  3. delayed unexpected respiratory insufficiency after the fortieth hour.

- Treatment of respiratory insufficiency is non-specific.

- Use R. H. Demling diagram (Figure 17.4) for decision making on intubation.

Electrical Burns

Electrical burns have some special features (they must be differentiated from arc burns due to high-voltage current which are flame burns).

- Skin injury may be minimal even when internal destruction is severe (sinews, muscle, nerves, blood vessels).

- Renal impairment is frequent (beware of hyperkalaemia).

- Cardiac, neurological, ocular, digestive, etc. involvement is possible.

- Surgical exploration for decompression is almost always necessary (fasciotomies).

Chemical Burns

Special first aid — Chemicals must be promptly diluted by prolonged washing (and not neutralized which produces heat); some specific treatments are required for:

- ***hydrofluoric acid:*** topical calcium gluconate gel 2.5 percent every hour; death from hypocalcaemia can happen for burned surface greater than 1 percent; give oral calcium 1-3 g and bring to the hospital quickly.

- ***phenol:*** cleansing with polyethylene glycol can be added to prolonged washing.

- ***phosphorus:*** must be kept wet until complete surgical removal (burns when in contact with air).

> *—by Jacques Latarjet (MD), Lyon, France,*
> *Co-chair, ISBI Prevention Committee.*

Chapter 18

Research Advances and Progress in Treating Burns

As long as there has been fire, people have managed to burn themselves. Every year more than 2.4 million Americans suffer burns. Fortunately, most burns are minor and can be treated at home, in a doctor's office, or hospital emergency room. But about 5 percent of burn injuries (120,000 annually) are severe enough to require hospitalization. Deaths from burns total some 12,000 each year.

Like other accidents, most burn injuries occur at home. Nearly 90 percent of the burn injuries that occur at home are caused by scalds, contact with a hot object such as an iron or a stove, or clothing that has caught on fire. About two-thirds of these burns involve the hands and arms while most of the rest are on the face and legs. Outside the home, the most common burn injury is that summer bugaboo sunburn, which probably predates even fire. Of more recent vintage are workplace burns caused by chemicals and electricity.

All burns, regardless of size, damage the skin, an effect that is usually visible. Even in the smallest burn—from a hot iron or a spatter of grease, for instance—the injured skin first becomes red, then turns brown. Burns also damage the capillaries, the tiniest of blood vessels. This, too, is visible, for the burn causes the capillaries to widen and fluids leak out of them more easily, resulting in a weepy appearance in more severe burns and a swelling of tissues around the burn. What is not visible is the injury burns cause to the body's immune system, making the victim more likely to develop infections.

FDA Consumer, February 1985.

205

How a burn is treated depends on how serious it is. One measure of severity is the percentage of the body that has been burned, usually estimated by what is called the "Rule of Nines." Under this system, the body is divided into eleven areas, each representing 9 percent or multiples of 9 percent of the total. An area equivalent to one side of the hand is about 1 percent of the body surface of an adult.

The Rule of Nines has to be modified for children under ten since their bodies have different proportions than adults. A child's head, for example, is larger in relation to the rest of the body than an adult's.

Another measurement of burn severity is the depth of the injury, described by the familiar terms "first," "second," "third" and "fourth" degree burns (see Table 18.1).

Table 18.1. Classification of Burns By Depth of Injury

Type	Amount of Skin Affected	Characteristics
First degree	Epidermis (top layer)	Redness, pain, no blistering.
Second degree	Epidermis, some dermis (underlying skin)	Red, mottled, blistered; weeping, wet surface; sensitive to air; severe pain.
Third degree	Full skin thickness	No blisters; leathery, white appearance; pain often absent because nerves in the skin have been destroyed.
Fourth degree	Full skin underlying and tissues, including muscle, tendon, joint and bone	Blackened appearance, dryness, severe pain.

First aid for small first degree burns is relatively simple. Nothing other than cool water may be needed. (Never mind what Aunt May said about using butter on a burn. The salt in the butter could make matters worse if the skin is broken.) Scientific studies have shown that cool water retards inflammation, blistering and tissue damage by reducing the heat of the burn. The burn should be kept in still (not running) water until the pain stops. Ice is not recommended. It may cause frostbite or other damage to the burned area.

In the majority of superficial burn cases, no further treatment is necessary, and the burn will heal by itself. If there is pain and discomfort it may be relieved by a number of nonprescription, or over-the-counter (OTC), topical drug products with ingredients such as benzocaine, menthol and diphenhydramine hydrochloride.

Skin protectants such as cocoa butter and petroleum jelly (e.g., Vaseline) may be used to cover the burn and protect it from the air. Topical antibiotics such as chlortetracycline hydrochloride and bacitracin may help prevent infection.

A complete list of OTC ingredients FDA considers safe and effective for the treatment of minor burns is given in Table 18.2.

A superficial burn that does not heal after seven days of self-treatment should be examined by a doctor. Any burn that is serious enough for a trip to the doctor should not be covered with medication. It probably would have to be removed during the doctor's examination, and the removal could be painful.

More severe burns require immediate medical attention. Not all will require hospitalization, however. Moderate and uncomplicated burns usually can be taken care of in the doctor's office or hospital emergency room. They are generally treated first by cleansing with soap and water and rinsing with a saline solution. Fluid is removed from unbroken blisters and the skin is left in place to provide a natural cover over the burn. Burns on the hands, legs, face, neck and thigh area are often left uncovered. This form of open treatment allows the wound to dry and prevents joint stiffness.

When closed treatment is necessary, however, the burn is covered with sterile, fine-mesh absorbent gauze impregnated with sterile petroleum jelly. Additional layers of gauze are piled on top and the whole is covered with a firmly applied bandage. To prevent infection, or fight it if it's already developed, prescription drugs such as 0.5 percent silver nitrate solution, mafenide or gentamicin ointment, or 1 percent silver sulfadiazine cream may be applied to the burn area before the wound is covered.

Table 18.2. Over-The-Counter Ingredients for Treatment of Minor Burns

External analgesics (painkillers) for the temporary relief of pain and itching associated with minor burns, sunburn:

Amine and "caine" type
local anesthetics

    Benzocaine Butamben picrate
    Dibucaine
    Dibucaine hydrochloride
    Dimethisoquin hydrochloride
    Dyclonine hydrochloride
    Lidocaine
    Lidocaine hydrochloride
    Pramoxine hydrochloride
    Tetracaine
    Tetracaine hydrochloride

Alcohols and ketones

    Benzyl alcohol
    Camphor 0.1 to 3 percent
    Camphor 3 to 10.8 percent and
        phenol in light mineral oil
    Camphorated metacresol
    Juniper tar
    Menthol
    Phenol 0.5 to 1.5 percent
    Phenolate sodium
    Resorcinol

Antihistamines

    Diphenhydramine hydrochloride
    Tripelennamine hydrochloride

Skin protectants for the temporary protection of minor cuts, scrapes, burns and sunburn:

Allantoin
Cocoa butter
Petrolatum (petroleum jelly)
Shark liver oil
White petrolatum

Topical antimicrobial (first-aid antibiotic) products to help prevent infection in minor cuts, scrapes and burns:

Chlortetracycline hydrochloride
Neomycin sulfate
Oxytetracycline hydrochloride
Tetracycline hydrochloride
Bacitracin
Bacitracin zinc
Polymyxin B sulfate (used only in combinations)

After about the third day, the wound can be soaked in water or a saline solution to help reduce inflammation.

Hospitalization is a must for all major burns. These include second degree burns involving more than 25 percent of the adult body surface (20 percent in children), third degree burns involving more than 10 percent of the body, and third degree burns on the hands, face or thigh area. Very young and very old patients should be treated in the hospital even when they have burns of lesser severity. The risk of death for any burn patient goes up in proportion to the total skin loss, and that risk is even greater for patients at the two ends of the age scale.

The initial concern in treating a severely burned patient is not the burn itself but the patient's general condition. The doctor must make sure that the patient can breathe, that intravenous fluid replacement has been started, and that other injuries have been given appropriate first aid. Once the patient is stabilized, appropriate treatment of the burn itself can begin. The goal is to replace the lost skin as quickly as possible, not only to prevent infection of the wound—the major cause of death from burns—but also to prevent further loss of fluids.

In times past, the burn patient was provided with fluids and nourishment, protected from infection as well as possible, and covered with bandages that required frequent and often painful changing. Left to heal on their own, burns treated in this manner usually resulted in disfiguring and disabling scars—if the patient survived. As recently as the early 1960s, doctors could not save a patient with burns over more than 30 percent of the body.

Today, a patient with burns covering more than 90 percent of the body has a chance for survival thanks to a better understanding of how burns affect body functions and to new methods for burn treatment.

Management of severe burns may involve any of a number of approaches, depending on the depth and extent of the burn. Most severe burns are ultimately covered with a skin graft, but a graft will not "take" on dead, burned tissue, called eschar. So the first order of business is to remove this tissue. In some cases a procedure of "total excision" is performed. This involves getting down to fresh, bleeding tissue.

Many burn experts recommend the immediate removal—within 24 hours—of the burned skin and prompt and total closing of the wound with a skin graft. Advocates of early removal say that the risk of death is reduced and the length of hospitalization is cut down by this method. The more conventional therapy involves covering the wound with dressings and antimicrobial medications until the burned tissue separates naturally from the healthy tissue when it is removed.

Whenever possible, the patient's own skin is used for grafting for the obvious reason that the body will not reject it. Grafts are obtained with dermatomes, devices that can remove skin at an even thickness. A split thickness graft, a slice of skin about ten fifteen-thousandths of an inch thick, includes the epidermis and a thin layer of dermis to provide cells for regeneration. A full thickness graft includes more of the dermis and may be used to cover a deep burn wound.

Thanks to its elasticity, skin can be stretched with specially designed instruments. Thus, grafts can be expanded as much as nine times their original size to get the maximum use out of the available skin. If the wound is large and the graft is small, the skin may be cut into postage-stamp-size pieces. These are interspersed over the wound, which is then covered with a dressing. New cells grow out from the edges of the unburned skin surrounding the wound and from the grafts.

When a burn is so extensive that there is little skin left for grafting, biological and synthetic materials can be used to close the wounds temporarily. Unlike gauze, these dressings can stay on the wound for several days at a time and can be removed without damaging new tissues.

Biological materials include human skin from a living donor or a cadaver. These are called allografts or homografts, meaning they are taken **from** the same species. The skin is an organ and, like the liver, kidney or heart, can be donated after death. Amniotic membrane—the lining of the placenta—is also used sometimes, but it is not very durable.

Pigs provide another source of biological graft material, because their skin is very similar to that of humans. However, porcine heterografts or xenografts (from a different species) don't stick to a wound and soon tend to be rejected.

Other biologic materials are sheets, mats, fabrics and sponges made from collagen. Collagen is the main protein in skin, tendon, bone, cartilage and other connective tissue. However, it is not elastic, it is hard to keep in place, and it does not control the growth of micro-organisms in the wound.

Burn dressings may also be made of synthetic materials such as thin silicone membranes and polyurethane and polyvinyl chloride plastics. These materials have the advantage of preventing moisture from evaporating while allowing oxygen to reach the wound, thus keeping it moist. One disadvantage, however, is that these materials do not stick well to the wound.

Another alternative is a composite dressing that combines a porous material, used against the wound, with a semipermeable membrane on the outside. The two layers are bonded with collagen peptides, polysaccharides or other proteins to improve adherence. This dressing permits water vapor transmission and appears to control bacterial growth in clean wounds. Drugs may be added to enhance the germ-killing effect. Such dressings also are used to cover the areas from which skin has been taken for grafts, as well as to add a protective layer over grafted areas.

While biological and synthetic dressings are useful in preparing burn wounds for grafting, experts say they are not a primary treatment for serious burn wound infection. What is needed is something as similar to real skin as possible.

The closest thing to artificial skin is being developed by researchers at Harvard University and the Massachusetts Institute of Technology. This experimental product consists of a meshwork made by combining two types of molecules found naturally in the body-collagen and chondroitin sulfate. The meshwork is laid over the wound to be used by the body as a scaffolding to build new skin. A layer of silastic (plastic) goes over the meshwork to provide a temporary seal, to be removed when the wound is healed. The researchers also are experimenting with "seeding" the material with skin cells to hasten the growth of new cells.

All types of dressings, from adhesive bandages and gauze to synthetic materials, as well as such devices as dermatomes to harvest grafts and expanders to stretch them, are regulated by FDA under the Medical Device Amendments of 1976.

The agency is presently classifying the dressings according to their intended use. For instance, those that are found equivalent to pre-amendment devices and those that simply provide a sterile covering—adhesive bandages and gauze—will be required to meet general requirements, such as Good Manufacturing Practices.

Occlusive dressings, such as the polyurethanes, that are found equivalent to pre-amendment devices used for the treatment of minor wounds and minor burns will be required to meet performance standards. Although they provide a greater degree of protection than the gauze dressings, these occlusive dressings do not actually aid in the healing of the wound. Until manufacturers can produce clinical evidence that they do, these products cannot be promoted for healing. Usually these dressings are applied for only two to three days. If they were to be on longer, there would be concern that some of their components might leach into the wound.

Dressings intended for major burns and "interactive" dressings that could play a part in the healing process, such as the Harvard-MIT product still under investigation, will have to be proved safe and effective before they can go on the market.

There are, of course, many other aspects to burn therapy besides repair of the wound. Maintaining adequate nutrition is of prime importance. To promote healing and prevent wasting of muscles, burn victims often need extra calories and protein.

In addition, there are the psychological, social and rehabilitation needs of severely burned patients who may face disfigurement, amputations, scarring, loss of feeling, lung problems and heat intolerance. Full recovery may take five to ten years.

Clearly, a burn can be a tragic event. What is more tragic is the fact that half of these injuries can be avoided by common sense preventive measures.

— by Annabel Hecht

Annabel Hecht is a member of FDA's communications staff.

Chapter 19

Burn Care Update

A set of white double doors opened to reveal a four-year-old elfin, blond boy whose hands and arms were obviously healing from a serious burn injury. His grandmother followed behind him. As the boy entered the lobby, he spied a tall, blonde nurse pulling a gurney toward him down a long corridor. He spontaneously yelled a boisterous greeting and ran to meet her as she knelt to catch him in her arms. Hugging the nurse and talking excitedly he reached up and gingerly extracted the stethoscope hanging around her neck. Remembering what she had taught him, he placed it properly in his ears and pressed the bell against her throat. Delighted with his observations, he then asked if she was to accompany him to have his pressure garment refitted. She answered. "Not this time," and as he proceeded down the hall with his grandmother to his appointment, he repeatedly turned, waved and shouted "Hi, Are you coming with me?" until he was out of sight.

According to Susan Camaret, RN, who heads the Sherman Oaks Community Hospital Burn Center Education Program in Los Angeles, scenes like these are not uncommon. "We have many patients we treated here nine or ten years ago who drop in when they happen to be in the area. They're always amazed at the fact that the same people are still working here—all their old buddies," Close relationships begin to develop here from the moment of admission. At that time, the entire Burn Care Team, including the discharge planner, begin coordinated treatment and planning.

©June 1984 *The Co-ordinator*. Reprinted with permission.

At the Burn Center, discharge planning is synonymous with patient and family education. This philosophy at the Center is reinforced by the fact that in severe cases, good education has been proven to be a main key to success.

Camaret explains that discharge planning is an ongoing educational role, encompassing much more than the hospital stay and getting them out of the hospital. It is a process of preparing the victim to make the transition from being an acute burn patient to becoming a rehabilitation patient, which may last many months.

The Sherman Oaks Burn Center is the largest private Burn Center in the United States. The Burn Team began about ten years ago. The discharge planning and patient education program materialized six years later when Camaret and her colleague, Linda Finlayson, RN, BA, began to explore educational and discharge needs. They developed the system as a natural adjunct to the Burn Center treatment. It has since evolved into a highly comprehensive, successful program.

Upon admission of a burn patient, the family is immediately called in to become active team members. Ann Liddell, MSW, LCSW, former Director of Social Services at the Burn Center states that due to this initial and continual family participation, the staff gets to know these people very well. They can identify various emotional and psychological stages which families experience because of their loved one's injury. The staff then nurtures the family's progress at the same pace as the patient's. Liddell noted, because of the development of such strong bonds between patient, family and staff "there is a tremendous amount of overlap in terms of the emotional aspects." Discharge planning and educational functions within the nursing and social work departments also overlap and are shared. A sharp delineation of duties is not noticeable within this total team structure.

Because of this family inclusion in the team, the staff can determine early who will be the major caregiver, who will be available at different times of the day, and other factors necessary to educate people to the right procedures. The majority of the patients at the Burn Center are released directly home with no intermediate institutionalization, largely due to such intensive screening and teaching.

Families naturally tend to interact with other families during the patient's stay and are encouraged by the staff to do so. This phenomenon of inter-family support works very well at the Center, allowing the families to air their feelings. Also, a previous patient who is returning for additional reconstructive surgery will occasionally take time to talk with a present patient and his or her family. Camaret mentioned she even has a few patients she can call on when necessary who are willing to come in to share their experiences.

Burn accidents are one of the most highly traumatic injuries for everyone involved: Lives can change drastically and may never return to pre-burn status. Families are given a descriptive booklet written by the Burn Center staff as soon as the primary trauma has been dealt with. It allows them to refer to something tangible if questions arise and a professional is not immediately available. The booklet is informative clinically as well as supportive emotionally. It facilitates staff teaching and commences with an understandable description of burn degrees and types:

"A burn is described according to its depth or its area of involvement on the body. First-degree burns are those to the most superficial skin cells and, in most cases, cause redness and sensitivity, but heal themselves. Second-degree or partial thickness burns are deeper than first-degree. They are open wounds characterized by blisters, redness and severe pain. In this type of burn, all but the deepest layer are damaged and recovery may take weeks or months. A third-degree or full thickness burn extends through all layers and may involve tissues beneath the skin. It is deep enough to damage muscles and bones. Skin is charred. There may be no pain, however, because nerve endings have been damaged. A third-degree burn will not heal, and the surface involved must fill in with inward growth of healthy skin around, it, or with grafts."

"Usually more important than the depth of the burn, is the size of the area it covers. First-or second-degree burns covering a large percentage of body area can be more serious than smaller third-degree burns."

"When you hear someone discussing percentage of burn on the body, they're usually referring to figures established on a chart called the "Rule of Nines." The surface area of the body is divided into the following percentages: arms, 9 percent each; head and neck, 9 percent; torso, 36 percent; perineum, 9 percent; legs, 18 percent each. The percentage of the burn will reflect the total of all the body areas affected."

"Burn severity is a combination of the percentage and the depth of the burn as well as the other injuries the patient may have sustained. Age and general physical health also play roles. Children heal more quickly than adults and older people take longer to recover."

"Burns are caused by fire and excessive heat; direct flames, flash explosions, hot steam blasts and hot water splashes: also by chemicals, alkalis, strong acids, electricity and radioactive substances such as X-rays or radioactive heat."

"Respiratory tract burns occur when a person inhales extremely hot air at the time of the accident, causing damage to membranes of the nose, throat, bronchial tubes and lungs. Tissues become swollen and secrete large amounts of fluid, mucus and serum which may interfere with breathing."

After education about the injuries themselves, families are taught about causes and treatments of shock, which is one of the most common results of a serious burn; edema; surgical treatment; skin grafts; contractures and the possibility of death, which may occur many weeks after the injury.

Rehabilitation techniques are commenced as soon as possible. Independence and participation in as many activities of daily living are vigorously encouraged. The staff will pad a fork or toothbrush for a patient whose wounds cannot tolerate a hard surface; families can bring clothing so the patient can get up in the morning and get dressed for the day. Camaret finds it amazing to observe her patients' tenacity in "the tremendous effort it takes to get themselves dressed; to zip up a jump suit when those hands don't really work well."

Occasionally, it's difficult to convince parents to allow their young children to do things for themselves. The parents understandably want to make life as easy and pleasant as possible in an attempt to right the wrongs which have befallen their children. Especially important, stresses Camaret, is that the home environment remain as close as possible to the pre-hospitalization status. Rules and routines should remain firm. "You can't make this up to them, doing everything for them and letting them have free reign." What they need is security in the form of familiarity, and consistent treatment and discipline.

Frequently, guilt is a major problem when a child is injured. The staff members at the Burn Center try to maintain a sense of this dilemma and strive to help the parents overcome these feelings and work toward independence. Both the patient and family must understand that by doing things for themselves, they are aiding the recuperative process.

Prior to the discharge date, a pre-discharge conference is held. At this time the home environment is analyzed. Situations such as a home containing only a shower stall when the patient is required to bathe in a tub must be resolved.

During this period questions and fears arise as to the ability of everyone involved to adequately perform care procedures. The family may have reservations about their capabilities, while the patient may express anxiety over leaving the safe, controlled hospital environment. All such reservations are openly discussed, and, when possible, assuaged.

All care techniques are demonstrated, explained, and then performed repeatedly by patient and caregivers under professional observation. Extensive, individualized, written instructions are provided. Camaret is presently in the process of completing a formulated discharge planning manual. However, she states, "I do not ever want to get to the point where I just walk in, hand them a book, show them how to do it, and leave it at that." Her premise is that if someone understands why they are doing a certain activity they are more apt to comply. As mentioned, discharge instructions are individualized according to patient status and complications. Topics vary, but a generic example of a written plan follows:

Discharge Instructions

A. DIET:

1. Eat three well balanced meals a day.
2. Include foods that are high in protein.
   a) Examples of foods high in protein are: beans, nuts, cheese, fish, eggs, meat, poultry, milk and milk products.
3. Between meal snacks should be nutritional.

B. WOUND CARE:

1. Cleanse wounds twice a day. Once in the morning and once at night.
2. Follow tub and shower guidelines for tub preparations and safety procedures.
3. Care for wounds as follows:
   a) Wash your hands well with soap and water.
   b) Bathe in bath tub.
   c) While in tub, wet wounds with water.
   d) Make a lather with soap in your hands. Use a mild soap such as Ivory, Safeguard or Dial.
   e) Gently, using your fingertips, wash hands and head.
   f) Rinse well using clean water.

g) Gently dry wounds using a 4 x 4.

   1. Open 4 x 4 halt way, lay on wounds, press gently and lift off gently. Be careful not to snag clips that are on wound.

h) Allow to air dry for about 45 minutes.

i) Wash your hands well.

j) Gently apply vitamin E oil with your fingertips.

   1. Apply vitamin E oil to all grafted areas and donor sites. This will prevent skin from becoming dry and cracking. It will also help decrease itching.

   2. The vitamin E oil should be applied so there is a thin layer over the wounds.

   3. It should be applied as often as necessary to keep wounds and donor sites lubricated.

   4. It should be applied before doing exercises.

k) After eating, if hands are slightly soiled, gently wash in warm soapy water.

   1. Be careful that the pressure from the faucet is not too hard.

   2. It will be necessary to dry hands using steps above for drying wounds.

   3. Apply vitamin E oil when air dry.

4. As time goes on he will become more and more able to do much of his own wound care with supervision. Just be very careful not to snag clips.

C. DRESSINGS:

1. During the day he is to have no dressings.

2. At night after cleaning wounds, he will have his splints applied as follows:

   a) Apply Adaptic to wounds. Wrap each finger separately. Place 4 x 4 over back of hand for padding and hold in place with a light kling wrap.

   b) Place splints in position.

   c) Hold in place with ace wraps.

      1. Ace wraps should be secure to hold splints in position but they should not be tight.

D. EXERCISES:

1. Follow exercise routine set up by occupational therapy.

2. He will be going for therapy daily for two weeks. Then two to three times a week for two weeks.

a) These appointments will be arranged by our occupational therapy department at a facility near your home.

3. You will also need to return here to be seen by our occupational therapy department once a week. These appointments can be made on the same day that his doctors visits are.

NOTE: It is *extremely* important to keep his appointments and for him to do his exercises as instructed.

E. SPECIAL INSTRUCTIONS:

1. No sun! The new skin will be more sensitive to sun and will tend to burn more easily.
   a) Protect areas that were burned with a wide brimmed hat and the gloves that will be specially made.
   b) This will be necessary for about a year.
2. He has been measured for a pressure garment, which is used to keep uniform pressure over the burned areas to help minimize scarring.
   a) This garment is only effective if worn as instructed.
   b) Come in when contacted by the P.T. Department to pick up the garment.
   c) If the gloves become loose fitting or too tight you will need to contact the P.T. Department and come in for refitting.
   d) Clean garment with mild soapy water every 24 hours and air dry.
3. The ace wraps should be cleaned each day using mild soapy water, rinse well and air dry.
4. Pets: Pets must be controlled. A misplaced paw may cause injury to newly grafted skin. Pet hair in the wounds may also cause damage. Pets should not be allowed to lick. Vacuum pet hairs daily.
5. Playing should be confined to indoors until otherwise instructed by your doctor.
   a) Be aware when he is playing with other children that they are not playing with objects that may be harmful.

F. APPOINTMENTS:

1. Call Doctor's office and make an appointment.
2. Call occupational therapy department here and set up appointment to be seen when you come for your appointment with your doctor.

NOTE: If you have any questions or problems, please feel free to call us anytime.

Other areas extensively covered are medications and skin changes.

Patients are thoroughly informed about their medications: Why they are taking them; What effects and side effects to watch for; When to take them; How to take them.

Skin changes should be anticipated as to color and sensitivity. Camaret observed that sometimes her shorter-stay patients have a more difficult time accepting the appearance of their skin during the healing process. This is because they are in the hospital for a short duration and have not undergone the numerous procedures; debridement, wound cleansing, dressing changes, etc. and seen the gradual change. They may get home, take a dressing off a foot and be horrified at the purple appendage. She tries to prepare them for the visual reality with slide presentations.

The child returns to his grandmother, happy and relaxed. As they leave through the double doors, the tall blonde nurse stands and watches them leave. She is smiling.

She knows that a trauma which began as something that could have ruined the child's life has been turned into an acceptable therapeutic experience by the specialist team at the Sherman Oak Burn Center.

—by Kimberly Staggs

Chapter 20

Initial Management of a Patient with Extensive Burn Injury

The burn patient is characterized as the universal trauma model.[14] The response to major burn injury affects all organ systems of the body, with the severity of this response proportional to the magnitude and duration of the extent of injury. To care for these traumatized patients, the nurse must have knowledge of the local and systemic manifestations of the burn injury to make a thorough assessment of the patient's condition and to evaluate the patient's response to planned interventions.

The clinical course of burn care is comprised of three phases: the resuscitative phase, the acute phase, and the rehabilitative phase. The resuscitative phase begins with the initial hemodynamic response to the injury and lasts until capillary integrity is restored and the repletion of plasma volume by fluid replacement occurs. The acute phase commences with the onset of diuresis of fluid mobilized from the interstitial space and continues through closure of the burn wound. Correction of functional deficits, contracture releases, and job retraining encompass the rehabilitative phase. This article focuses on the resuscitative phase. Primary nursing care considerations discussed include initial stabilization at the scene and in the hospital, assessment of burn depth, and monitoring of the patient's response to the initial therapy.

©June 1991 *Critical Care Nursing Clinics of North America* Vol. 3, No. 2. Reprinted with permission.

Anatomy and Functions of the Skin

The integumentary system consists of two major layers: the epidermis and the dermis (Fig. 20.1).[7] The epidermis varies from 0.07 mm to 0.12 mm in thickness with the deepest layers found on the palms of the hands and the soles of the feet. Although the epithelial layer is subdivided into five separate layers, each with their own functions, the most important layers are the stratum corneum and the stratum germinativum. The stratum corneum is composed of dead keratinized cells and surrounding lipids that inhibit the passage of physical, chemical, and noxious agents found in the environment. This layer also protects the body against invasion of micro-organisms. The innermost layer of the epidermis, the stratum germinativum, is responsible for the reproduction of new epithelial cells that migrate toward

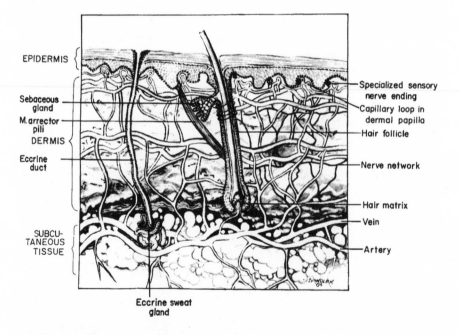

Figure 20.1. *The integumentary system is composed of three skin layers, appendages, nerves, and blood vessels.* From *Heigel EB: The skin: Basic considerations. In Criep LH (ed): Dermatologic Allergy: Immunology, Diagnosis, Management. Philadelphia, WB Saunders, 1967, p 7; with permission.*

the surface to replace the outer layers. Without the presence of the stratum germinativum cells, new epithelium will not be produced.

The dermal layer ranges in thickness from 1 mm to 2 mm and lies below the epidermis. This layer is composed primarily of connective tissue and collagenous fiber bundles and provides a nutritional supportive bed for the epidermis. Within the dermis is a highly vascular network, called the rete subpapillare, which is composed of venules and capillaries that nourish the avascular epidermis. Nerve fibers, called Meissner's corpuscles, also originate in the dermis and are specific to the sensation of touch.

Additionally, the corpuscles of Vater-Pacini (pressure), Ruffini (heat), and Krause (cold) are located in the dermal and underlying subcutaneous layers. Of particular note in the dermal layer are the sweat glands and hair follicles, which, with their epithelial lining, serve in the re-epithelialization of partial-thickness wounds.

Beneath the dermis is the hypodermis, which contains the fat, smooth muscle, and areolar tissue. This layer is irregular in shape, varies in thickness from one part of the body to another, and is anchored by connective tissue originating in the dermis. The hypodermis acts as a heat insulator, shock absorber, and nutritional depot that is mobilized during starvation.

Depth of Burn

The degree of cellular injury is determined by the temperature and duration of heat exposure.[12] The longer the skin is in contact with the heat source and the higher the temperature, the deeper the cell destruction will be. In the past, the depth of burns was classified as first, second, and third degree. Today, first and second degree burns are referred to as partial-thickness burns and third degree burns as full thickness injury (Table 20.1). First-degree partial-thickness burns involve injury to the outermost layer of the epidermis and are usually caused by a minor flash or a sunburn. The skin is pink or light red, dry without blister formation, painful to touch, and usually heals within five days. Systemic reaction is absent or mild. These patients do not require hospitalization and may have an exfoliation of the superficial epidermal layer several days after exposure. The percentage of this type of burn injury is not used in fluid resuscitation calculations.

Second-degree partial-thickness burns are further subdivided into superficial partial-thickness and deep dermal partial-thickness injury. These burns are usually caused by brief contact with hot liquids, flames, or exposure to dilute chemicals. Superficial partial-thickness burns involve the epidermis and a limited portion of the dermis. Wounds are bright red or mottled in appearance, contain bullae, are wet and weeping, and are exquisitely painful to touch (even to a current of air). Blanching will be followed with capillary refill, and hair follicles remain intact. Healing occurs with minimal scarring in ten to twenty-one days.

Deep dermal partial-thickness burns involve destruction of the epidermis and most of the dermis, with only the epidermal cells lining the hair follicles and sweat glands remaining intact. The injured tissue is dark red or yellow-white in color, has large, often ruptured bullae, is slightly moist, and has decreased skin sensation to a pinprick but intact sensation for deep pressure. Although these deep dermal burns will heal, they will do so only after a prolonged period with friable epithelium and are prone to hypertrophic scarring and marked contracture formation. Current treatment usually involves excision and skin grafting to these areas.

Table 20.1. Depth of Burn Injury

	SUPERFICIAL PARTIAL THICKNESS (FIRST DEGREE)	SUPERFICIAL PARTIAL THICKNESS (SECOND DEGREE)	DEEP DERMAL PARTIAL THICKNESS (SECOND DEGREE)	FULL THICKNESS (THIRD DEGREE)
Predisposing Cause	Sunburn, ultraviolet exposure	Brief exposure to flash flame and liquid spills	Hot liquids or solids, flash flame, direct flame, intense radiant energy	Prolonged contact with flames, hot liquids, hot objects; steam; chemicals; electric current
Morphology	Minimal epithelial damage	Epidermis; minimal damage to dermis	Entire epidermis and varying levels of dermis; intact epidermal lined appendages (hair, sweat)	Epidermis, dermis, epidermal appendages; portion of subcutaneous fat; possible involvement of connective tissue, muscle, bone
Characteristics	Red, dry, tender, slightly erythematous, painful	Moist, bright pink or mottled red, blisters, intact blanching, intact tactile and pain sensors	Pale, waxy, absent blanching, mostly dry, sensitive to pressure but not pinprick	Dry, leathery, insensate, avascular; pale yellow to brown to charred; thrombosed vessels
Healing Time	Approximately 5 days	Within 21 days with minimal scarring	Prolonged healing period; unstable epithelium, late hypertrophic scarring, marked contracture formation; possible conversion to full-thickness injury	No longer capable of self-regeneration; requires grafting

Full-thickness burns are caused by flame, high-voltage electric current, concentrated chemical exposure, or contact with hot metal or liquids. These burns involve destruction of all layers of the skin down to or past the subcutaneous tissue to include fat, fascia, muscle, and/or bone. They display a charred or pearly white, parchment-like appearance, are dry and leathery, and frequently have thrombosed vessels visible through the burned tissue. Despite the dry appearance, the surface of the wound will leak fluids absorbed from the underlying tissue. The wounds are insensate to touch and, by definition, require grafting for wound closure.

Zones of Injury

Thermal burns are additionally classified into three concentric zones of tissue injury, with the central zone being the most severe and the peripheral zone being the least damaged (Fig. 20.2).[5, 10] The outermost zone is termed the zone of hyperemia and is analogous to a first-degree burn that heals in approximately five days. Adjacent to the zone of hyperemia is the zone of stasis, in which tissue perfusion is compromised. If resuscitation promptly restores tissue blood flow, this tissue typically survives. The innermost zone of burn injury is the zone of coagulation, which has the most intimate contact with the heat source. This area is characterized by cellular death.[9, 10]

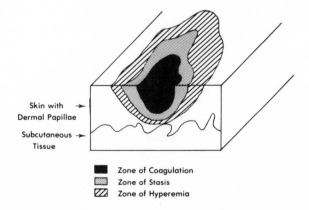

Skin with → Dermal Papillae

Subcutaneous → Tissue

■ Zone of Coagulation
▨ Zone of Stasis
▨ Zone of Hyperemia

Figure 20.2. Zones of injury showing the three layers of tissue damage. From *Moncrief JA: The body's response to heat. In Artz CP, Moncrief JA, Pruit BA, Jr (eds):* Burns: A Team Approach. Philadelphia, WB Saunders, 1979, p 25; with permission.

Systemic Manifestations of Burn Shock

Burn injury affects all organ systems and is manifested by a biphasic pattern of early hypofunction followed by hyperfunction.[15,16,18]

The incidence, magnitude, and duration of the systemic manifestations of burn shock are proportional to the extent of burn and reach a plateau at approximately 50 percent to 60 percent total body surface area (TBSA) involvement.[15, 16]

Cardiovascular Response

Following the burn injury, there is a release of catecholamines, resulting in a decreased cardiac output and an increased peripheral vascular resistance. With this initial response, fluids shift from the intravascular to the extravascular space through burn injured capillaries, leading to edema formation in the burned tissue. This "leak," which is comprised of the loss of sodium, water, and plasma proteins, is followed by a decrease in cardiac output, hemoconcentration of red blood cells, diminished perfusion to major organs, and generalized body edema. In patients receiving adequate fluid resuscitation, the cardiac output returns to normal in the later part of the first twenty-four hours after burn.[3] As plasma volume is replenished during the second twenty-four hours, the cardiac output increases to hypermetabolic levels and slowly returns to more normal levels as the burn wounds are closed.[13]

Renal Response

A similar biphasic renal response occurs. With the decreased intravascular volume following burn injury, the kidneys experience a reduction in renal plasma flow and glomerular filtration rate, resulting in a low urine output.[13] If fluid resuscitation is inadequate to meet the intravascular requirements or if resuscitation is delayed, acute renal failure can occur. By the end of the first post-burn day, the capillary vascular integrity is restored. Following resuscitation, interstitial fluids are pulled back into the intravascular compartment, and a modest renal diuresis occurs.[15]

Pulmonary Response

The response of the pulmonary vasculature is like that of the peripheral circulation; however, the pulmonary vascular resistance is greater and lasts longer than the peripheral vascular resistance.[16] During this early period, the patient may exhibit a transient, modest pulmonary hypertension. A decrease in oxygen tension and lung compliance also may be evident, even in the patient without inhalation injury.[2] Immediately following burn injury, the minute ventilation may be unchanged or slightly decreased in the hypovolemic patient without inhalation injury. Following the resuscitative phase, minute ventilation increases in a manner relative to burn size.[16]

Gastrointestinal Response

A common response to patients with burn wounds over 20 percent TBSA is a decrease in gastrointestinal activity.[12] This decrease in function is caused by a combination of the effect of hypovolemia and the neurologic and endocrine response to the injury.[16] This response prohibits resuscitation by the oral route and necessitates the insertion of a nasogastric tube to prevent abdominal distention, emesis, and potential aspiration. With adequate fluid resuscitation, gastrointestinal activity returns to normal within twenty-four to forty-eight hours.

Immunologic Response

The immunologic response may be divided into two categories: the mechanical barrier response and the cellular immune response. As a mechanical barrier, the skin functions as an important defense mechanism against invading organisms. Any alteration in the skin integrity provides an opportunity for invasion of microorganisms. Although the exact mechanism of the cellular immune response is unclear, it is hypothesized that the complex interaction of the components of the immune response may be caused by either an altered host environment and/or an injury-induced host-deficiency state. The eventual result is complement activation and a depression of other components, such as T-helper and T-killer cell activity and polymorphonuclear leukocyte activity.[20]

Types of Burn Injury

There are three main types of burn injuries: thermal, chemical, and electric. Thermal injury, the most common type of burn injury, is caused when the skin comes in contact with a source of sufficient temperature to cause cell injury and cell death by protein coagulation.

227

The severity of injury is directly related to heat intensity and duration of contact. A chemical injury is caused by thermal energy produced when strong acids or alkalies react with tissue.[16] As with other thermal injuries, the amount of tissue necrosis is proportional to the duration of exposure and the concentration of the agent. Because alkalis have a higher binding affinity to the tissue and thus are more difficult to remove, they frequently cause greater damage than the acidic compounds. A search for a neutralizing agent wastes valuable time, but, more importantly, the increased heat of the neutralizing reaction may cause further tissue damage. Therefore, copious water lavage is the treatment of choice for chemical injuries. Although a thirty-to sixty-minute water lavage is recommended for most acid burns, alkali injuries may require hours of lavage to remove the compound from the skin.[16] Initial estimation of the depth of the chemical burn may be difficult because of the potential for further tissue necrosis during the first twenty-four hours following injury.

Although water lavage is the universal treatment for chemical burns, specific interventions are required for certain chemicals. Agricultural chemicals, such as limes, should be brushed from the skin prior to lavage, as the application of water to the powder on the wound may produce a strongly alkaline solution that increases injury. With limited solubility in water, phenols, which are found in deodorants, sanitizers, and disinfectants, should be removed with solvents, such as glycerol, polyethylene glycol, or propylene glycol. Water, however, should be used in the absence of these compounds.[11, 16]

Chemical burns from hydrofluoric acid, a compound commonly used in industry, occur when the fluoride ion penetrates the skin and surrounding tissue. Current treatment involves copious lavage with water or benzalkonium chloride. Persistent pain is indicative of continuing tissue necrosis and warrants consultation with a burn referral center. Further treatment may include subcutaneous injection of 10 percent calcium gluconate directly into the burn site or calcium gluconate soaks to decrease symptoms and limit local tissue destruction.[12]

Tar burns are contact burns that require immediate cooling with cool water. Removal of the compound is not an emergency. The urgency consists of stopping the burning process. Following this treatment, adherent tar should be covered with a petrolatum-based ointment and dressed to promote emulsification of the tar. Following tar removal, the wound may be assessed for depth and severity of burn.[12, 15]

Chemical injury to the eye deserves special attention because of the potential for permanent damage to the cornea. Early signs of

ı, tearing, local irritation, and
ı, iritis, lens damage, and in-
ators of possible strong alkali
thirty minutes or more is re-
the eye. Use of cycloplegic eye
ɔrmation of synechia. Addition-
enerously applied to the eye to

ırn injury, occurs when electric
ion of electric energy into heat.[16]
include current voltage, type of
·ay of the current, and duration
;rarily classified as low voltage
reater than 1,000 V).[15] Alternat-
direct current and is frequently
·y arrest, tetanic muscle contrac-
vertebral bodies, and long bone
.e damage usually is associated
ɔlve the hands or feet or the cor-
.ren.

With high-voltage injury, the differences in the conductivity of various tissues, such as bones and nerves, are of relatively little importance, as all areas of the body act as volume conductors.[16] Higher temperatures are produced by the passage of current through segments of the body with small cross-sectional areas as opposed to segments of larger cross-sectional areas. Therefore, injury to the digits of the hand are usually more severe than damage to the trunk. Whereas injury is more severe at the contact points of higher current density, resistance rises with voltages lower than 1,000, resulting in limited passage of current and decreased tissue heating.

At greater than 1,000 V of electricity, relatively constant levels of current are maintained, which may arc across the patient's skin surfaces, particularly at the flexion surfaces of joints. These arc burns tend to be more severe when associated with decreased skin resistance from water on the skin surface. Arcing also may cause additional thermal injury as a result of the ignition of clothing. After the flow of current has ceased, the layers of tissue cool unevenly, with the superficial layers cooling more rapidly than the deeper tissue. As a result, the deeper tissues often sustain more damage due to prolonged heat exposure, resulting in extensive subfascial edema and tissue necrosis not evident on external examination.

The formation of cataracts is a common complication of electric injury and may occur from one or two days to three or more years following injury. An ophthalmologist should examine the patient after admission and frequently throughout the hospital stay to document the status of the cornea.[16]

Nursing Care Considerations

Initial Care at the Scene

First-responder care at the scene of the injury should focus on stopping the burning process while, at the same time, preventing self-injury. With a flame injury, the patient should be placed in a supine position to prevent the spread of flames to the head and upper torso. The flames should be extinguished with water or smothered with a blanket, or the patient should be rolled on the ground. Smoldering clothing should be removed to prevent further thermal injury. In the event of a chemical burn, all clothing, to include the socks, shoes, and gloves, should be removed, and the wound should be flushed with copious amounts of water to stop the burning process. With an electrical injury, the patient should be removed from the current with a nonconducting object, such as a dry stick, to ensure that the rescuer does not become part of the electrical current pathway.

The initial assessment of the burn patient at the scene consists of a primary survey followed by a secondary survey.[12] The primary survey consists of those interventions used on any trauma patient: assessment of airway, breathing, and circulation, as well as immobilization of the cervical spine when indicated. As stated earlier, the need for cardiopulmonary resuscitation is greatest with electric injury because of the potential passage of current through the heart or the respiratory center.

Carbon monoxide poisoning is a leading cause of death at the scene and should be suspected in any patient burned in a dwelling fire, particularly those burned in a closed space.[12] Carbon monoxide possesses an affinity for hemoglobin that is 200 times that of oxygen and competes with oxygen for available binding sites on the hemoglobin molecule.[8] To accelerate the dissociation of carbon monoxide from hemoglobin, the patient should be treated with 100-percent oxygen administered through a tight-fitting, non-rebreathing mask.[15] This treatment is thought to be effective, because laboratory data show a fifty percent reduction in the carboxyhemoglobin level in forty minutes on 100-threatening injuries. Following this examination and stabilization, the patient should be promptly transported to the hospital for further care. Unless indicated by other associated injuries, insertion of an intravenous catheter is not necessary if the patient is to arrive at a medical facility within 30 to 45 minutes.[15, 16] If a delay in care is expected, an intravenous catheter should be inserted, preferably in an unburned extremity, and an infusion of a crystalloid solution, such as lactated Ringer's, begun. A record of the type and amount of fluids administered should be maintained. Transport should not be delayed, however, if immediate venous cannulation is unsuccessful. Due to ensuing edema formation, all jewelry should be removed, and burned extremities should be elevated. The head and chest also may be elevated unless contraindicated due to severe hypotension or cervical spine injury. The patient should be wrapped in a clean sheet and blankets to conserve body temperature. Cold-water soaks should be used only for the temporary relief of burn discomfort. Prolonged applications of ice may further impair the microcirculation in already damaged tissue and are therefore not recommended for use. Additionally, it is important to avoid interventions leading to hypothermia, which, when combined with burn shock, may lead to circulatory embarrassment.

Emergency Department Care

On arrival in the emergency department, the care described above should be started for those patients who have not received prehospital assessment, and treatment should be extended for those who received initial care in the field. If intravenous cannulation was not initiated, the nurse should insert a large-bore cannula in a peripheral vein, or a central line should be started by the physician. For accurate urinary output measurements, an indwelling urethral catheter should be placed. A nasogastric tube should also be inserted in all patients at risk for intestinal ileus (TBSA greater than 25 percent) and connected to continuous low suction to prevent emesis and aspiration.[15, 19]

The administration of humidified 100-percent oxygen should be maintained on all patients suspected of carbon monoxide poisoning or inhalation injury. A carboxyhemoglobin level should be obtained, and oxygen therapy continued until levels less than 15 percent are achieved.[12] The nurse should continue to monitor the patient for signs and symptoms of impaired oxygenation, such as hypoxemia (agitation, tachypnea, anxiety, stupor, and cyanosis), and impending upper airway obstruction (hoarseness, stridor, wheezing, and rales).

At this point, the extent of burn should be calculated using one of two methods: the rule of nines or the Lund and Browder age versus area diagram. This calculation provides the basis for determining fluid requirements during the resuscitation phase.

A major nursing responsibility during the fluid resuscitation phase includes the measurement of hourly urine output. Because the infusion rate depends on the patient's response to the burn injury, the nurse should monitor the patient for adequate urine output, with 30 to 50 ml/h as the desired range for the adult and one ml/kg/h as the preferred range for the child under 30 kg.[12, 15] Measurements outside these parameters should be brought to the physician's immediate attention. Hourly volumes of 75 to 100 ml are the expected ranges in patients with high-voltage electric injury.[12, 15]

Monitoring of the patient's vital signs also may be used to judge the adequacy of fluid resuscitation. A heart rate of 100 to 120 beats per minute in the adult patient is an expected physiologic response to a major burn during the resuscitation period.[3,15] In the older patient, the heart rate becomes a less reliable monitoring tool because of the inability of the heart rate to increase in response to a hypovolemic state. Blood pressure measurements taken on a burned extremity may be exceedingly low and a false indication of hypovolemia, if the auditory signal is attenuated by excessive edema and vasoconstriction.[15] Frequently, the patient with extensive burns will have an indwelling arterial cannula for blood pressure monitoring. Such pressure measurements are most accurate if the cannula is placed in a central artery as opposed to an artery in a distal extremity with decreased flow rate. A decreased blood pressure is a late finding of inadequate resuscitation.[3]

Continued Emergency Department Care

While care is ongoing, the nurse should obtain a brief history from the patient, the emergency medical technicians, or persons in attendance at the scene of the injury. Pertinent information includes the time of the incident; whether the injury occurred in a closed or an open space; possibility of inhalation injury; the presence of additional associated injuries; and, in the event of electric injuries, the source of electric current. Obtaining a past medical history is important, particularly relating to cardiac, pulmonary, and renal problems, as well as the presence of diabetes and central nervous system disorders. A knowledge of the presence of allergies and the patient's current medication regimen also may be helpful. A tetanus toxoid booster should be administered if the patient has been previously immunized but has not received tetanus toxoid within the last five years. If a tetanus immunization history is not known, the patient should receive 250 units of human tetanus-immune globulin and the first of a series of active immunizations with tetanus toxoid.[13, 21] The burn wounds should be covered with a clean, dry dressing or sheet, and the patient should be kept warm with blankets or heat lamps.

Burn Center Referral

Following initial treatment and stabilization in an emergency department, consideration should be given to consulting with a burn referral center for further care and transfer. The American Burn Association has identified specific injuries that usually require referral to a burn center (Table 20.2).[1, 12] These criteria alert the professional staff to those patients who may have special burn care considerations and, thus, require the expertise of staff specially trained in the care of the burn patient. The United States and Canada are divided into 12 regions, each with one or more tertiary burn-care centers.[17] Referring hospitals should contact one of the burn centers in their region for burn consultation.

Patient Transfer Procedures

The transfer of the burn patient should be coordinated between the referring physician and the receiving physician at the burn center. Transfer is best accomplished during the resuscitative phase before the patient encounters complications, such as pneumonia, sepsis, cardiac dysrhythmias, and major organ complications, which could serve as contraindications to patient movement.

When the burn center is contacted regarding the potential transfer of a burn patient, the receiving physician records current information about the patient's clinical status (Fig. 20.4). Included in this record is such information as the fluids infused, laboratory values, cardiac parameters, and the circulatory status of the extremities with circumferential burns. Any recommendations for change in the therapeutic regimen are given to the referring physician during this initial contact.

During the transfer procedure, all patients with major burns should be accompanied by a physician, if possible, to ensure adequate monitoring. A nurse experienced in burn care and patient transport also should be in attendance. Additionally, a respiratory therapist

Table 20.2. Burn Center Referral Criteria

1. Second-and third-degree burns >10 percent BSA in patients < 10 years and >50 years of age.

2. Second-and third-degree burns >20 percent BSA in other age groups.

3. Second-and third-degree burns that involve the face, hands, feet, genitalia, perineum, and major joints.

4. Third-degree burns >5 percent BSA in any age group. 5. Electrical burns, including lightning injury.

6. Chemical injuries with serious threat of functional or cosmetic impairment.

7. Inhalation injury with burn injury.

8. Circumferential burns of the chest or extremity.

9. Burn injury in patients with pre-existing medical disorders that could complicate management, prolong recovery, or affect mortality.

10. Hospitals without qualified personnel or equipment for the care of children should transfer burned children to a burn center with these capabilities.

11. Any burn patient with concomitant trauma (e.g., fractures) in which the burn injury poses the greatest risk of morbidity or mortality. If the trauma poses the greater risk, however, the patient may be treated in a trauma center initially, until stable, before being transferred to a burn center. Physician judgement will be necessary in such situations and should be in concert with the regional medical control plan and triage protocols.

BSA = body surface area. Data from *Nebraska Burn Institute: Advanced Burn Life Support Course Manual. Nebraska Burn Institute, Lincoln, NE, 1990.*

```
Date and time of call_____

Referring MD_____Telephone_____

Hospital_____City_____State_____

PATIENT INFORMATION

Name_____SSN_____Status:  Active Duty_____
                                                      Retired    _____
Age_____Sex_____Pre-Burn Weight_____             Dependent  _____
                                                      VAB/BEC    _____
Date of Burn_____Cause_____              PHS        _____
                                                      Civilian   _____
Extent of Burn_____3rd Degree_____

Areas burned_____

Inhalation injury_____Allergies_____

Associated injuries_____

Pre-existing injuries_____

TREATMENT CHECK-LIST

Resuscitation:  Calculated need (2ml/Kg/%TBS)_____

        Fluid in_____Urine Output_____

Airway_____Blood gases_____ET Tube_____

Medication:  Analgesics or sedatives_____Tetanus_____

             Antibiotics_____Other meds_____

Escharotomies:  Arms_____Legs_____Chest_____

Wound care:  Wash and debride_____Topical agent_____

Lab tests:  HCT_____Electrolytes_____BS_____BUN_____

Request:  Insert NG tube; avoid general anesthesia or IM meds;
          Keep I&O

INFORMATION FOR FLIGHT PLAN

Burn Team_____Family to accompany patient_____

Location of nearest airport with jet traffic_____

Transportation for team at destination_____
```

Figure 20.3. *US Army Institute of Surgical Research Patient Transfer Sheet.*

Table 20.3a. Nursing Care Plan: Burn Injury Resuscitative Phase, continued on next page.

NURSING DIAGNOSIS	EXPECTED OUTCOMES	INTERVENTIONS
Fluid volume deficit related to increased capillary permeability, increased intravascular hydrostatic pressure, increased evaporative losses	Urine output maintained at 30–50 mL/h for adults and 1 mL/kg/h for children less than 30 kg body weight Presence of weight gain during the resuscitative phase (intake > output) Vital signs within expected parameters based on age and medical history; BP adequate in relation to pulse and urine output Cardiac output WNL latter part of postburn day 1 and at hyperdynamic levels during postburn day 2 Electrolytes WNL (sodium approaching 130 mEq); Hct moderately elevated Negative urine sugar and acetone Clear sensorium	Vital signs q1h. I and O q1h and evaluate trends. Weight qd or bid (unless contraindicated by trauma injury). Monitor BUN, Hct, electrolytes every 12 h or as ordered. Assess LOC hourly. Titrate fluids per MD order; monitor response according to desired volume of urine output.
Impaired gas exchange related to carbon monoxide poisoning or inhalation injury; ineffective airway clearance related to tracheal edema and airway epidermal slough	Unlabored respirations 16–24/min $Po_2 > 90$ torr $Pco_2 < 40$ torr; O_2 sat >95% Clear bilateral breath sounds Clear to white pulmonary secretions Ability to mobilize secretions	Assess and document breath sounds every 4 h, LOC hourly. Cough, deep breathe, and incentive spirometry hourly. Administer humidified O_2 therapy as ordered. Elevate HOB to facilitate lung expansion. Monitor O_2 sat hourly; evaluate ABGs prn. Monitor carboxyhemoglobin levels as ordered. Turn every 2 h to mobilize secretions. Assess and document pulmonary secretions with suctioning procedures. Suction every 1–2 h prn; monitor sputum characteristics. Monitor for indications of impending airway obstruction, i.e., stridor, wheezing, rales, hoarseness, O_2 desaturation. Prepare for endotracheal intubation and mechanical ventilation as ordered.
Potential for injury related to stress response, impaired vascular perfusion in extremities with circumferential burns, corneal drying, and immobility	Absence of gastrointestinal bleeding Gastric pH > 5 Presence of adequate arterial perfusion to all extremities with circumferential burns BP cuff removed from extremity between readings Absence of corneal ulcerations due to increased environmental temperature, delayed blink reflex, and severe eyelid edema Absence of decubitus ulcer formation No evidence of decreased joint function	Measure NG pH every 2 h. Administer antacids per MD orders to keep gastric pH >5. Monitor NG drainage for presence of active bleeding. Remove all jewelry and constrictive clothing at the scene or in the emergency department. Elevate burned extremities continuously above the level of the heart. Monitor extremities hourly for signs and symptoms of limited blood flow. Monitor arterial pulses with ultrasonic flow detector hourly for 72 h on all extremities with circumferential burns. Prepare for escharotomy or transfer of the patient to the OR for fasciotomy.

Table 20.3b. Nursing Care Plan: Burn Injury Resuscitative Phase, continued from previous page; continued on next page.

NURSING DIAGNOSIS	EXPECTED OUTCOMES	INTERVENTIONS
		Apply eye lubricating ointment every 2 h.
		Loosen facial ties on ET and NG tube to accomodate edema formation; protect ears, nasal septum, and alae from pressure exerted by facial ties.
		Pad footboard and siderails continuously.
		Pad pressure areas, such as ankles, elbows, feet, ears, and scapulae.
		Provide active and passive ROM hourly; apply positioning splints as needed.
		Maintain urinary output at 75–100 mL/h in the presence of urinary hemochromogens.
		Monitor for increase or decrease in urine pigmentation.
Potential for injury related to presence of urinary hemochromogens and electric conductivity through the heart and respiratory system	Absence of visible urinary hemochromogens ECG and respirations WNL	Monitor cardiac rhythm of the electric injury patient for 24 h following cessation of cardiac dysrhythmias.
Potential for infection related to impaired skin integrity from burns, impaired immune response, and numerous invasive procedures	Absence of burn wound microbial invasion Temperature 99–101°F rectally Absence of redness, swelling, and purulence at invasive line insertion sites Absence of bacteria and yeast in blood, urine, and sputum	Cover wounds with a clean sheet during patient transfer. Administer tetanus toxoid prophylaxis as ordered. Continually monitor temperature with soft rectal probe. Apply heat lamps to maintain body temperature. Cleanse wound with surgical detergent disinfectant; shave hair remaining in and around burn wound; gently debride. Cover wound with topical antimicrobial agent as ordered. Use sterile technique when performing invasive procedures; assess invasive catheter sites bid.
Alteration in comfort related to acute burn injury and exposed nerve endings	Patient verbalizes increased level of comfort VS return to baseline after medication administration Patient uses alternative pain control measures, if possible, to supplement pharmacologic control Adequate VSs following narcotic administration	Assess need for analgesia as evidenced by verbal statements of pain, changes in vital signs, and increased state of agitation. Administer intravenous analgesia as ordered for painful procedures and other needed times per assessment, and monitor and document response. If possible, teach patient alternative methods of pain control, i.e., music therapy, relaxation therapy, and imagery; assist with use of these methods. Reduce anxiety level through explanation of procedures, talking to patient while performing nursing interventions.
Potential for ineffective patient/family coping due to emergent critical illness	Verbalization of goals of treatment regimen Verbalization of emotional stressors, concerns, and behaviors Verbalization of understanding and knowledge of available support service	Prior to family's initial visit, communicate with family the patient's extent of burn and physical appearance changes Provide family with visitation information within 24 h of admission. Provide emotional support during visiting times.

Table 20.3. Nursing Care Plan: Burn Injury Resuscitative Phase, continued from previous page.

NURSING DIAGNOSIS	EXPECTED OUTCOMES	INTERVENTIONS
		Allow family uninterrupted visitation as possible.
		Provide family with daily updates and major changes in patient condition.
		For impending patient transfer, provide family with available support services to assist with their travel.
		Encourage family attendance at family group meetings.

WNL = within normal limits; Hct = hematocrit; I & O = intake and output; bid = twice a day; BUN = blood urea nitrogen; LOC = level of consciousness; ABG = arterial blood gas; O_2 sat = oxygen saturation; HOB = head of bed; NG = nasogastric; MD = medical doctor; OR, operating room; ROM = range of motion; ECG = electrocardiogram; HR, heart rate; BP, blood pressure; Po_2, partial pressure oxygen; Pco_2, partial pressure carbon dioxide; ET, endotracheal.

should be available for the transfer should the patient require ventilatory support. The transfer may be accomplished by ground ambulance, rotary wing aircraft, or fixed wing aircraft, depending on the patient's status, distance to the transferring hospital, and availability of air support. If the patient is transferred by helicopter, the medical team must ensure stability of the patient, as interventions are difficult to institute in the noisy, poorly lighted, cramped, and turbulent environment of that aircraft.

Before leaving the referring hospital, the transferring team must accomplish a rapid but thorough patient assessment. Prior to air transport, the nurse must insert a nasogastric tube to accommodate the expansion of intestinal gases that occurs as atmospheric pressure decreases. The team should ascertain proper placement of intravenous cannulae or catheters and should suture all lines in place to avoid accidental dislodgement during movement. Adequacy of the patient's pulmonary status should be determined by arterial blood gas values and physical examination. The patient should be intubated prior to transfer if respiratory complications are thought to be an impending problem. Wounds should be wrapped in protective dressings, and the patient should be wrapped in heat-reflecting aluminum wrap and blankets to maintain body temperature. Circulation to the extremities should be assessed as previously described, and escharotomies should be performed if impaired blood flow is documented.

Critical Care Unit

The critical care nurse plays a vital role in the assessment of patient needs and in the determination of a realistic plan of care for the burn trauma patient (Table 20.3). When the patient is received in the critical care unit, the nurse should continue to monitor for complications related to fluid therapy. Because the fluid requirements are based on body weight prior to injury, the patient should be weighed on admission. If the patient cannot be weighed, an estimated weight should be obtained from the patient or a reliable family member. Vital signs and urine output should be assessed and recorded hourly, and fluids should be adjusted according to these hourly assessment parameters. Because of the early release of adrenal hormones that may cause hyperglycemia, the urine should be tested for sugar and acetone. Pulmonary artery pressure monitoring is reserved for those patients with complicating heart disease, those who do not respond to resuscitation in the anticipated manner, or those who require more than twice the estimated fluid needs.[15,18]

Electrocardiographic monitoring should be instituted on all major burns and on patients with suspected myocardial trauma, electric injury, and patients with a cardiac history. Because of the potential of high-voltage damage to the cardiac muscle or conduction system disturbances with any type of electric injury, the cardiac rhythm should be monitored for twenty-four hours following the cessation of dysrhythmias.[15, 16]

As the patient receives resuscitation fluid, the resulting edema may constrict the arteries in extremities with circumferential full-thickness burn. The best means for assessing arterial perfusion is by the use of an ultrasonic flow detector. Preferred arterial detection sites are the palmar arch vessels in the upper extremities and the posterior tibial artery in the lower extremities.[13, 15] In the instance of burned digits, flow is assessed in the digital blood vessels. Other signs of altered perfusion, although not as reliable as the ultrasonic flowmeter method, include cyanosis of the unburned extremity distal to the circumferential involvement; delayed capillary refilling; paresthesia; deep tissue pain; and progressive diminution or absence of the pulse. Swelling and coolness of the extremities are not reliable indicators of decreased peripheral perfusion.[13]

In the presence of these signs, an incision may be made through the eschar (termed escharotomy) to release the constricting tissue and allow for swelling to occur without inhibiting tissue perfusion (Fig. 20.4). This procedure may be performed at the bedside. Anesthesia

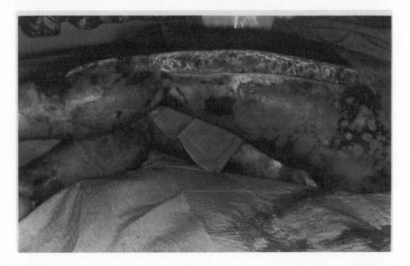

Figure 20.4. Escharotomy performed on the lateral aspect of the circumferentially burned left leg and extended from the upper thigh across the knee joint to the lower margin of the full thickness burn at the midcalf level. Note the wide separation of the incisional margins indicating the magnitude of subeschar edema formation.

is not required, because the eschar of a full-thickness burn is insensate. The incision should be placed along either the medial or lateral aspect of the extremity and should be extended over involved joints avoiding the major vessels, nerves, and tendons. The incision should extend through the involved eschar to the subcutaneous fat to permit separation of the edges of the incision. If circulation is still felt to be inadequate, another escharotomy incision along the contralateral aspect should be performed. Because of the risk of permanent tendon damage to the fingers, finger escharotomies should not be performed without consultation with a burn referral center.[12] In patients in whom a circumferential truncal burn limits chest excursion and impairs ventilatory exchange, a chest escharotomy also may be required.

With high-voltage electric injuries or burns involving the deep muscles, edema of the deep muscle may occur, resulting in the need for a fasciotomy. Fasciotomies are done in the operating room under general anesthesia and often involve the debridement of dead tissue at the same time.

Pain management becomes a primary nursing consideration as most patients exhibit intense pain following burn injury. Even patients with deep tissue injury may require large doses of analgesics, as wounds are often a combination of partial-and full-thickness burns. During the resuscitation phase, pain can be well controlled with intravenous morphine. The dosage should be titrated to the patient's response and may be administered by intermittent intravenous injection or by continuous intravenous infusion. Because hypovolemia impairs soft-tissue circulation, analgesics should not be given subcutaneously or intramuscularly, because the patient may experience a profound episode of hypotension and decreased respirations with the reabsorption of the interstitial fluids containing the medication. When muscle relaxation is needed to provide adequate ventilation, depolarizing blocking agents, such as pancuronium bromide, may be used.[15]

Following hemodynamic and pulmonary stabilization, initial burn wound care should be instituted. The nurse should cleanse the patient's wounds with a surgical detergent disinfectant. For partial-thickness wounds, the current practice is to excise bullae greater than two cm in diameter to rid the wound of the protein-rich blister fluid, an excellent environment for bacterial proliferation. Bullae less than two cm can be left intact.[15] Body hair should be shaved from the wound and from a generous margin around the wound periphery. Particular attention should be given to the scalp, as burns beneath the hair may remain undetected unless the head is adequately shaved. The patient's wounds then should be covered with a topical antibiotic agent. Because of the burn patient's impaired immune status, protective isolation is the recommended dress code for all members of the health care team.

The formation of gastroduodenal ulcers, frequently referred to as Curling's ulcers, used to be a major complication in the burn patient. Today, this pathologic phenomenon is largely preventable with the prophylactic administration of H2 histamine receptor antagonists and antacids. At the Institute of Surgical Research, the routine practice is to alternate the administration of aluminum hydroxide and magnesium hydroxide antacid preparations every two hours to titrate the gastric pH above five. Because magnesium hydroxide predisposes the burn patient to diarrhea, the alternate administration of aluminum hydroxide helps to prevent this complication.[6] An H2 receptor antagonist is given intravenously or by mouth every four to six hours.[15]

Patients with inhalation injury require frequent auscultation for decreased breath sounds, wheezing, or rales. The nurse should also assess for the onset of hoarseness, stridor, or increasing facial and neck edema. All patients with inhalation injury should be encouraged to cough on a regular basis and should be repositioned frequently. For the intubated patient, frequent suctioning is mandatory for the removal of secretions, soot, and sloughed mucosal debris and to maintain arterial blood gas values within acceptable limits.

On the day of burn, examination of the eyes should be performed by the physician to detect and document global or corneal injury. Although swollen lids usually protect the globe and cornea during the resuscitation period, instillation of sterile ophthalmic lubricant or artificial tears is required to protect any exposed cornea.[15]

The nurse should ensure functional body alignment of the burn patient at all times. To facilitate edema reabsorption, the patient should be placed in Fowler's position, and burned upper extremities should be elevated above the level of the heart with slings or foam wedges. The foot of the bed also should be raised to elevate burned lower extremities. Footboards should be used to prevent footdrop complications. Extreme caution should be exercised to protect pressure areas during the resuscitation phase, as decubitus ulcer formation may occur quickly. Bedrails may have to be padded, and foam wedges or pads used to protect the heels and elbows from breakdown. In lieu of a pillow, a small foam donut is useful to keep the head midline and to protect burned ears from the pressure of the mattress. The nurse should perform range of motion exercises at least five minutes every hour to decrease edema and maintain pre-burn mobility and function. Endotracheal tubes and nasogastric tubes should be secured midline in the nares to prevent erosion of the nasal septum or alae. With the loss of fluid and heat through the burned tissue, the patient must be provided with a warm environment to maintain body temperature. This may be done by increasing the temperature of the patient's room and by directing heat lamps or shields toward the patient.

The nurse plays a vital role in assisting the patient and family to cope with the burn trauma. During the resuscitative phase, the nurse works closely with the physician to prepare the family for their first visit after the burn incident. The nurse should be available for nursing-related questions during family visiting hours and for assisting the family to interact with the critically ill burn patient. Additionally, if the patient was transferred to a burn center away from the family's home, the nurse may determine the need for social work referral and assistance with temporary lodging.

Summary

During the resuscitation period, a knowledge of burn pathophysiology assists the nurse in conducting thorough assessments and providing effective nursing interventions in the acutely ill patient. The many variables associated with the burn injury contribute to the presentation of each burn patient as one with a unique injury that requires the most vigilant nursing care and expertise. The total dedication required of health care workers as members of a multidisciplinary burn team provides a significant professional challenge. Meeting that challenge appreciably strengthens the chances of burn patient survival.

References

1. American Burn Association: Hospital and prehospital resources for optimal care of patients with burn injury: Guidelines for operation and development of burn centers. *J Burn Care Rehabil* 11:97,1990.

2. Demling R H: Fluid and electrolyte management. *Crit Care Clin* 1:27, 1985.

3. Demling R H: Fluid replacement in burn patients. *Surg Clin North Am* 67:15, 1987

4. Demling R H: Post graduate course: Respiratory injury, Part III. *J Burn Care Rehabil* 7:227, 1986.

5. Freeman J W: Nursing care of a patient with a burn injury. *Crit Care Nurs* 6:52, 1984.

6. Gottschlich M M, Warden GD, Michel M, et al: Diarrhea in tube-fed burn patients: Incidence, etiology, nutritional impact, and prevention. *J Parent Enter Nutr* 12:338, 1988.

7. Heisel E B: The skin: Basic considerations. In Criep L H (ed): Dermatologic Allergy: Immunology, Diagnosis, Management. Philadelphia, W B Saunders, 1967.

8. Kenner C V: Burn injury. In Kenner C V, Guzzetta C E, Dossey B M (eds): Critical Care Nursing: Body-Mind-Spirit, ed 2. Boston, Little, Brown, 1985, p 1101.

9. Mikhail J N: Acute burn care: An update. *Journal of Emergency Nursing* 14:9, 1988.

10. Moncrief J A: The body's response to heat. In Artz C P, Moncrief J A, Pruitt B A, Jr. (eds): Burns: A Team Approach. Philadelphia, W B Saunders, 1979, p 23.

11. Mozingo D W, Smith A A, McManus W F, et al: Chemical burns. *J Trauma* 28:642, 1988.

12. Nebraska Burn Institute: Advanced Burn Life Support Course Manual. Nebraska Burn Institute, 4600 Valley Road, Lincoln, NE 68510, 1990.

13. Pruitt B A Jr: The burn patient: 1. Initial care. In Ravitch M M (ed): Current Problems in Surgery. Chicago, *Year Book Medical Publishers*, 1979, p 1.

14. Pruitt B A Jr: The universal trauma model. *Bull Am Coll Surg* 70:2, 1985.

15. Pruitt B A Jr, Goodwin C W Jr: Thermal and environmental injury. In Moore E E (ed): Early Care of the Injured Patient, ed 4. Philadelphia, B C Decker, 1990, p 286.

16. Pruitt B A Jr, Goodwin C W Jr: Thermal injuries. In Davis J H, Druker W R, Foster R S, et al (eds): Clinical Surgery. St. Louis, C V Mosby, 1987, p 2823.

17. Pruitt B A Jr, Mason A D Jr, Goodwin C W Jr: Epidemiology of burn injury and demography of burn care facilities. *Prob Gen Surg* 7:235, 1990.

18. Pruitt B A Jr, Treat R G: The burn patient. In Dudrick S J, Bave A E, Eiseman B, et al (eds): Manual of Preoperative and Postoperative Care, ed 3. Philadelphia, W B Saunders, 1983, p 697.

19. Wachtel T L: Epidemiology, classification, initial care, and administrative considerations for critically burned patients. *Crit Care Clin* 1:3, 1985.

20. Warden G D: Immunologic response to burn injury. In Boswick J A (ed): The Art and Science of Burn Care. Rockville, Aspen, 1987, p 113.

21. Warden GD: Outpatient care of thermal injuries. *Surg Clin North Am* 67:147, 1987.

—by Molly C. Burgess, RN, MS

Lieutenant Colonel, Army Nurse Corps, and Head Nurse, Burn Critical Care Unit, US Army Institute of Surgical Research, Fort Sam Houston, Texas.

Chapter 21

Management of the Pediatric Patient with Burns

Abstract

Two million people in the United States receive medical treatment each year for burn injuries. One hundred thousand of these patients are hospitalized, and 7,800 die as a direct result of their injuries.[1] Of the patients hospitalized 30 percent to 40 percent are under 15 years of age. Sixty-seven percent are male. The average age of children with burns is 32 months.[2] Flame burns account for approximately 13 percent of accidents, scalds account for 85 percent, and electrical and chemical burns account for approximately 2 percent. The majority of scald injuries are small. Sixteen percent of burn injuries are not accidental, and approximately half of these are a result of documentable, inflicted abuse.[3] (J Burn Care Rehabil 1993; 14:3-8).

Emergency Management

Burns covering greater than 10 percent to 15 percent total body surface area (TBSA) in children require immediate institution of fluid resuscitation, as do any burns associated with smoke inhalation. Even very small burns affecting hands, feet, face, perineum, or joint surfaces and burns resulting from electrical injuries where deep-tissue involvement is suspected should be treated as emergencies, and the patient should be hospitalized.[4] After the patency of the airway is established, any smoldering clothing should be removed. If chemical injury is suspected, copious irrigation with water should be performed. The burns should then be covered with clean, dry sheets. Cold, wet compresses may be applied to small injuries but not to large injuries, because severe hypothermia may result. Under no circumstances should ice be applied to injuries. The evaluating team should be prepared to immediately and simultaneously evaluate cardiopulmonary status, establish intravenous access, and insert a nasogastric tube and an indwelling urinary catheter. Fluid therapy must be started immediately on infants who have burns covering 10 percent TBSA and on older children who have burns covering 15 percent TBSA.

Fluid Resuscitation. Fluid resuscitation should be initiated with an isotonic electrolyte solution (e.g., lactated Ringer's) while precise calculations for resuscitation are carried out. The rate of fluid administration should be approximately 450 ml/m^2 body surface area or should be a quantity sufficient to maintain a urine output of 1 ml/kg/hr. The wound should be cleaned and debrided, and assessment should be made of the size of the burn. This assessment should be done with the use of body proportion charts specific to children, with the body surface area calculated from standard nomograms. Fluid resuscitation in children should be based on body surface area with the formula of 5000 $ml/m^{2'}$ burned area and 200 ml/m^2 total body surface for maintenance; half the total volume should be infused over the first eight hours after burn injury, and the remainder should be infused over the succeeding sixteen hours.[5]

Controversy exists over whether and when to add colloid to the resuscitation fluids. Intravasvascular protein loss from increased vascular permeability after burn injury has definitely been shown to decrease the colloid oncotic pressure of plasma.[6] Most recent animal studies show that this loss of protein is most marked during the first six to eight hours after uncomplicated injuries.[7-9] The addition of albumin to resuscitation fluid does decrease after burn edema.[10] Colloid treatment should be instituted from eight to twenty-four hours after burn injury; 12.5 gm human serum albumin/L D_5 lactated Ringer's solution has served to maintain stable intravascular albumin levels.[11] Note that in children 1 year of age lesser quantities of sodium are required because of their peculiar renal function; a solution containing 70 to 80 mEq sodium/1 should be considered.

The adequacy of resuscitation must be continually assessed by a variety of clinical parameters beginning with urine output, which should be maintained 0.5 ml/kg/hr. The state of sensorium, pulse,

pulse pressure, and the adequacy of capillary filling with arterial blood gases are usually sufficient monitors to determine whether acidosis is occurring. In only very complicated cases are arterial, central venous, and pulmonary artery pressure monitors required.

After the first 24 hours after burn injury, fluid requirements decrease to a constant that remains as long as the burn wound is open. Fluid is properly replaced with 3750 ml/m^2 burned area and 1500 ml/m^2 total body surface area/day. The sodium requirements are low after the first 24 hours after burn injury, with 50 mEq sodium and 20 to 30 mEq potassium/day being required. Our solution of choice is D$_5$ 0.33 percent normal saline solution with 20 to 30 mEq potassium phosphate (phosphate replaces chloride because of frequent hypophosphatemia).[12]

The transition from intravenous to oral fluids can be accomplished during the first few hours after burn injury. Homogenized milk infant formulas for infants, or soy-based products for infants who have lactose intolerance can be given by constant infusion via nasogastric tube or small-bowel feeding tube. The amount of milk is increased at four hour intervals, depending on the patients tolerance as determined by hourly gastric residuals, and the intravenous fluids are decreased proportionately. The objective is to keep fluid intake constant.[11] Ideally, oral fluid replaces intravenous therapy by the end of 24 hours after burn injury. When full nutritional requirements are taken enterally, a liquid diet is instituted and is gradually advanced to a regular diet with supplements. The milk program reduces the incidence of stress ulcers and also helps meet the caloric requirements of the patient with burns. Because the concentration of sodium in homogenized milk is only 25 mEq/L most patients with burns covering greater than 20 percent TBSA require sodium supplementation in the form of sodium chloride tablets or 3 percent sodium chloride elixir (four to six divided doses). The risk of hyperosmolality is low, but patients on high-calorie, high-protein feedings who sustain extensive evaporative water losses must be monitored frequently for this possibility.

Energy Requirements. The burn injury instigates a hypermetabolic response characterized by protein and fat catabolism. Children with burns covering 40 percent TBSA treated with early excision and grafting experience resting energy expenditures of approximately 50 percent above predicted levels. These energy expenditures increase with the physiologic demands of pain, anxiety, and mobilization. Additional caloric demands are made with cold stress, especially because children have a larger surface area-to-mass ratio, which allows proportionally more heat loss than adults.

Caloric demands can be decreased by providing environmental temperatures of 28° to 33° C, blankets during transport, and the liberal use of analgesia and anxiolytics. Uninterrupted sleep intervals are especially important to the child with burns.

Despite these measures the increased metabolic rate, urinary nitrogen excretion, and lipolysis add to a steady erosion of lean body mass. The objective of any caloric supplementation program should be to maintain body weight ±5 percent of pre-admission levels. Children with preexisting nutritional deficits will present the burn team with a particular challenge.

Many formulas to achieve this end have been proposed. Most were derived for adults and do not address the specific needs of children. As previously stated children have a greater surface area-to-mass ratio than do adults, so caloric demands can be more accurately calculated through formulas based on surface area. A series of such formulas has been developed specifically for children. Infants should receive 1000 kcal/m² body surface area burned + 2100 kcal/m² body area per day. Children aged two to fifteen years should receive 1300 kcal/m² body surface area burned + 1800 kcal/m² body area per day.[13] Adolescents, although similar to adults in size, still require additional calories for growth and should be replaced according to the formula 1500 kcal/m² body surface area burned + 1500 kcal/m² body area per day.[14] Alternately, caloric requirements can be calculated from resting energy expenditures as measured by indirect calorimetry, adding 40 percent to 50 percent (REE x 1.4) for activity.

Children, like all patients with burns, should receive supplements of Vitamins C and A, zinc, and multivitamins. Because of the immaturity of their renal systems children more frequently require sodium supplementation, and they should be closely monitored for both hyponatremia and hypochloremia.

It is preferable that alimentation be initiated within six to eight hours after burn injury. It has been noted the hypermetabolic response may be diminished[15] and intestinal integrity may be maintained[16] with the early implementation of enteral nutrition. Sufficient oral calories can be provided to children with small injuries, but those with burns covering 40 percent TBSA should have a small-bowel (duodenal) feeding tube placed to facilitate continuous delivery of calories. Parenteral hyperalimentation should be avoided because of the potential infectious complications and increased mortality associated with its use.[17]

Failure to reach caloric requirements needed for weight maintenance, positive nitrogen balance, and energy equilibrium will result in delayed or abnormal wound healing, in addition to multiple immunologic derangements. Maximal use of provided calories can be achieved with exogenous supplementation of growth hormone. Recombinant human growth hormone administration has been associated with increased rates of donor site healing,[18] earlier achievement of positive nitrogen balance,[19] and decreased rates of protein breakdown.[20]

Early work in small animal models implicated catecholamines as a major mediator of postburn hypermetabolism.[21] Consequently, we have examined the effect of nonselective P-adrenergic blockade on hemodynamic and metabolic responses in patients with burns. Propranolol significantly decreased heart rate and left-ventricular work but did not change cardiac index or metabolic rate.[22] However, there was an increase in net urea production that could be minimized by dietary supplementation. Propranolol has been shown to reduce peripheral perfusion and lactate production.[23] Further work revealed that patients undergoing P-blockade were able to increase their metabolic rates when subjected to cold stress.[24] Isoproterenol-challenge tests were shifted to the right, but patients responded in a parallel fashion to controls. This response was absent in patients whose metabolic rates were already maximal (e.g., patients with sepsis). We have used propranolol therapeutically in forty-three patients over four years for 19.5 ± 13.6 days (mean $\pm$ SD). In this period one patient died with the cause of death being pneumonia and mucus plugs obstructing the upper airway. No patients developed hypotension, azotemia, bronchospasm, hyperglycemia, or hypoglycemia.

Prevention of Infection

Early Excision and Grafting. The burn eschar presents a constant potential reservoir of microbes and their byproducts. The ultimate protection to be afforded to the child with burns is the removal of this reservoir before its colonization. Early excision and grafting within the first 24 hours after burn injury is an especially attractive therapy. We excise the entire wound and cover as much of it as possible with autograft meshed 4:1. We obtain physiologic closure with cadaveric allograft meshed 2:1. Those wounds for which there is insufficient autograft to definitively close are covered with 2:1 meshed cadaveric allograft, which is replaced as donor sites heal. Tangential excision is the preferred procedure, and fascial excisions are reserved for deep, extensive burns. Excising the wound within the first twenty-four hours has a blood loss of approximately 0.4 ml/cm^2, which is similar to the blood losses associated with procedures performed at sixteen days after burn injury.[25] Excisions first performed between these time points has twice the blood loss.[25] Early excision can be safely carried out by an experienced burn team if the anesthesiologist is knowledgeable with postburn fluid resuscitation requirements. We reserve early total excision to flame injuries of obvious full-thickness depths, and we believe our survival statistics for massive burns is documentation of its efficacy.

Many burn centers do not routinely resuscitate children with full-thickness burns covering greater than 80 percent to 90 percent TBSA. However, as we have demonstrated,[26] these patients can be routinely salvaged with the use of the early excision and grafting technique. Such children with massive burns who are given appropriate psychologic and social support can and do participate in society. In fact, these children show no significant differences from their age-matched peers in terms of psychologic adjustment, social adjustment, and self-esteem parameters as measured by standardized psychologic tests. Given the opportunity to survive their debilitating injuries, these children differ from their peers only in appearance. They participate in life in the same manner as other children; they go to school, play sports, date, get jobs, get married, and start families just as would be expected had they not been burned.

Scald injuries are notoriously difficult to assess during the early postburn period. These are generally conservatively treated for seven to ten days, after which they have matured and have truly declared their depth. In a randomized study of children with scalds of indeterminate depth, we reported that almost 50 percent of these children healed without surgical intervention, obviating the risks of anesthesia and blood transfusions without unduly lengthening hospital stay.[27]

It is virtually impossible to completely eradicate the bacterial flora present on and in the burn wound, but the number and character of these indigenous inhabitants can be controlled. This end is accomplished through the use of various topical antimicrobial agents. It is important to realize that no single agent is totally effective against all burn wound pathogens and that topical therapy should therefore be guided by in vitro results. Wound surfaces should be routinely cultured starting at the time of admission. This practice allows for the observation of the evolution of microbial populations and provides the burn team with objective data from which appropriate therapeutic decisions can be made.

Currently, the topical agent of choice is silver sulfadiazine. This water-soluble cream is easy to apply, is painless on application, has a broad bacteriostatic spectrum, and is readily available. The most common adverse reaction to this agent is a transient leukopenia, which is believed to be due to the margination of white blood cells rather than to be a true allergic response. Silver sulfadiazine can be applied with the use of fine mesh gauze dressings and can be wrapped with bulky absorbent gauze wraps and tubular net elastic bandages.

Mafenide acetate cream has been demonstrated to be a very effective, broad-spectrum bacteriostatic agent. It is the only agent demonstrated to diffuse through burn wound eschar and is therefore frequently used to treat injuries to cartilaginous surfaces such as ears. Mafenide acetate cream is painful upon application and may cause acid-base imbalances resulting from carbonic anhydrase inhibition, particularly if large surface areas are treated. A second form of mafenide acetate, a 5 percent solution, has been used effectively on burn wounds,[28] split-thickness skin graft sites,[29] and excised wound beds.[30] This agent has not been reported to cause the pain or acidosis[31] associated with the cream form of mafenide acetate.

Biologic and Synthetic Dressings

Biologic dressings, when applied to fully debrided, relatively uncontaminated wounds, have been shown to adhere to the wound surface[32] reduce wound bacterial colony counts, limit fluid and protein loss,[33] reduce pain, and increase the rate of epithelialization. Traditionally, biologics were represented by porcine heterograft and human skin allograft and were used exclusively for temporary closure. Currently, the biologics would also include the homologous cultured skin replacements and autologous cultured epithelium, which may provide permanent closure.

Porcine (pigskin) was one of the first biologic dressings used, and good results can still be achieved with its use, particularly when it is applied to a fresh, clean, partial-thickness scald burn. We rarely use porcine skin any longer and have replaced it with cadaveric allograft, which is harvested and stored by our local tissue bank. Allograft is used not only on partial-thickness injuries but also as a temporary cover for the excised wounds of patients who have insufficient donor sites to provide autologous tissue to close their extensive wounds. Additionally, we use homograft to physiologically close our widely meshed autografts, which is a technique described by Alexander.[34]

The use of homograft, however, may present the patient with the risk of contracting sero-transmitted diseases, and so many physicians have abandoned its use in favor of the synthetic dressings. Many of these dressings have been used with results that may rival those of homograft, but as yet no comparison studies have been performed.

Children are more easily treated with biologic or synthetic dressings as opposed to the more traditional gauze and topical agents. Biologics are painless to apply (unless staples are being used to secure them), and they decrease the pain of the dressed wound. Additionally, most biologics and synthetics are a onetime application that remains in place until the wound is healed. This greatly reduces the pain and trauma associated with daily dressing changes as well as the frequent tissue disruptions resulting from the removal of adherent dressings.

Inhalation Injury

The presence of an inhalation injury is the primary determinant of mortality in the patient with burns, particularly the infant and children with preexisting pulmonary conditions. Mortality estimates vary depending on the differing criteria for diagnosis of inhalation injury, but they are typically 45 percent to 60 percent in adults.[35-37] The development of more sophisticated and sensitive methods of airway evaluation has led to an increase in the early identification of the inhalation injury. Serial bronchoscopic evaluation of the large airways is a routine procedure that is performed each time the child is anesthetized. In this way it becomes easy to identify changes to the mucosa of the airways and to initiate prompt treatment.

Treatment of the inhalation injury should begin at the scene, starting with the assessment of the burn's cause. Oxygen should be administered by face mask if there is any question of smoke exposure. Carbon monoxide has a much higher affinity for hemoglobin than does oxygen, impairing oxygen delivery to already anoxic tissues. Supplemental oxygen is able to clear the carbon monoxide more rapidly, increasing oxygen delivery to the tissues. Several elements of a fire are capable of producing injury to the respiratory tract. The most obvious element, heat, has been repeatedly demonstrated to cause little damage unless conveyed by steam (which is capable of carrying 4,000 times the heat of dry air). The upper-respiratory tract is an extremely efficient heat exchanger. Acute asphyxia and carbon monoxide poisoning are common causes of early death in house fires, because the fire consumes all the available oxygen. However, the majority of the damage to the airways is caused by the chemical reactions undergone by the products of incomplete combustion. These substances, such as aldehydes and oxides of sulfur and nitrogen, mix with the endogenous water of the lung to produce corrosive chemicals that erode the mucosa and cause sloughing of the epithelium.

Histologic changes in the larynx, trachea, and major bronchi range from mild erythema to charring, marked congestion, and complete desquamation of the epithelium. There is some evidence to suggest that exposure to smoke causes degradation of surfactant and decreases its production, resulting in atelectasis.

Traditionally, the child with an inhalation injury was immediately intubated and was placed on mechanical ventilation. After several days a tracheostomy was performed, and mechanical ventilation was continued. General anethestics were administered to perform surgical procedures, the child was restricted to bed rest, and fluids were restricted to decrease the development of pulmonary edema. With this approach mortality rates and the incidence of pneumonia were very high, and weaning from the ventilator was difficult. Over the past decade we have initiated the practice of aggressive nonintervention, viewing nasotracheal intubation as a major source of iatrogenic morbidity. A nasotracheal tube allows a direct route for bacteria into the major airways and prevents the body's own homeostatic mechanisms from functioning properly. Fluid restriction paradoxically increases rather than decreases pulmonary edema probably because of the trapping of activated neutrophils within the microcirculation of the lung.

If an inhalation injury is suspected on admission or during the first operative procedure, all children have their airways bronchoscopically examined. Surgical procedures are performed with the patients under ketamine anesthesia without intubation and frequently with ongoing duodenal feeding. Humidified oxygen is administered by face mask during the procedure, and the patient is awakened before leaving the operating room. Our patients are not intubated for tachypnea (up to respiratory rates of 80 breaths/minute), but only for deteriorating blood gases. Children are mobilized early. Active range of motion is initiated on the fifth post-graft day and ambulation, if there are no lower extremity grafts, is initiated as early as the second postoperative day. Even if ambulation is not possible, children sit in bed to receive their meals or watch television. Aggressive pulmonary toilet with deep breathing, incentive spirometry, and nebulized solutions of heparin (5,000 in 5 ml normal saline solution every six hours) and n-acetyl cysteine liquefy casts and secretions, thereby facilitating their expectoration. Neither prophylactic antibiotics nor steroid therapy are useful in the treatment of inhalation injuries and may instead promote detrimental effects.

Aggressive surgical removal of devitalized tissue, early enteral nutrition, and cautious use of endotracheal intubation and mechanical ventilation have allowed the survival of children with massive thermal injuries. The size of burn that results in death of half of the patients under eighteen years of age treated at our hospital with or without inhalation injury is now 98 percent TBSA. Over thirty patients with burns >80 percent full-thickness have survived in the last three years and are prospering. At this time our attention is now focused on the long-term rehabilitation and psychosocial adaptation of these children.

References

1. Report on the epidemiology and surveillance of injuries. No. F472-R7. Rockville, Maryland: Health Services and Mental Health Administration; 1972. US Department of Health, Education, and Welfare publication F472-R7.

2. Feller I, Keith J C. National burn information exchange. *Surg Clin North Am* 1970; 50:1423-36.

3. Feldman K W. Child abuse by burning. In: Kempe C, Helfer R E, eds. The battered child, 3rd ed. Chicago: University of Chicago Press, 1980:147-62.

4. Curreri P W, Luterman A, Braun D W Jr, et al. Burn injury: analysis of survival and hospitalization time for 937 patients. *Ann Surg* 1980; 192:472-8.

5. Carvajal H F. Acute management of burns in children. *South Med J* 1973; 68:129-31.

6. Roberts J C, Courtice F C. Measurement of protein leakage in the acute and recovery stages of the thermal injury. *Aust J Exp Biol Med Sci* 1969; 47:421-33.

7. Brouhard B H, Carvajal H F, Linares H A. Burn edema and protein leakage in the rat. I. Relationship to time of injury. *Microvasc Res* 1978; 15:221-8.

8. Carvajal H F, Linareas H A. Effect of burn depth upon edema formation and albumin extravasation in rats. *Burns* 1981; 7:79-84.

9. Carvajal H F, Linares H A, Brouhard B H. Relationship of burn size to vascular permeability changes in rats. *Surg Gynecol Obstet* 1978; 147:161-6.

10. Stone H H. The composite burn solution. IN: Polk H C Jr, Stone H H, eds. Contemporary burn management. Boston: Little Brown Co, 1971; 93-104.

11. Carvajal H F. A physiologic approach to fluid therapy in severely burned children. *Surg Gynecol Obstet* 1980; 150:379-84.

12. Kreusser W, Ritz E. The phosphate-depletion syndrome. *Contre Nephrot* 1978;14:162-74.

13. Hildreth M A, Herndon D N, Desai M H, et at. Current treatment reduces calories required to maintain weight in pediatric patients with burns. *J Burn Care Rehabil* 1990; 11:405-9.

14. Hildreth M A, Herndon D N, Desai M H, et al. Caloric needs of adolescent patients with Burns. J Burn Care Rehabil 1989; 10:523-6.

15. Wood R A, Caldwell F T, Bowser-Wallace B H. The effect of early feeding on postburn hypermetabolism. *J Trauma* 1988; 28:177-83.

16. Inoue S, Epstein M D, Alexander J W, et al. Prevention of yeast translocation across the gut by a single enteral feeding after burn injury. *J Parenteral Ent Nutrition* 1989; 13:565-71.

17. Herndon D N, Barrow R E, Linares H A, et al. Increased mortality with intravenous supplementation in severely burned patients. *J Burn Care Rehabil* 1989; 10:309-13.

18. Herndon DN, Barrow RE, Broemeling LD, et al. Effect of exogenous growth hormone on the rate of donor site healing in pediatric burn patients. *Ann Surg* 1990, 212:424-31.

19. Wilmore D W, Moylan H A, Bristow B F, et al. Anabolic effects of human growth hormone and high caloric feedings following thermal injury. *Surg Gynecol Obstet* 1974;138:875-88.

20. Gore D C, Honeycutt D, Jahoor F, et al. Effect of exogenous growth hormone on whole body and isolated-limb protein kinetics in burned patients. *Arch Surg* 1991;126:38-43.

21. Herndon D N, Wilmore D W, Mason A D, et al. Humoral mediators of nontemperature-dependent hypermetabolism in 50 percent burned adult rats. *Surg Forum* 1977; 28:37-9.

22. Herndon D N, Barrow R.E, Rutan T C, et al. Effect of propranolol administration on hemodynamic and metabolic responses of burned pediatric patients. *Ann Surg* 1988; 208:484-92.

23. Gore D C, Honeycutt D, Jahoor F, et al. Propanolol diminishes extremity blood flow in burned patients. *Ann Surg* 1991; 213:568-74.

24. Honeycutt D, Barrow R, Herndon D. Cold stress response in patients with severe burns after B blockade. *J Burn Care Rehabil* 1992; 13:181-6.

25. Herndon D N, Desai M H, Broemehing L D, et al. Early burn wound excision significantly reduces blood loss. *Ann Surg* 1990; 211:753-62.

26. Herndon D N, Gore D, Cole M, et al. Determinants of mortality in pediatric patients with greater than 70 percent full-thickness total body surface area thermal injury treated by early total excision and grafting. *J Trauma* 1987; 27:208-12.

27. Desai M H, Rutan R L, Herndon D N. Conservative treatment of scald injuries is superior to early excision. *J Burn Care Rehabil* 1991; 12:482-4.

28. Harrison H N, Bales H W, Jacoby F. The absorption into burned skin of sulfamylon acetate from five percent aqueous solution. *J Trauma* 1972; 12:994-8.

29. Lee J J, Marvin J A, Heiinbach D M, et al. Use of percent five sulfamylon (mafenide) solution after excision and grafting of burns. *J Burn Care Rehabil* 1988; 9:602-5.

30. Shuck J M, Thome L W, Cooper C G. Mafenide acetate solution dressings: an adjunct to burn wound care. *J Trauma* 1975; 15:595-9.

31. Harrison H N, Shuck J M, Caldwell E. Studies of pain produced by mafenide acetate preparations in burns. *Arch Surg* 1975; 110:1446-9.

32. Burleson R, Eiseman B. Nature of the bond between partial-thickness skin and wound granulations. *Surg* 1972; 72: 315-22.

33. Lameke L O, Nilsson G E, Reithner H S. The evaporative water loss from burns and the water-vapour permeability of grafts and artificial membranes used in the treatment of burns. *Burns* 1978; 3:159-65.

34. Alexander J W, MacMillan B F, Law E, et al. Treatment of burns with widely meshed skin autograft and meshed skin allograft overlay. *J Trauma* 1981; 21:433-8.

35. DiVincenti F C, Pruitt B A, Jr., Reckler J M. Inhalation injuries. *J Trauma* 1971; 11:109-17.

36. Stone H H, Martin J D Jr. Pulmonary injury associated with thermal burns. *Surg Gynecol Obstet* 1969; 129:1242-6.

37. Venus A, Matsuda T, Capiozo J B, et al. Prophylactic intubation and continuous positive airway pressure in the management of inhalation injury in burn victims. *Crit Care Med* 1981; 9:519-23.

—by David N. Herndon, M D,
Randi L. Rutan, RN, BSN, and
Thomas C. Rutan, RN, MSN
Galveston, Texas.

Chapter 22

Pain in Burn Patients

Framework for Pain Management in the Burn Patient

Critical care nurses make a crucial difference in patient outcomes, and nowhere is this more clearly evident than in the burn intensive care environment, where patients experience intense pain related to injury and treatment. The elimination of all or even some of the pain of burn injury has been shown to have a significant effect on a positive outcome for the patient, both physiologically and psychologically (Murray, 1972).

Although the goal of any pain management program is to eliminate pain, there is a necessity for a compromise among pain perception, the pain state, and safe medical practice (Loeser, 1987). This compromise helps prevent physiological complications. Psychological morbidity is a problem in burn patients, however, and presents as several syndromes with consistent patterns of symptoms. Such morbidity is significantly more likely to develop in patients with pain-management problems than in patients with controlled pain (Ehleben & Still, 1985).

There are four factors present in pain: nociception, pain perception by the individual, suffering, and pain behavior (Loeser, 1987). Of the four, nociception is the easiest to understand. It has been described as the perception by the system of potential tissue damage caused by thermal or mechanical energy that impinges on specialized nerve endings (A-delta and C fibers; Loeser, 1987).

Pain perception by the individual is best described as what the individual says the pain is like and when he or she says it occurs (McCaffery, 1979). At the National Institutes of Health (NIH) consensus conference, pain was described as:

- [a] subjective experience that can be perceived directly only by the sufferer. It is a multidimensional phenomenon that can be described by pain location, intensity, temporal aspects, quality, impact and meaning.

- [b]Pain does not occur in isolation but in a specific human being in psychosocial, economic and cultural contexts that influence the meaning, experience, and verbal and non-verbal expression of pain. (NIH, 1987, p. 36).

Inherent in this definition is the concept of suffering, an affective response generated by pain at higher nervous centers (Loeser, 1987). Suffering is affected by stress, anxiety, fear, depression, and loss, all of which are exaggerated by the very nature of an acute burn injury. The language of pain is used to describe suffering. Therefore, "I hurt" may be an expression of an affective state rather than of actual pain stimuli.

Suffering leads to pain behavior. All behaviors are real and perceived by patients to be expressions of real pain; therefore, the caregiver must ask why the patient is exhibiting pain behavior rather than whether the pain is real. One group of investigators found that there were no significant relationships between variables such as total body surface area burned, depression, or days since burn injury and expressed pain behavior (Charlton, Klein, & Gagliardi, 1981). Nevertheless, environment strongly influences pain behavior, leading some clinicians to advocate controlling pain in the burn unit by modifying the environment to control manifestations of pain behavior (Fagerhaugh, 1974). The major environmental stressors in the critical care burn unit include temperature, noise, and fatigue from continuous monitoring.

There are a number of other stressors, both physiological and psychological, that lead to pain in the burn patient. As a result of damage to skin, exposed nerve endings, and the release of chemicals in response to injury, physical pain exists (Kibbee, 1984). Burn pain is acute in nature and most often subsides with healing (Merskey, 1986).

It is often intermittent as a result of operative procedures and other painful treatment regimens, but it has an underlying persistent background component that contributes to an overall perception of nearly constant pain (Perry, Heidrich, & Ramos, 1981). Chronic pain can develop as a result of complications related to scar formation as well as functional deformities (Freund et al., 1981).

Major psychological stressors associated with burn injury involve the real threat to survival and fear of disfigurement (Davidson & Noyes, 1973; Noyes, Andreasen, & Hartford, 1971). Often, depression results from guilt related to the cause of the burns, forced dependency on others, and impaired emotional gratification as life plans are disrupted. Cultural influences, fatigue, repeated surgeries, painful procedures, and anxiety related to the ability to cope with pain are major influences on how pain is perceived. Such stressors, coupled with the need to interact with and depend on staff who both inflict and relieve pain, can be overwhelming to even the emotionally strongest of individuals.

There are three phases of burn care associated with pain-control requirements: resuscitative, acute, and rehabilitative (Marvin, 1987). All three phases require a combination of pharmacological and nonpharmacological therapy, but the balance between the two changes as physical healing takes place.

This chapter discusses the role of the critical care nurse in pain management of the adult burn patient. The nursing process provides the framework for the discussion of the applications and implications of research findings for nursing practice primarily in the resuscitative and acute phases, when patients are the most critically ill. Future research considerations are explored.

Assessment of Burn Pain

Pain in the burn patient is difficult to assess accurately. The perception of pain by the burn patient is multidimensional and varies considerably, as it does in all patients with acute pain (NIH, 1987). There will always be some manifestations of pain behavior unless the patient is pharmacologically paralyzed. The nurse may make some judgments of the amount of pain that the patient is experiencing on the basis of the extent of injury and previous experience of pain in other patients, but intensity and severity of injury are not adequate indicators of the severity of pain (Kibbee, 1984; Perry et al., 1981). Suffering obviously occurs, but its nature is unique to each patient's physiological and psychological stressors.

261

If the operational definition of pain in the clinical area is that it is whatever the patient says it is and occurs when the patient says it occurs, then theoretically the health care team should be able to base interventions on the patient's own assessment of his or her pain. In reality, even if the patient is well oriented, this is difficult to do while ensuring safe medical practice during burn therapy. Although pain management should be a cooperative effort among all health care team members, the patient, and the patient's family, often the nurses'subjective assessments of pain behaviors are the only assessments made (Kibbee, 1984). The assessment of burn pain has been the topic of a number of research studies focusing on the patients' perceptions, the nurses' assessments, or the correlation of the two.

In a comprehensive descriptive study of how patients assessed their burn pain, patients' descriptions of pain intensity varied little despite heterogeneity in the group related to extent of burn, age, ethnicity, and socioeconomic background (Perry et al., 1981). Background as well as procedural pain was evaluated, and findings indicated that most patients had extended periods of mild or no pain. Despite these periods, patients rated their overall pain as high because of its intensity during procedures and because the milder pain affected movement and sleep. Often the patients did not complain of pain or request more frequent medication administrations. Perry et al, (1981) were unable to correlate the severity of the patients' pain with dosage, type, and frequency of analgesics given, emphasizing a possible lack of accurate or thorough assessments as a basis for individualizing pain management.

A study of the pain experience of patients with posttraumatic stress disorder (PTSD) revealed that such patients reported higher levels of procedural and nonprocedural pain than other burn patients but had a tendency to manifest fewer behavioral cues (Perry, Cella, Falkenberg, Heidrich, & Goodwin, 1987). This patient population was drawn from a sample of 134 adult patients in a broader analgesic study. Of the 104 subjects whose records were complete enough for review, 43 (41 percent) had untreated PTSD. If these patients do give fewer cues, these findings indicate that there may be a significant group of undermedicated patients unless careful assessments are done on all patients.

Burn patients have demonstrated more positive than negative adaptive behaviors during painful treatments (Klein & Charlton, 1980). Observations of positive adaptive behaviors included patient discussions of progress and future plans, statements of well-being or ability to manage pain, and compliance with instructions. Negative behaviors most often were reflected in statements of physical discomfort rather than signs and symptoms of psychological problems such as depression. There was no correlation between differences in frequency of positive and negative adaptive behaviors related to burn variables such as extent of burn, days since onset of injury, and site of burn (Klein & Charlton, 1980).

There is a great deal of disparity in research findings concerning nurse characteristics and their influences on assessment of patient pain. Some research findings in this area are noteworthy, however. Amnad, Perry, and Genovese (1982) found that nurses significantly underestimated the intensity of nonprocedural pain compared to their patients. In contrast, Walkenstein (1982) reported a positive correlation between the nurses' and patients' overall perceptions of pain, although she could find no significant correlation when procedural pain assessment was analyzed. It has been shown that new graduates, new burn nurses, associate and bachelor degree graduates, and nurses older than 30 years of age tend to overestimate the patient's procedural pain, whereas veteran nurses, diploma graduates, and nurses younger than 25 underestimated pain (Iafrati, 1986). Although the difference was not statistically significant, Walkenstein (1982) found that nurses licensed for three to five years assessed pain more accurately than nurses with less than two years of experience or those with more than six years of experience. Fagerhaugh (1974), on the other hand, did not find that length of stay in nursing or burn nursing affected pain perception or intervention. Perry and Heidrich (1982) did find a statistically significant overestimation of pain perception by staff members who had spent less time in burn care. They found no discrepancy between how physicians and nurses assess pain, however.

In summary, the research findings indicate that pain assessment principles are difficult to generalize in the burn patient population but that application of such principles to the individual patient is essential to effective pain management. Findings conflict about correlations between patients' and nurses' assessments of pain. It may well be that only the patient can serve as the true control for assessing pain. The use of pain flow charts may be the only reliable way to determine the effectiveness of management through continuous assessment and analysis. The validity and reliability of pain assessment scales are well established, but nurses and other health care team members must have the knowledge and confidence to treat pain on the basis of assessed data.

Future research is needed to establish pain-assessment parameters for noncommunicative patients. Physiological signs may be the only factor available, but such parameters need to be evaluated closely in light of the maximal physiological stress that the burn patient undergoes.

The incidence of routine documentation of pain assessments is not reported in the literature. Empirical evidence indicates that usually only verbal expressions of pain with occasional general comments mentioning restlessness are documented. What criteria nurses use to document assessments, and the thoroughness of the documentation, need to be described. If patients and nurses are reporting under-treatment of pain, then perhaps assessments are not adequate, especially as they relate to evaluation of pain therapy. Nurses must be patient advocates for appropriate pain therapy. They cannot fulfill this responsibility, however, without accurate assessments based on knowledge of the patient's response to therapies.

Planning for Intervention

There is no universally accepted treatment for the relief of pain and suffering (NIH, 1987), but five factors are essential to a plan of care for effective pain management:

- adequate assessment (already discussed),
- establishment of a therapeutic goal,
- knowledge of therapeutic modalities,
- documentation and communication of the plan, and
- evaluation of the plan.

Who is accountable for pain management? In determining the goal of therapy, the issue of accountability for pain management must be addressed. It is an integrated approach involving patient, family, physician, nurse, and allied health care professionals (NIH, 1987). It must be emphasized that each plan must be individualized on the basis of adequate assessment.

Nurses are able to predict which experiences will be painful. These are most commonly related to the following burn care procedures: debridement; dressing changes; occupational and physical therapy procedures such as ambulation, positioning, and immobilization of grafted limbs; care of donor sites; second-degree burns; regeneration of nervous tissue; underlying chronic discomfort without environmental stimuli; and emotional suffering (Heidrich, Perry, & Amnad, 1981). As previous discussion has indicated, correlations between nurses' and patients' perceptions of pain vary. Such discrepancies can lead to differences in goals and result in ineffective care plans.

Establishment of a Therapeutic Goal

Although the goal of total pain relief within safe parameters is verbalized by many, contemporary science cannot ensure the relief of all pain. This fact can, and does, lead to unclear goals for pain management in the critically burned patient.

Fagerhaugh (1974) undertook the study of pain expression and control with the premise that total relief of pain is not possible and, therefore, that patients must be helped to tolerate the pain. Pain was evaluated from an organizational-work-interactional perspective. The investigator believed that the primary aspects of management for both patients and staff are the endurance of pain and the controlling of pain expression. Several key assumptions were delineated that could affect the goal of therapy:

- The degree and duration of pain depend on the extent and location of the burn as well as other factors. (This assumption was not supported in other studies [Kibbee, 1984; Perry et al., 1981.])

- Expressions of pain such as crying out, moaning, and screaming are intolerable and devastating to patients and staff.

- Staff members must control their own responses to pain expression.

The investigator drew many interesting conclusions that could have a significant impact on determining the goal of therapy and thus interventions chosen to effect that goal:

- Staff give a high priority to technical competence, which prevents them from thinking about a patient's tragic future. Staff use pride in technical competencies and the reputation of the burn unit to control the patient's pain behavior.

- Patients with less severe and extensive burns feel that they have less right to complain.

- If staff neglect pain therapy, then patients feel that they have a right to complain.

Because the goal of therapy is the philosophical foundation for the plan of care, it must be clearly defined. Without a goal of total relief of pain, then such an outcome does not exist in the minds of the patients or the staff. If such a goal becomes the target, then adequate pain relief always becomes possible through effective cooperation between the critically ill patient and the critical care nurse in an environment conducive to achieving this mutual goal.

Knowledge of Therapeutic Modalities

The third step in planning for adequate pain control in the burn unit is selecting effective therapeutic modalities. This requires knowledge of the psychological and physiological changes in the three phases of burn care as well as how to implement the actual modalities.

The paradox of pain management in burn nursing is that nurses inflict pain and then must relieve it (Heidrich et al., 1981; Walkenstein, 1982).

The paradox causes conflicting emotions that often lead nurses to minimize the severity of the patient's pain or to become outwardly unresponsive to the patient while inflicting pain. As one nurse stated, "If it's for long periods, I sometimes get headaches or stomach cramps. If it's when I'm behind schedule or my assignment is very difficult, or I'm finishing off a long work stretch, I get angry or intolerant," (Heidrich et al., 1981; p. 261).

Some nurses believe that the unsatisfactory management of burn patients' pain is due to burn patients' being a difficult group of patients with many personality problems (Heidrich et al., 1981). They stated that they would use placebos to see "how much pain the patient is really having," (Heidrich et al., 1981, p. 260). Although misconceptions related to the use of placebos is documented, one may hope that such punitive use is waning with increased education.

There are several other major reasons for undertreatment of pain in burn patients (Kibbee, 1984). The most common reasons are fear of addiction to drugs, fear of respiratory depression, fear of nutritional consequences of constipation, and lack of knowledge of the pharmacology of pain medication. Although these factors have been studied and reported in the general literature as well as in the burn pain-management literature, health care providers continue to have such fears, and they are reflected in clinical pain management. No studies could be found that evaluated the effectiveness of continuing education about pain therapies in terms of changing or improving staff interventions for pain management.

Documentation and Communication of the Plan

Documentation and communication of the plan is the fourth factor to be considered when establishing a plan for pain management.

Such documentation and communication is often inadequate. This is inferred from the number of patients who complain about inadequate pain relief. No studies could be found in the literature that actually investigated the prevalence of a documented plan for pain management or what components of the nursing process most frequently are documented. The nursing diagnosis proposed by the North American Nursing Diagnosis Association for acute pain is unclear and not well researched. Burn pain is not addressed at all and should be investigated as a separate diagnosis because it has components of both acute and chronic pain syndromes (Merskey, 1986).

Evaluation of the Plan

Without adequate documentation and communication of the plan, evaluation cannot occur. This fifth and crucial component of the plan must be considered at the beginning of the planning process. Evaluation provides the feedback loop for the critical care nurse to reassess the patient and environment, in light of the observed responses to implemented therapies, and to determine whether the goal is being met.

Summary of Intervention Planning

There is clearly a need for individualized nursing care plans for acute pain management (NIH, 1987). Without adequate planning, consistent and effective pain management is not possible. Such planning is the foundation for the implementation and evaluation of this most crucial aspect of burn care.

Implementation of the Plan of Care

There are three phases of burn care, all requiring analgesia therapy as well as other pain-management techniques (Marvin, 1987). Throughout all three phases, two components of the burn pain experience are present: background or nonprocedural pain and procedural pain. Both these components must be addressed in each phase to achieve the goal of total pain relief. Both pharmacological and nonpharmacological pain relief measures must be considered.

Phase 1: The Resuscitation Plan

In this phase, pain is generally injury related (i.e., thermal and associated injuries), acute, and often severe at first (Marvin, 1987).

It is described as throbbing, stinging, and smarting and increases in intensity with movement or procedures (Merskey, 1986). Often this pain is continually present in some degree and is exacerbated by the application of antimicrobial topical creams.

Phase I lasts approximately 72 hours and is characterized by marked vascular instability and severe fluid shifts resulting in massive edema. Narcotic medication is universally used in this phase, but absorption of medication is unpredictable unless it is given intravenously. There are three methods for administering intravenous narcotics: intermittent bolus, fixed-rate continuous infusion, and continuous modified variable-dose infusion (Wolman, 1988). The most common narcotics used in this phase are meperidine and morphine. The choice of narcotic used should reflect planning according to deposition factors described in studies with burn patients. Meperidine (Demerol) has widely varying peaks of effects that do not gradually decline predictably in the burn patient (Goodfellow, Bloedow, Marvin, & Heimbach, 1981). Morphine also has been shown to be more rapidly eliminated in burn patients even though it has a rapid and extensive distribution (Inturrisi, Perry, & Genovese, 1982; Perry & Inturrisi, 1983).

Although drug administration by intermittent bolus allows for increasing titration to control for adverse effects such as respiratory depression or cardiac instability, this method results in unstable blood levels of the drug and increased nursing time. Boluses usually begin at the equivalent of approximately 5 mg of morphine and are increased until background pain relief is obtained or significant respiratory depression occurs. Any respiratory depression that will occur usually does so within seven minutes of intravenous administration (Jaffe, 1980).

Hypotension can be a significant consideration in this phase when evaluated in the context of the burn patient's altered capillary dynamics. If rapid adjustment of drug level becomes necessary as a result of overmedication, then naloxone can be used to control the side effects. The patient must be monitored closely after the administration of naloxone because of its short half-life compared to narcotics.

The fixed-rate continuous infusion method provides stable drug levels and consistent pain control with decreased nursing time. There is a delay in action onset and a risk of accumulation with resulting overdose as pain requirements change. Disadvantages of this method are negated with the use of a continuous variable-dose infusion, which allows the nurse to modify the dose of the infusion according to the patient's response (Wolman & Luterman, 1988).

A comparison study of continuous modified variable-dose infusion and intermittent boluses indicated that the continuous variable-dose infusion group required less morphine sulfate and fewer narcotic administrations per hour of hospitalization than the intermittent bolus group. Patients in both groups did receive supplemental intermittent boluses of narcotics, anxiolytics, and sedatives as needed. No significant differences were, noted in the total amount or number of administrations of anxiolytics between groups (Wolman & Luterman, 1988).

In a study of continuous methadone infusion in patients, results indicated good pain control in the resuscitative phase (Miller, Denson, Concilus, & Warden, 1988). These findings were predicated on patient perception of pain relief. If the patient was unable to respond because of mental status changes, then subjective assessments of pain relief were made by the medical and nursing staff. Caution must be exercised with methadone because of its extended half-life and the difficulty in rapidly reversing its adverse effects.

The important concepts in administering narcotics in the resuscitative phase are related to the dynamics of capillary changes, sustained control of background pain, and recognition of additional requirements related to procedural pain. Intermittent bolus administration of narcotics to control nonprocedural pain is ineffective and reinforces negative pain behavior.

The critical care nurse's thorough knowledge of the pharmacokinetic properties of the drug chosen is essential to the safe implementation of the pain-management plan in this phase. As nurses gain knowledge in drug dosages and pharmacokinetics, fears about addiction, drug tolerance, and respiratory depression will not interfere with the implementation of a well-planned pain-management program titrated to the patient's specific response.

Phase 2: The Acute Phase

This Phase Ranges from 72 hours after the burn in patients with extensive burn injuries until healing or closure of the burn wound. Pain-management modalities begun in this phase often are the initial pain therapies for burn patients with less than 20 percent burns (Marvin, 1987). In phase 2, capillary dynamics are stabilized and analgesic medications can be given safely by intravenous, intramuscular, or oral routes, depending on the size of the burn and stage of healing.

Intravenous narcotic medications continue to be used in this phase for pain control because of the numerous operative and treatment procedures required at this time. As healing begins, other methods of narcotic administration can be used effectively and in combination with other therapies. There are a number of side effects that can result from narcotic analgesia, but they can be minimized with careful planning. Although development of tolerance poses a minimal risk, it can occur. To decrease this problem, medication can be titrated for effect and then weaned as need decreases (Kibbee, 1984). Fear of constipation in patients who have an increased need for nutritional intake can be managed effectively by the use of stool softeners and bulk laxatives (Kibbee, 1984). The method chosen to administer the narcotic and careful assessment of the patient can reduce the risk of respiratory depression.

Procedural and nonprocedural pain remains a problem until all wounds are healed and may continue after wound healing as a result of physical therapy, scar maturation, and psychological manifestations. Procedural pain related to wound management is severe and usually produces extreme anxiety, which exacerbates the pain.

Control of anxiety is acknowledged to be important in pain relief, but treating anxiety with medications increases pain behavior and physical tolerance to analgesics (Halpern, 1974). In addition, sedation can decrease the patient's ability to cooperate with treatment regimens while masking the symptoms of inadequate pain control. It therefore becomes important, even in the early stages of burn care, for nurses to use some form of nonpharmacological antianxiety measures along with pharmacological measures to mediate pain relief.

Stress reduction is beneficial in dealing with acute burn pain management. In a study by Wernick, Jaremko, and Taylor (1981), patients and nurses were given training in procedures for developing patients' cognitive coping skills, cognitive restructuring, and application. The treated subjects showed improvement in terms of decreased unauthorized pain medication requests, physical and emotional self-ratings, control of pain during hydrotherapy and wound debridement, compliance with hospital routine, and decreased anxiety.

In a second study, a patient group trained in three treatment methods (relaxation; imagery, desensitization, and sensory information; and biofeedback) was compared with a control group (Kenner & Achterberg, 1983). Significant improvement on measures of subjective pain, state anxiety, and peripheral temperature was seen in the imagery and biofeedback groups. There were no differences among measurements of these variables in the control group. Measurements in the relaxation group were inconsistent.

It was demonstrated in another experimental study that patients who received a standardized debriefing about burn care and pain and a short training program in relaxation and imagery techniques had better pain control than patients who did not receive such interventions (Tobiasen, Hove, Mani, & Hiebert, 1984). One hundred percent of the experimental group stated that their coping strategies reduced their pain, compared to only 50 percent of the control group's perceptions of pain relief. In addition, the nurses perceived that the experimental group patients were more compliant with the treatment regimen than the control group.

Such nonpharmacological methods appear to be effective for both background pain and procedural pain, particularly when combined with pharmacological pain management. More definitive studies related to relaxation techniques are indicated. The following case study illustrates my personal use of such procedures.

John was a 25-year-old man who attempted suicide by turning on the gas oven in his apartment. When he awoke the next morning, he was dismayed to find that he had been unable to kill himself and automatically lit his morning cigarette. The apartment exploded, and John received partial-and full-thickness burns over 70 percent of his body. In the burn unit, his anxiety precluded effective pain relief. He cried and yelled continuously.

One night I attempted to use imagery and relaxation techniques to assist John. I had never attempted these techniques and was very busy, but I felt that the effort would be worth it if John could be helped to relax. I asked John to imagine that he was on a cloud floating peacefully over the countryside. In approximately 20 minutes, he was relaxed and quiet.

John remained comfortable for almost an hour, when he suddenly started screaming for me (apparently he was failing off his cloud). Despite this setback, imagery and relaxation remained useful techniques to assist John as long as he was guided to a peaceful place that was on the ground.

The question remains, How extensively are such techniques used by nurses in acute pain management? No studies could be found that describe the extent of use of such techniques or how to train nurses to use the techniques effectively. It may be a perception on the nurses' part that such methods are time consuming and produce inconsistent results or that they require extensive training to learn.

During phase 2 many procedures are carried out that can be extremely painful. In fact, procedural pain related to debridement is described by patients as being the most painful burn care experience (Perry et al., 1981). Perry and Heidrich (1982) surveyed 151 American burn units to determine how burn pain is assessed and managed during debridement. Table 22.1 indicates their findings related to analgesic preferences, dose, and administration route during debridement for adults.

Methods of controlling pain described in their study are still being evaluated. They include narcotics, nitrous oxide, ketamine, hypnosis, transcutaneous electrical nerve stimulation, variations in procedural techniques, and supportive psychotherapy and relaxation training. Many of these studies are being conducted by nurses as the primary investigators. Despite the volume of research, there continues to be no documented definitive analgesic method for burn pain management.

In more recent years investigators have explored the role of ß-endorphins and their relationship to pain management in burns. Goosen (1986) identified peaks and sudden elevations in ß-endorphin levels associated with specific clinical events. She was not able to show any significant relationships between ß-endorphin levels and the following variables: time interval after burn, burn severity, required analgesic dosage, or a combination of burn severity and the required analgesic dosage. In contrast, Osgood, Carr, Kazianis, & Kemp (1988) found that lowered plasma ß-endorphin levels were even lower in burned rats

Table 22.1. Analgesic Preference, Dose, and Administration Route during Debridement in Adults

Route	Analgesic	N	Dose (mg, mean ± standard deviation)	Range (mg)
Intramuscular (IM)	Morphine	50	10.7 ± 4.5	2– 35
Intravenous (IV)	Morphine	32	8.9 ± 5.4	2– 25
IM	Meperidine	37	75.7 ± 52.9	25–375
IV	Meperidine	8	70.5 ± 14.1	50–100
Oral	Codeine	30	63.0 ± 22.7	30–130
IM	Codeine	3		
Oral	Oxycodone	5		
IM	Alphaprodine	2		
IV	Alphaprodine	1		
Oral	Pentazocine	2		
Oral	Methadone	1		
	None	6		

Source: From "Management of Pain during Debridement: A Survey of U.S. Burn Units" by S. Perry and G. Heidrich, 1982, *Pain, 13,* 269. Copyright 1982 by Elsevier Science Publishers BV. Reprinted by permission.

two days after burn while the rats were receiving exogenous opioids. This finding was in agreement with their clinical findings. Although the data from the two studies appear to conflict, the possibility that narcotics may contribute to low plasma endorphin levels by competing with endorphin at μ receptor sites should continue to be explored carefully.

A new category of drugs, endorphin releasers, shows promise in the area of pain relief. One of these is Ceruletide, a synthetic decapeptide closely resembling cholecystokinin and gastrin. When this drug was administered intravenously over 30 minutes once or twice a day, powerful analgesia was obtained that lasted up to 12 hours (Dolecek et al., 1983). It was accompanied (after several days of administration) by a euphoric mood and persistent increased elevations of ß-endorphins in the blood.

Phase 3: The Rehabilitative Phase

This phase covers the period from closure of the wound to complete scar maturation (Marvin, 1987). It lasts approximately six to twelve months. Although this phase is rarely encountered by critical care nurses, it is helpful to understand the pain control issues that patients face to prepare them for the transition from acute burn care. Generally there are more behavioral manifestations of pain in this phase as patients begin to assimilate some of the life changes required as a result of their devastating injury.

Even after the burn wound has healed, pain can result from the return of nerve function. The return of nerve function can be accompanied by active vasodilation, vasoconstriction, and return of tactile sensation. The reflex neuronal function may be restored within five or six weeks of excision and grafting, or return may take up to six months in wounds healed by granulation and contracture or late grafting (Freund et al., 1981). It has been demonstrated that neuronal tissue can be trapped in the scar and cause pain in a wound that is completely healed (Ponten, 1960).

Scar tissue produced by an inflammatory process also may be painful because of persistent activity of tissue enzymes. As scar tissue matures, itching and pain with exercise occur. Itching in particular is a mentally and physiologically fatiguing symptom. When patients compared the effects of the three most commonly used medications to relieve the symptom of itching, hydroxyzine (Atarax) was perceived to be the most beneficial (Vitale & Luterman, 1988). The critical care nurse also will be required to assist patients with this annoying symptom when patients with extensive burns require grafting procedures

273

over a period of several weeks. In this situation wound or donor sites in various stages of healing are present in different areas of the body.

Pharmacological management of pain in the rehabilitative phase usually consists of acetaminophen and nonsteroidal anti-inflammatory agents. Antidepressants or mild analgesics may be useful.

During the rehabilitative phase the patient faces many psychological problems, with depression and anxiety frequently manifested (Marvin, 1987). Pain perception is exacerbated by these emotions and complicates the diagnosis and management of pain symptoms. Group therapy and other psychological modalities may be necessary to prevent the extensive development of pain behaviors that may develop into a chronic problem. Such therapies often begin in the acute phase, and the critical care nurse must be cognizant of the influences of depression and anxiety on pain management even in the early stages of care of patients with extensive burns.

As many clinicians have often stated, the only safe way to administer narcotic analgesia is to titrate the dose to the patient's response. In burn care, this axiom can be extended to all forms of pain therapy. The pain involved is usually severe, continuous at some level of intensity, and associated with several confounding psychological and cultural variables. It is not possible to assume that one particular protocol will benefit most patients in a particular phase of care. It is the critical care nurse who must continually assess the patient's responses and then mobilize the entire health care team to modify the plan of care.

Evaluating the Plan of Care

In evaluating the effectiveness of a pain-management plan for critically burned patients, several questions can be posed. First, is the patient satisfied with the level of pain management? If not, the nurse must assess the following:

- What does the pain mean to the patient? Is the goal of the caregiver the same as that of the patient?

- Is pain control ineffective for background pain? Procedural pain? Both? Is some other factor involved, such as an inflamed intravenous site or hidden injury?

- What is the balance between pharmacological and nonpharmacological pain relief modalities? Is the balance appropriate for the phase of burn care? Is anxiety a major factor, and is it being managed appropriately?

- How and when does the patient express pain? Does the pain correlate with inappropriate dosage intervals for the analgesic used? Is the dosage appropriate? What method of administration is used? Would a flow sheet be helpful to collate and analyze data (for example, to correlate symptoms with therapies and results)? What environmental factors may be affecting the patient?

- What does the patient think will control the pain better?

The nurse also must ascertain whether there are physiological side effects with the current medication plan. If so, he or she must reassess the type and method of delivery of analgesic and then weigh the benefits of the current analgesic therapy against the risks of side effects.

There is an obvious need to continue studies and to explore combinations of therapies for both procedural and background burn pain. Both physicians and nurses must examine their attitudes toward pain management and work collaboratively to develop safe and effective approaches to pain management in the critical care environment. Old myths and misconceptions must be replaced by personal accountability for continued education related to pharmacological and nonpharmacological pain therapy advances.

Much more patient, nursing, and physician education is needed to maintain sensitivity and to promote greater use of the full spectrum of pain-control modalities that have already been studied and found effective. The patient and family must be actively involved in the implementation of the plan of care through honest feedback as to the effects of medication and control of the medication dosage and by participating in nonpharmacological methods to reduce pain.

As Heidrich and colleagues (1981) write, burn pain is "not a single entity but a kaleidoscopic experience, a series of discrete severely painful procedures punctuating the day and night and superimposed upon an underlying pervasive physical and psychologic discomfort," (p. 260). Nurses are at the bedside 24 hours a day; therefore, they must take the initiative to evaluate and ensure the adequacy of burn pain management. They are the only health care providers available continuously to evaluate the plan. The following guideline summarizes the responsibilities of the nurse regarding pain management:

P—place the patient in as much control as possible
A—assess and analyze continuously the response to pain therapy
I—individualize the approach to pain control for each patient
N—never give up.

References

Amnad, R., Perry, S., & Genovese, V. (1982). Non-procedural pain as perceived by burn patient and nurse. *Proceedings of the American Burn Association,* 14, 64.

Charlton, J.E., Klein, R., & Gagliardi, G. (1981, September). *Assessment of pain relief in patients with burn.* Paper presented at the third World Congress on Pain at the International Association for the Study of Pain, Edinburgh, Scotland.

Davidson, S.P., & Noyes, R. (1973). Psychiatric nursing consultation on a burn unit. *American Journal of Nursing,* 73, 1715-1718.

Dolecek, R., Jezek, M., Adamkovi, M., Polivka, P., Kubis, M., Sajnar, J., Doleckovi, D., Kurkcova, J., & Zavada, M. (1983). Endorphin releasers: A new possible approach to the treatment of pain after burns—A preliminary report. *Burns,* 10, 41-44.

Ehleben, C., & Still, J. (1985). Psychological morbidity and pain. *Proceedings of the American Burn Association,* 17. (Abstract 104).

Fagerhaugh, S. (1974). Pain expression and control on a burn care unit. *Nursing Outlook,* 22, 645-650.

Freund, P.R., Brengelmann, G. L., Rowell, L.B., (1981). Vasomotor control in healed grafted skin in humans. *Journal of Applied Physiology,* 51, 168-171.

Goodfellow, L.C., Bloedow, D., Marvin, J., & Heimbach, D. (1981). Meperidine disposition following burn trauma. *Proceedings of the American Burn Association,* 13, 66.

Goosen, G. (1986). ß-Endorphin levels in burned patients. *Proceedings of the American Burn Association,* 18. (Abstract 127).

Halpern, L. (1974). Treating pain with drugs. *Minnesota Medicine,* 57, 176-184.

Heidrich, G., Perry, S., & Amnad, R. (1981). Nursing staff attitudes about burn pain. *Journal of Burn Care and Rehabilitation,* 2, 259-261.

Iafrati, N. (1986). Pain on the burn unit: Patient vs nurse perceptions. *Journal of Burn Care and Rehabilitation,* 7, 413-416.

Inturrisi, C., Perry, S., & Genovese, V. (1982). Morphine: Pharmacokinetics and pain relief in burn patients. *Proceedings of the American Burn Association*, 14, 45.

Jaffe, J.H. (1980). Drug addiction and drug abuse. In A.G. Goodman, L.S. Goodman, & A. Gilman (Eds.), *The pharmacological basis of therapeutics,* (6th ed., pp. 535-584). New York: Macmillan.

Kenner, C., & Achterberg, J. (1983). Non-pharmaceutical pain relief for burn patients. *Proceedings of the American Burn Association,* 15, 100.

Kibbee, E. (1984). Burn pain management. *Critical Care Quarterly,* 7, 54-62.

Klein, R., & Charlton, J.E. (1980). Behavioral observation and analysis of pain behavior in critically burned patients. *Pain,* 9, 27-40.

Loeser, J. (1987). Conceptual framework for pain management. *Journal of burn Care and Rehabilitation,* 8, 309-312.

Marvin, J. (1987). Pain management. *Topics in Acute Care Trauma Rehabilitation,* 1, 15-24.

McCaffery, M. (1979). *Nursing management of the patient with pain,* (2nd ed.). Philadelphia: Lippincott.

Merskey, D.M. (Ed.). (1986). Classification of chronic pain: Descriptions of chronic pain syndromes and definitions of pain terms. *Pain,* 3, s43-s44.

Miller, A., Denson, D., Concilus, R., & Warden, G. (1988). Continuous infusion of methadone in severely burned patients. *Proceedings of the American Burn Association,* 20. (Abstract 149).

Murray, J. (1972). The history of analgesia in burns. *Postgraduate Medical Journal,* 48, 124-127.

National Institutes of Health Consensus Development Conference. (1987). The integrated approach to the management of pain. *Journal of Pain and Symptom Management,* 2, 35-44.

Noyes, R., Andreasen, N.J.C., & Hartford, C.E. (1987). The psychological reaction to severe burns. *Psychosomatics,* 12, 416-442.

Osgood, P., Carr, D., Kazianis, A., & Kemp, J. (1988). Exogenous opioid analgesics may suppress ß-endorphin release in the normal and burned rat. *Proceedings of the American Burn Association*, 20.

Perry, S., Cella, D., Falkenberg, J., Heidrich, G., & Goodwin, C. (1987). Pain perception in burn patients with stress disorders. *Journal of Pain and Symptom Management*, 2, 29-33.

Perry, S., & Heidrich, G. (1982). Management of pain during debridement: A survey of U.S. burn units. *Pain*, 13, 267-280.

Perry, S., Heidrich, G., & Ramos, E. (1981). Assessment of pain by burn patients. *Journal of Burn Care and Rehabilitation*, 2, 322-326.

Perry, S., & Intunisi, C. (1983). Analgesia and morphine disposition in burn patients. *Journal Of Burn Care and Rehabilitation*, 4, 276-279.

Ponten, B. (1960). Grafted skin: Observation on innervation and other qualities. *Acta Chirurgica Scandinavica* 257(Suppl.), 1-178.

Tobiasen, J., Hove, G., Mani, M., & Hiebert, J. (1984). Coping with pain: Training strategies for the burn-injured patient. *Proceedings of the American Burn Association*, 16, 38.

Vitale, M., & Luterman, A. (1988). Severe itching and the burn patient. Proceedings of the *American Burn Association*, 20. (Abstract 46).

Walkenstein, M. (1982). Comparison of burned patients' perception of pain with nurses' perception of patients' pain. *Journal of Burn Care and Rehabilitation*, 3, 233-236.

Wernick, R., Jaremko, M., & Taylor, P. (1981). Pain management in severely burned adults: A test of stress inoculation. *Journal of Behavioral Medicine*, 4, 103-109.

Wolman, R. (1988, March). *Concepts*. Paper presented at the 20th annual meeting of the American Burn Association, Seattle, WA.

Wolman, R., & Luterman, A. (1988). The continuous infusion of morphine sulfate for analgesia in burn patients: Extending the use of an established technique. *Proceedings of the American Burn Association*, 20. (Abstract 150).

— by K.A. Puntillo (Ed.) and Nancy C. Molter

Chapter 23

Topical Agents in Burn and Wound Care

Abstract

With any open wound, infection may occur. Many factors such as age and general health status may increase the likelihood of infection, but the size and depth of the wound are critical factors in determining the chronicity of any wound. Infection greatly adds to the morbidity associated with open wounds. An infected wound not only heals more slowly, there is also the risk of systemic infection and even death. Infected wounds also scar more severely and are associated with more prolonged rehabilitation. Topical therapeutic agents have been shown to be effective in the management of open skin wounds. These agents may assist less complicated healing and decrease the conversion of a partial-thickness injury to a full-thickness injury, and thereby reduce wound related morbidity. Common topical agents with suggestions for application are discussed in this review. [Ward RS, Saffle JR. Topical agents in burn and wound care. *Phys Ther*. 1995; 75:526-538.]

Introduction

Physical therapists are often involved with direct treatment of open wounds, including the application of topical agents and dressings. The severity of a wound, its location, and its depth and size can affect

279

healing time and generate problems of pain, malaise, and disability. Knowledge of the status of a wound, and its effect on the patient, is useful in making decisions about the application of appropriate topical agents.[1(pp.145-146)].

Wound treatment protocols vary, and competent wound care requires an understanding of the rationale for numerous treatment techniques that include the application of topical agents. Such treatments often use fixed protocols. The purpose of this chapter is to provide information on which sound judgment can be rendered in the selection of topical agents in the care of burns and other skin wounds.

Wound Assessment

Depth

Wounds are often described in terms of depth of injury. Burns and some other skin traumas, for example, are classified as superficial (first degree), partial-thickness (second degree), or full-thickness (third degree) injuries.[2] Superficial injury involves the epidermis, and such wounds are erythematous and mildly painful.[3] Partial-thickness injury involves some degree of damage to the dermis and may be further classified as superficial partial-thickness or deep partial-thickness injury.[3] Superficial partial-thickness injury, which disrupts the epidermis and the superficial portion of the dermis, is manifested as painful, red, blistered, and moist when the blisters are broken, whereas deep partial-thickness injury involves deeper layers of the dermis and can present as pale or red wounds that can also be painful or relatively anesthetic.[3] Full-thickness injury involves destruction of the entire dermis, which results in a relatively painless wound with a leathery, dry, and often tan or brown texture and appearance.[3]

Depth of injury for skin or pressure ulcers is commonly described by using a staging system.[4] A stage 1 ulcer (or nonblanching erythema) is characterized by red, unbroken skin in which the erythema at the site does not fade with elimination of pressure. A stage II ulcer exhibits disrupted epidermis, often with some invasion into the dermis. Stage III ulcers demonstrate dermal injury. Stage IV ulcers include exposed subcutaneous tissue and may penetrate even deeper.

Size

Burn wounds, and other large wounds, are described according to percentage of body surface area involvement.[5] Smaller wounds, such as pressure ulcers, are characterized by measurements that often include the circumference or the distances between the borders of the wound.[4,6] The size of the wound is important partly because, in general, large wounds are at greater risk for infection than smaller wounds. Some topical agents should not be used for extended periods of time over large open wounds because of the risk of toxicity secondary to systemic absorption. [7(pp. 1165-1166)].

Location

Because skin responds to injury by contracting, wounds that are located over joints may lead to limitation of movement and eventual contracture. Topical agents, and a dressing that is minimally restrictive, can be important in allowing motion. Many topical agents also are not recommended for the face because of concerns that the agent may enter the eye or be unintentionally ingested.

Reassessment of the Wound

Documentation of the depth and size of injury is important in measuring the progress of wound healing. Depth, size, and location of injury will also help in making a determination of an appropriate topical agent. Wound evaluation is necessary to make decisions about the efficacy of, or the potential for modifying the choice of, a topical agent. If the chosen topical agent does not appear to be successful, another topical agent may be substituted. Table 23.1 outlines conditions related to wound care that should invite medical consultation.

Common Infections

Common bacterial skin infections include gram-positive bacteria (eg, *Streptococcus, Staphylococcus aureus*) and gram-negative bacteria (eg, *Pseudomonas aeruginosa*).[12] *Candida* is a common source of fungal infections in skin wounds.[13] Because the stratum corneum is normally too dry to support microbial growth, infections on the skin rarely occur unless the skin is broken. Topical wound therapy provides treatment against severe infection, and, if infection does occur, another topical agent should be selected. A wound that appears to be regressing (Table 23.1) should be cultured. The infecting agent should be identified, and the wound should be treated with debridement and application of an appropriate topical agent and dressing.

Table 23.1. Circumstances That Should Involve Medical Consultation

Suitable treatment has been unsuccessful (delayed wound closure, infection)

Signs of widespread infection or inflammation (redness, warmth, pain, swelling, fever, malaise) are present (particularly outside the borders of the wound)

The condition of the wound appears to be worsening (signs of infection, increased size or depth)

A predisposing trauma or illness or symptoms of an illness exist that have not been treated or followed by a physician

The lesions cover a large surface area and/or are deep

Large-area wounds have been treated with certain topical chemical agent for several days

There is uncertainty as to what is the organism infecting the wound

The manifestation of symptoms that may indicate systemic infection (eg, malaise, fever)

Techniques of Wound Care

Antiseptics

The use, or misuse, of antiseptics that are used to cleanse and prepare wounds for application of a topical agent should be recognized. Antiseptics are used to reduce bacterial contamination by inhibiting the growth of microorganisms, and antiseptics should be applied to intact skin and not used directly on wounds as topical agents.[14] Antiseptics may increase the intensity and duration of inflammation,[15,16] and they have also been shown to be toxic to human keratinocytes[17] and fibroblasts[18,19] and to retard epithelialization.[20]

Iodine solutions and iodophors are often used as antiseptics. Diluted iodine solutions (iodine solution *USP* [*United States Pharmacopeia*] [2 percent iodine, 2.5 percent sodium iodide] and iodine tincture *USP* [2 percent iodine, 2.5 percent sodium iodide, 50 percent alcohol]), though bactericidal, may irritate tissue, stain the skin, and cause sensitization. [21(p781)] Iodine solutions have a broad spectrum and rapid germicidal action. Iodophors (such as povidone-iodine), which are compounds of iodine and carriers or solubilizing agents, are not as problematic as other iodine solutions with regard to irritation, skin staining, and sensitization.[20] As germicidal agents, however, iodophors are not as effective as the sodium-iodine solutions.[22,23.]

Hydrogen peroxide is very commonly used as an antiseptic on wounds; however, it has limited bactericidal effectiveness,[20,24] is toxic to fibroblasts[20] and impairs the microcirculation of wounds.[17] The mechanical cleansing effect of hydrogen peroxide, often attributed to the "fizzing" (which is caused by its decomposition to oxygen and water when it comes in contact with blood and tissue fluids), is questionable. Given the concerns about the detrimental effects of hydrogen peroxide on tissue at the wound site, it is not recommended as an antiseptic.[14]

Wound Dressings

Wounds require periodic washing, debridement, and observation. Because the effectiveness of topical agents is time limited[25(PP137-139)] these agents must be reapplied to enhance their therapeutic effects. Washing the wound and reapplying the topical agent before there is an infection will reduce the risk of infection. After it has been thoroughly cleansed to remove any loose eschar or debris as well as old topical medications, (Figure 23.1 to 23.8) the wound should be dried to afford better adherence before topical agents are applied to the wound surface. Topical antibiotics are applied to the wound site to the appropriate thickness and covered with a dressing. The dressing is applied to prevent removal of the topical agent by contact with objects and to maintain a moist wound environment. The comfortable, moist covering for the wound afforded by topical agents will increase patient acceptance of the dressing application, and the moist environment may also enhance wound healing and decrease the stiffness frequently associated with dry wounds.

A discussion of all of the dressings that are currently available to help with wound care is beyond the scope of this chapter. Nevertheless, the proper combination of topical agents with either biologic or synthetic wound coverings can decrease the likelihood of infection and enhance wound healing.

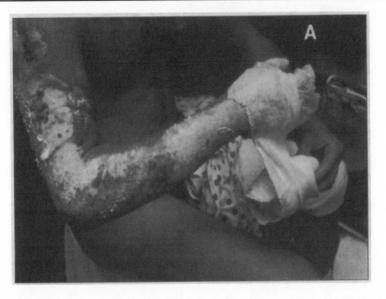

Figure 23.1. *Dressing change with silver sulfadiazine. (A) Patient with deep partial-thickness and full-thickness burns to the right arm, shoulder, and back removing dressings in preparation for washing.*

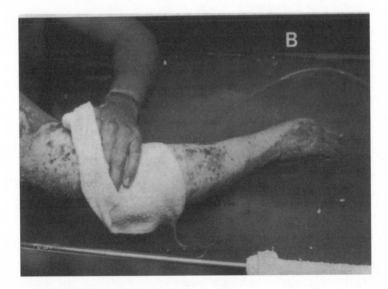

Figure 23.2. *(B) Patient washes the wounds in the hydrotherapy tank to remove old cream and to perform gentle debridement.*

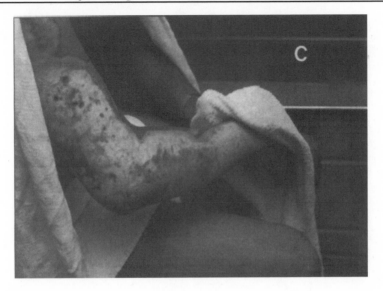

Figure 23.3. (C) The wounds are gently dried with a clean towel.

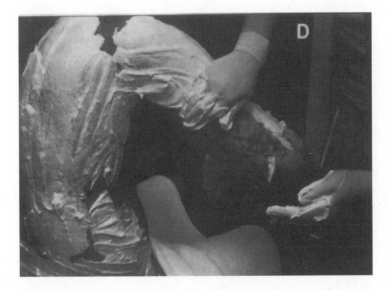

Figure 23.4. Silver sulfadiazine is applied with a gloved hand.

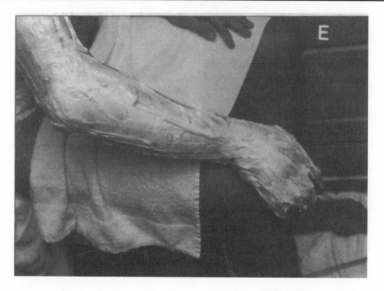

Figure 23.5. *(E) A consistent layer of silver sulfadiazine is placed over the entire wound; the cream is applied thickly enough that the wound cannot be visualized through it.*

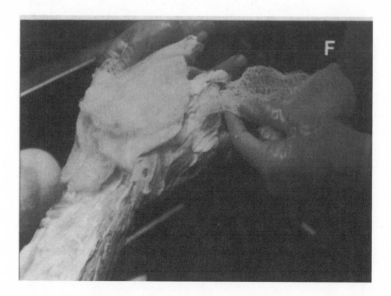

Figure 25.6. *(F) Dry gauze is applied over the silver sulfadiazine.*

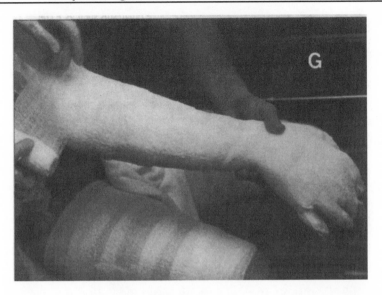

Figure 25.7. (G) The dressing is applied proximal to distal on the extremity.

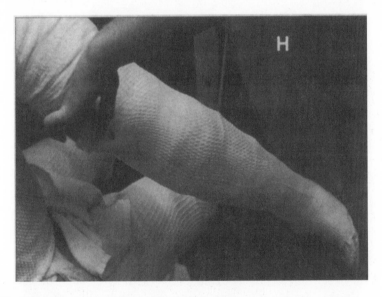

Figure 25.8. (H) The gauze is held in place with elastic netting.

(Figures 25.1-25.8 reproduced with permission from Saffle JR, Schnebly WA. Burn wound care. In: Richard RL, Staley MJ, eds. Burn Care and Rehabilitation: Principles and Practice. Philadelphia, Pa: FA Davis Co; 1994.137-139, 174.)

Topical Agents

The term "topical agent" implies the use of an antimicrobial applied to the surface of the wound. The importance of a topical application is particularly apparent in ischemic wounds, in which dependable dispatch of a systemic (ie, bloodstream) antimicrobial to the damaged tissue cannot be assured.[25(PP137-139)] Further, the loss of the stratum corneum decreases the resistance of percutaneous absorption of the chemical agents.

The following section provides information on currently used topical agents, but is not exhaustive. A list of the topical agents is provided in Table 23.2.

Table 23.2. Common Topical Agents Used in Wound Care.

Type of Topical Agent	Proprietary or Nonproprietary Name
Ointments	Bacitracin
	Polymyxin B sulfate
	Neomycin
	Polysporin
	Neosporin
	Povidone-iodine 10% ointment[a]
Creams	Silver sulfadiazine 1% cream[a]
	Mafenide acetate 0.5% cream[a]
	Nystatin[a]
	Nitrofurazone 0.2% compound[a]
	Gentamicin 0.1% cream[a]
Solutions	Acetic acid 0.5% solution
	Sodium hypochlorite (Dakin's) solution
	Silver nitrate 0.5% solution[a]
	Chlorhexidine gluconate 0.05% solution

[a]Physician's prescription required.

Ointments

Techniques/Indications for Use.

Ointments are water-in-oil preparations in which the amount of oil exceeds the amount of water in the emulsion.[26] The ointment base of these topical agents is comfortable and soothing, and although these agents can be used successfully on both partial-and full-thickness wounds, they are most commonly applied on partial-thickness injuries. Ointments are typically more occlusive and lubricating than other preparations. Ointments should be applied just thickly enough to cover the wound and to keep the wound moist. A petrolatum gauze is often placed over the ointment-covered wound. The dressing should be changed routinely, because the antibacterial action of the ointments will last for only approximately twelve hours. In addition, the ointments eventually dry and the dressings will then stick to the wound, leading to pain and damage of cells with removal. Because of the lubricating properties of ointments, they may be useful as topical agents for wounds such as exposed tendons.

Though some hypersensitivity reactions (eg, itching, rashes, swelling) have been reported, these incidents are uncommon and mainly occur over areas of normal skin exposed to the agent for an extended period.

Bacitracin. Bacitracin is a polypeptide antibiotic that is generally available in a white petrolatum base (ointment). This ointment is effective against gram-positive cocci and bacilli. The mechanism of action for bacitracin is inhibition of cell-wall synthesis.[21(p779)] The development of bacitracin-resistant organisms is rare. Bacitracin promotes wound healing indirectly by controlling the level of infection on a wound surface. Bacitracin may also enhance reepithelialization of the wound,[27,28] although bacitracin has been shown either to have no affect on keratinocyte proliferation or to slightly decrease it in vitro.[29] The uncommon incidence of resistant strains is unlikely to increase, because bacitracin acts on the properties of the bacterial plasma membrane and not on molecular synthesis.[30] Bacitracin augments the antimicrobial action of polymorphonuclear leukocytes (PMNs).[31] Although this antimicrobial action may act to enhance the bactericidal properties of bacitracin, the significance of this to wound healing is not fully understood. Bacitracin has been shown to be safe for topical application in infants and children, as well as adults, with rare occurrence of hypersensitivity reactions (itching, swelling, anaphylaxis), and is unlikely to result in contact dermatitis.[32] A recent survey of burn centers showed that bacitracin was used in 43 percent of these facilities.[33] When topically applied, the absorption of bacitracin is minimal and systemic toxicity is unusual. Topical nonprescription bacitracin has a concentration of 400 U/g to 500 U/g of ointment. Bacitracin is typically applied one to three times daily. In burn and wound care, bacitracin is often used on superficial partial-thickness wounds and burns to the face.

Polymyxin B sulfate. Polymyxin B is a simple, basic peptide antibiotic that is generally available in an ointment base (white petrolatum). This ointment is effective against gram-negative organisms such as *Enterobacter* and *Escherichia coli* and may mildly inhibit most strains of *P aeruginosa*.[34] Interaction of polymyxin B with phospholipids allows penetration and disruption of bacterial cell walls and therefore affects membrane permeability. The phospholipid content of certain bacterial cell walls may preclude entrance of the drug.[35] The formation of polymyxin B-resistant organisms is infrequent. As with bacitracin, polymyxin B encourages healing by containing surface bacteria. Polymyxin B caused a greater reduction of keratinocyte proliferation in vitro than does bacitracin.[29] According to Hansbrough et al,[31] polymyxin B inhibited the ability of PMNs to destroy ingested microorganisms, which may suppress the ability of the wound to restrain bacterial proliferation. Hypersensitivity reactions (itching, swelling, anaphylaxis) occur infrequently with topical application. The absorption of topically applied polymyxin B is negligible, and systemic toxicity is rare and is often related to use over a large area for an extended period of time. Combinations of either 5,000 U/g or 10,000 U/g of ointment are available in nonprescription form. This ointment is generally applied one to three times per day to superficial partial-thickness injuries and to burns of the face.

Neomycin. Neomycin is available in an ointment base for topical application. This broad-spectrum antibiotic is particularly effective against gram-negative organisms such as *E coli*, *Enterobacter*, and *Klebsiella pneumoniae*, but may also inhibit gram-positive organisms such as S *aureus*.[7(PP1165-1166)] The bactericidal activity appears to result from the inhibition of protein synthesis of bacteria by binding to a ribosomal subunit.[7(PP1152-1153)] Resistant organisms are more common with neomycin than with polymyxin B or bacitracin. Neomycin influences wound healing by controlling the proliferation of bacteria on the wound surface. It appears that neomycin has no negative affect on keratinocyte proliferation in vitro,[29] but it has demonstrated inhibitory action on PMNs.[31] Hypersensitivity reactions, particularly skin rashes, also occur more frequently with neomycin (occurring in 5 percent,-8 percent of patients) than with bacitracin or polymyxin B.[7(pp1165-1166),32] Ototoxicity and nephrotoxicity have been reported following application to large area wounds.[7pp1165-1166)] The common concentration is 3.5 mg of neomycin per gram of ointment. Neomycin may also be prepared in a cream. This ointment is generally applied one to three times per day to superficial partial-thickness wounds.

Polysporin or Neosporin. Polysporin is a combination of polymyxin B sul- fate and bacitracin in an ointment base. Neosporin is a blend of neomycin, bacitracin, and polymyxin B sulfate, also in an ointment. The combination of these agents produces no untoward interactions, side effects, or hypersensitivities different than those mentioned for the individual drugs. The combination, however, has advantages and disadvantages. For example, hypersensitivity may be more common with the use of Neosporin than Polysporin because of the presence of neomycin in the ointment. Although the mixtures of antimicrobials in these ointments may be used to provide a broader spectrum antibiotic, no data exist that establish the superiority of the combination of ointments over any of the individual agents discussed previously.

Povidone-iodine. The ointment form of povidone-iodine can be used as a topical agent. The bactericidal spectrum of povidone-iodine includes gram-positive and gram-negative bacteria in vitro, *Candida*, and fungi. The mechanism of action appears to relate to the capability of iodine to oxidize microbial protoplasm. Information about the development of resistant organisms could not be found. Povidone-iodine fosters healing by restricting the number of infective organisms on a wound. The value of the antimicrobial effects of this topical agent must be weighed against reports of delayed wound healing.[36,37] Povidone-iodine at clinical concentrations has been shown to be toxic to human fibroblasts and keratinocytes in vitro.[38,39] Polymorphonuclear leukocytes are inhibited by this topical agent.[31] Povidone-iodine is not a commonly utilized topical agent for burn care in the United States.[33] Contact dermatitis has been reported with prolonged exposure of the ointment to uninjured skin,[40] and metabolic acidosis has also been described with extended exposure to this topical agent,[8-10] although these reports do not establish povidone-iodine as the absolute cause of the acidosis.[41] Povidone-iodine has also been reported to be inactivated by wound exudate.[42,43] This topical agent may "harden" wound eschar rather than soften it, thus increasing the difficulty, and discomfort of wound debridement. This topical agent should not be applied during pregnancy, or on a newborn, on small children, or on patients with suspected or known thyroid disease.[41] Povidone-iodine ointment should be applied once or twice daily. The ointment may also temporarily stain skin or linens. Povidone-iodine may be best suited, but may not be the first choice, for use on full-thickness tissue injuries.

Creams

Techniques/Indications for use. An assortment of antibacterial agents are available in cream bases. Creams are oil-in-water emulsions in which the amount of water exceeds the amount of oil, and the term "creams" is most commonly used for water-miscible products.[44(p2839),45] Each of the agents is potent and useful for the appropriate wound and infective organisms. Creams are usually easy to apply, are often soothing to the patient, and are useful on varying depths of wound (Figure 23.2). Following removal of old dressings, creams from previous treatments are washed off and the wound is lightly debrided. The cream is then applied to the gently dried wound. A cream should be applied so that the wound cannot be visualized through it.[25(137-139)] A dry gauze wrap should then be placed over the treated wound. Regular dressing changes are encouraged to avoid the drying of the topical agent and because the creams are effective against organisms for only eight to twelve hours. The following topical agents are commonly available in cream form.

Silver sulfadiazine 1 percent cream. Silver sulfadiazine is a topical sulfonamide compound of silver nitrate and sodium sulfadiazine introduced by Fox[46], and prepared in a 1 percent water miscible cream. Silver sulfadiazine is effective against a wide range of flora, particularly gram-negative bacteria (eg, *E coli, Enterobacter; Klebsiella* species, *P aeruginosa*), but including gram-positive bacteria (eg, *S aureus*) and *Candida albicans*.[42,47] The formation of resistant organisms and superinfection to silver sulfadiazine is rare.[42] Superinfection occurs when a new organism, which is resistant to the current treatment, infects the wound. Bactericidal effects are likely due to modification of the cell membrane and alteration of the cell wall. This topical agent promotes wound healing because of its bactericidal properties. There is evidence that silver sulfadiazine is toxic to human

keratinocytes and fibroblasts in vitro.[39,48,49] The rate of reepithial-
ization in a porcine wound model, however, was enhanced when the
wound was treated with silver sulfadiazine.[28,50] Silver sulfadiazine also
appears to inhibit the effect of PMNs in killing microorganisms as well
as local lymphocyte function,[31,51] although whether this has an influence on wound healing is yet unknown.

Silver sulfadiazine is currently the most extensively used topical
agent for burn care in the United States.[33] Although transient leukopenia has been reported after the first few days of use,[52-54] the leukopenia is typically not severe,[52] remits even with continued use of the
drug,[52] occurs in only 5 percent to 15 percent of patients,[53] and is not
correlated with septic episodes.[47,54] Allergies to the sulfa in the cream
are unusual, and very mild cutaneous sensitivity (typically a rash)
occurs in less than 5 percent of patients and seldom requires discon-
tinuance of topical therapy.[42] Because of the possibility of kernicterus
(associated with sulfonamide therapy), silver sulfadiazine should be
avoided during pregnancy, on premature infants, or on infants younger
than two months of age.[55] The cream itself causes no pain. This cream
is easy to apply, comfortable and soothing for patients, and is readily
removed with washing. Though the silver may oxidize to a gray color,
this cream does not stain skin or linen. Silver sulfadiazine should be
applied one to two times daily. This agent is indicated for use with
deep partial-thickness and full-thickness injuries. Its use on superficial partial-thickness injuries may be indicated if the wound is large
and the patient is at risk for systemic sepsis or for comfort and ease
of dressing a smaller wound. Some retardation of healing time is likely
to be expected.

Mafenide acetate 0.5 percent cream (Sulfamylon). Mafenide
acetate 0.5 percent cream (mafenide) is a methylated topical sulfonamide compound. Mafenide was introduced prior to silver sulfadiazine and was widely used for the treatment of burns.[56] Until silver
sulfadiazine was marketed, mafenide was the most widely used topical agent for burns. This drug has a wide range of antibacterial activity against most gram-negative and gram-positive pathogens (its
activity may be limited against some *S aureus*).[42-57] The formation of
resistant organisms is rare, but superinfection with *Candida* may
occasionally develop.[58] The mechanism of mafenide is not fully understood. Mafenide assists with wound healing by providing control of
superficial infection. This topical agent has been shown to inhibit
human keratinocytes and fibroblasts in vitro.[39,48,49] McCauley et al[59]
suggest that the use of mafenide may be more inhibitory to

293

reepithelialization than silver sulfadiazine. Mafenide suppresses PMN and lymphocyte activity.[31,51]

Although mafenide is available in many burn centers in the United States, it is used with much less frequency than silver sulfadiazine.[33] The drug is readily absorbed into the eschar and may therefore be a useful alternative to silver sulfadiazine for an invasive wound infection.[42] The chance of sulfa allergy is higher with mafenide acetate than it is with silver sulfadiazine. Rashes may be seen in about 50 percent of patients receiving mafenide treatment.[42] In addition, secondary tachypnea and hyperventilation may result as a consequence of a drug-induced metabolic acidosis (secondary to inhibition of carbonic anhydrase).[60] Metabolic acidosis induces the respiratory compensation, and elevated minute ventilation has been reported to extend to 50 L/min.[42] When mafenide is being used, respiratory status, blood gases, and pH levels should be monitored regularly. Moncrief[11] reported that toxicity may increase in correlation with the duration of treatment and size of area treated. The drug is considerably painful upon application.[61] Because of the risk of toxicity and the associated pain, the agent is indicated for full-thickness tissue injury, either on small wounds or for as short a time as possible on large wounds. Further, the topical agent should not be applied more often than every twelve hours because of the absorption of the drug.

Mafenide acetate may also be made into a solution from powder (5 percent concentration) for use in "wet-to-moist" dressings. Its bactericidal activity is comparable to that of the mafenide cream and causes less pain on application.[11,57,62] The risk of toxicity-related acidosis may also be decreased with the use of the 5 percent mafenide solution.[62]

Nystatin. Nystatin is an effective fungicide against *Candida*. *Candida albicans* develops little resistance to the drug, but other strains of *Candida* may develop resistance.[63] Increased cell-wall permeability is thought to be the mechanism for nystatin's fungicidal action. If a fungal infection is present on the wound surface, nystatin may aid healing by containing the contagion. No reports could be found describing the effect of nystatin on human keratinocytes or fibroblasts. Dermal hypersensitivity reactions are rare even with extended use, and the cream does not stain skin or linen. Nystatin cream should be applied one to three times each day on wounds with fungal invasion.

Though often used in cream form, nystatin is also available as ointment. Nystatin can also be mixed into solution from its powder form for use in "wet-to-moist" dressings. It may also seem reasonable to combine nystatin in solution with other agents such as bacitracin, polymyxin B sulfate, neomycin, or mafenide acetate to increase the spectrum of activity of the solution. Though reasonably intimated, mixtures may not guarantee an increase in antibacterial efficacy. Kucan and Smoot[63] reported that adding nystatin powder (5,000,000 U/L) to 5 percent mafenide solution did not adequately control fungal growth in studied burn wounds. Any of these solutions must be prescribed by a physician and mixed by a pharmacist.

Nitrofurazone 0.2 percent Compound. Nitrofurazone displays a broad antibacterial spectrum, including being effective against *S aureus*, *Enterobacter*, and *E coli*, but it is less effective against *P aeruginosa* than silver sulfadiazine or mafenide acetate and has no significant fungicidal activity. The formation of resistant organisms is rare, but bacteria may develop a mild resistance with prolonged use. The mechanism of action appears to be by inhibition of bacterial enzymes. Wound healing is likely augmented by the control of surface infection. Nitrofurazone has been shown to have a detrimental effect on the growth and migration of keratinocytes in culture.[39] Nitrofurazone is not frequently used in burn centers in the United States.[33] The cream causes no pain following application. The development of usual symptoms of contact dermatitis (rash, local edema, and pruritus), though rare, have been reported. This topical agent should be applied once daily and is indicated more for use on full-thickness injuries.

Nitrofurazone may also be mixed in solution for application with "wet-to-dry" dressings. Information about the bactericidal effects, wound healing, and hypersensitivity reactions of the cream applies equally to the solution.

Gentamicin 0.1 percent cream. This drug is very effective against gram-negative organisms such as *Enterobacter*, *Klebsiella*, and *P aeruginosa*.[7(pp1161-1163)] The mechanism of action of this agent appears to be inhibition of protein synthesis and messenger ribonucleic acid translation.[7(pp1161-1163)] Resistant organisms can be expected, and this resistance certainly limits the use of this medication. Gentamicin may not be excessively toxic to keratinocytes,[29] but has been shown to inhibit the activity of PMNs.[31] Skin hypersensitivity has been reported with gentamicin. Ototoxicity and nephrotoxicity can occur, particularly when the drug is used in large volumes or for an extended period of time.[7(pp1161-1163)] Gentamicin should be applied to small wounds or larger full-thickness injuries once a day.[7(pp1161-1163)] Because of the development of resistant bacterial strains and the risk of toxicity, it is suggested that this topical agent be used only when treatment with other topical medications has been unsuccessful, that it not be used prophylactically, and that it be discontinued when the wound colonization is controlled.

Solutions

Techniques/Indications for Use.

Topical agents in solution are useful if the choice of dressing is "wet-to-moist."[44(p2838)] The drug of choice is generally added in its powder form to distilled water or physiologic saline. Solutions are a useful form for topical agents, especially when applied to wounds with cavities or fissures, because they can easily be cleansed by rinsing.[44(p2838)] The wound should be thoroughly rinsed following removal of old dressings to ensure removal of previously applied agents. The wound may then be gently debrided, and a gauze soaked in the solution of choice is then placed on the wound. If the gauze is being placed in a deep wound, care must be taken to not disrupt healing tissue by overaggressive insertion of the dressing. All exposed parts of the wound should be covered by the soaked gauze.[44(p2838)] This type of dressing is often held in place by an elastic wrap because the occlusiveness of the wrap helps prevent leakage of the solution. Gauze soaked with the solution form of a topical agent is easily applied and removed from most wounds unless the gauze is allowed to dry out, at which time it can be damaging because of the associated removal of newly forming tissue.[44(2838)] The solutions should be applied often enough to keep the dressing from drying.

Topical agents in solution generally provide safe and effective treatment of infected wounds, but the requirement that dressings not be allowed to dry out undoubtedly increases the cost of the technique. These solutions are necessarily unstable, and therefore they must be mixed fresh. Topical solutions must be prescribed by a physician and should be mixed by a pharmacist to ensure appropriate concentrations and antiseptic preparation. The following topical solutions are frequently used in the treatment of cutaneous wounds.

Acetic acid 0.5 percent. Acetic acid at this concentration is bactericidal to many gram-negative and gram-positive microorganisms but is especially effective against *P aeruginosa*.[64-65] Solutions of 0.25

percent acetic acid have also been reported, but they appear to be less effective in reducing microorganisms on wounds.[38] This weak acid penetrates the cell wall and disrupts the cell membrane to establish its bactericidal effects. Any wound-healing assistance provided by this solution would be in curbing growth of inhibitory infective organisms on the surface. Acetic acid has demonstrated toxicity to fibroblasts in culture.[38] Reduced epithelial cell proliferation in culture[29] and delayed healing of cultured epithelial autografts have been reported at 0.25 percent strength.[66] It may be that 0.5 percent concentrations are more toxic to regenerating epithelium, but this has not been reported. Gruber et al[67] described no adverse effect on reepithelialization of donor sites when comparing 0.25 percent acetic acid with saline. Acetic acid has been shown to reduce PMN function.[31] Skin irritation may occur if acetic acid is used at, or higher than, the 0.5 percent concentration. Acidosis may result from protracted use over large surface-area wounds. This solution should be applied frequently enough to keep the wound moist, and it should be rinsed of thoroughly between applications. This topical agent in solution is a good choice for small infected wounds.

Sodium hypochlorite (Dakin's Solution). This sodium hypochlorite (0.5 percent or 0.25 percent NaOCl) solution is considered a general bactericidal (eg, *Staphylococci* and *Streptococci*), fungicidal, and virucidal agent. Concentrations as low as 0.025 percent have also demonstrated bactericidal effects.[68] The bactericidal effects are the suggested rationale for aiding wound healing. Sodium hypochlorite at 0.25 percent, however, has displayed toxicity to fibroblasts[38,39,68,69] and keratinocytes[29,39] in culture. Polymorphonuclear leukocyte viability is also inhibited by this topical agent.[31,69] Sodium hypochlorite solutions of 0.5 percent would be expected to demonstrate at least these same levels of toxicity. Tissue toxicity was not observed at concentrations of 0.025 percent.[68] Delays in epithelialization and neovascularization might be expected.[29,39] Sodium hypochlorite dissolves blood clots and may also delay clotting. Bleeding may ensue, and the wound should be carefully monitored when using this solution. Acidosis may result following continuous use over large-area wounds. This solution may also cause pain. A diluted sodium hypochlorite solution is frequently used to irrigate wounds. In any dilution, the solution should be thoroughly rinsed off the site between dressings, as prolonged exposure can lead to skin irritation. The soaked dressing should be changed often enough to avoid drying of the dressing. As with acetic acid, this sodium hypochlorite might be considered as an alternative for treating small, infected wounds. Because of its level of tissue toxicity at typical concentrations, this solution may not be a suitable choice for treatment of partial-thickness injuries that are sparsely colonized. Less concentrated solutions such as 0.025 percent should be considered for clinical use.[68]

Silver nitrate 0.5 percent. Silver nitrate in solution provides bactericidal activity against a wide range of bacterial flora, but is probably more effective against gram-positive bacteria (eg, *S aureus*). Silver nitrate solution has demonstrated invulnerability to resistant organisms.[70] Wound healing may be enhanced by control of local infection with this topical agent. There are conflicting reports about the toxicity of silver nitrate solution to epithelium.[39,71] The solution is extremely hypotonic, and electrolytes (eg, sodium and potassium) leach into the dressing. This leaching can lead to electrolyte imbalances, especially with prolonged use over large-area wounds. Use of silver nitrate on large wounds requires monitoring of electrolytes.[72] Bacterial reduction of nitrate to nitrite may lead to methemoglobinemia with use of this topical agent.[73] This potential complication, though rare, should be suspected if skin around the wound appears gray or cyanotic, and the diagnosis can be confirmed with blood methemoglobinemia measurement.[42] No reports of hypersensitivity reactions in the skin have occurred with the use of silver nitrate solution. Because of potential toxicity, silver nitrate has been suggested to be more effective on smaller surface-area wounds.[47] Although silver nitrate is a reasonable choice as a topical agent for smaller wounds, frequent soaking of the dressings (about every two hours) is required for the agent to remain effective and application of the solution may be slightly painful. Further, the solution stains skin, wounds, dressings, linen, and clothing a dark brown or black. The agent does not penetrate eschar readily and therefore should not be the first choice for treatment of established infections.[42]

Triple antibiotic solution. Bacitracin (50,000 U), polymyxin B (200,000 U), and neomycin (40 mg) can be combined in 1 L of saline to produce a triple antibiotic (TAB) solution to use as a "wet-to-moist" dressing for infected wounds of several types.[25(p174)] This solution shows at least a moderate level of activity against a variety of gram-negative and gram-positive organisms, with activity against *P aeruginosa* being poor.[74] No data on resistant organisms were available. The components of the solution, when in ointment form, showed limited toxicity to keratinocytes.[39] Nystatin, in powder form, may be added to the solution if there is a combined bacterial/fungal infection. This TAB solution may be indicated for fresh, poorly colonized wounds such as new skin grafts or donor sites because of its potentially low level of tissue toxicity.

Chlorhexidine gluconate solution. Chlorhexidine gluconate solution (0.05 percent in distilled water) affords antibacterial activity against gram-positive bacteria, including *P aeruginosa* and *Klebsiella*, and against gram-positive bacteria such as *S aureus* and *E Coli*.[74] Local infection control may assist wound healing. No data could be found that discussed the tissue toxicity of this solution, and systemic toxicity appears to be rare.[42,75] This solution rarely causes skin reactions; however, with prolonged, repeated use, contact dermatitis may develop.[76,77] The apparent low toxicity and high bactericidal properties of this solution indicate that it may be a useful option as a topical therapeutic solution for different depths and sizes of injury. The solution should be used often enough to keep the wound moist.

Moisturizers

Although moisturizers are not typically discussed in the context of "topical agents," a brief discussion is warranted, particularly as it relates to sensitivity reactions and to antipruritic agents. Dryness, flakiness, and pruritus are typical in freshly epithelialized wounds and result from the loss of production of skin oils. Superficial wounds and true partial-thickness wounds will eventually recover the ability to produce skin oils; however, deeper wounds will not. Topical moisturizers, used as needed (often more frequently than twice a day), will relieve most complaints of flakiness and itching. Hypoallergenic moisturizers that are not alcohol based, and contain no perfumes, are preferred. Patients may develop sensitivity reactions to moisturizers that contain perfumes.[78] These reactions often occur as skin rashes or increased pruritus. If such a reaction occurs, the use of that moisturizer should be discontinued, the rash should be allowed to clear, and the patient should then explore other moisturizers to find one that will not produce an irritation. If the rash persists following a change of topical agent, a medical consultation should be obtained.

There are some mild antipruritic creams that may be acquired without prescription, and these creams should be applied as infrequently as will allow for control of itching. There are also several choices of topical corticosteroids that are used as antiinflammatory and antipruritic agents. These corticosteroids, which require physician prescription, should be applied as prescribed and seldom require prolonged use. Adverse reactions of burning, itching, erythema, and skin and papular rashes have been reported, and topical corticosteroids should be discontinued if any of these symptoms occur. Systemic effects of topical corticosteroids are considered reversible.

Other Considerations

General contraindications. Any known sensitivities, or the development of sensitivities to the pharmaceutical components of each of these preparations in ointment, cream, or solution, should be considered a standing contraindication for a particular topical agent.

Resistant strains. Although resistant strains of organisms may develop against some of the topical agents discussed, this has not created a major barrier to treatment of wound infection by the available choices of agents provided in this review. Methicillin-resistant *Staphylococcus aureus* (MRSA) is a reasonably common gram-positive species of bacteria that can cause a number of infections, including bacteremias, pneumonias, and soft tissue and bone infections. Because most cases are nosocomial, infection control and isolation precautions should be a part of any wound care measures along with the use of topical agents. In the case of MRSA, silver sulfadiazine, mafenide acetate, and nitrofurazone (as well as mupirocin, a topical agent not described in this chapter) may be effective in treating this resistant strain.[79-81] Smoot et all[81] report that in their burn unit mafenide acetate has limited activity against MRSA. This may be the result of their frequent use of this agent, which may have produced an MRSA resistance in their particular center.[81] If there is a topical agent of choice in a clinic and a resistance to a particular organism develops, the resistance may be clinic specific and other topical agents should be used in attempts to subdue the resistant pathogen.

Other. Incorrect medication can result in delayed healing, discomfort, increased scarring, progression of the infection, or toxicity. For example, delayed healing may lead to proliferation of fibroblasts and an increase in scarring. A large-area wound treated with the same topical agent for several days also has a potential for systemic toxicity.[7(pp1165-1166)-11] A therapist who is aware of recurring wounds or infections should refer the patient to a physician.

Patients should be taught the appropriate application of topical agents and dressings, as well as the signs of infection. Patients should also understand that such drugs are never to be taken internally.

Topical Agents and Wound Healing

Any human tissue requires oxygen to remain viable. The importance of blood supply to the skin can be easily illustrated with the example of a pressure ulcer. Though there are other contributing factors to the formation of pressure ulcers, it is clear that local ischemia caused by pressure-induced constriction of capillaries leads to death of the involved skin. Capillary regrowth and associated wound remodeling are hampered by decreased oxygenation.[82-84] Additionally, infection is enhanced by an ischemic environment because bacteria require little oxygen compared with the associated cells.[85] Further, by consuming oxygen, bacteria decrease the amount of oxygen available to the tissue.[86] Inadequate wound healing with concurrent inflammation and increased scarring is another consequence of bacterial proliferation and related tissue hypoxia.[87] A diabetic ulcer is a classic example of a poorly perfused wound that demonstrates substandard wound healing along with chronic inflammation.[88] Burn wounds are ischemic as a result of the thrombosis caused by the injury. Full-thickness burns display this thrombosis through all layers of affected skin, whereas partial-thickness burns demonstrate incomplete thrombosis. Topical agents are used to fight wound infection related to decreased tissue vascularity.

Controlling infection in open wounds will enhance wound healing. Topical agents reduce the number of germs but do not obliterate them. Improved wound healing decreases the pain and scarring that contribute to wound related physical impairment.

By removing bacteria and necrotic debris, debridement and cleansing are important components of any wound care program to prevent infection.[1(pp150-156)] Necrotic tissue present on a wound surface promotes infection by providing nutrients for bacteria. Besides fighting superficial infection, most topical agents will help soften wound eschar, which will assist with debridement of tissue. Removing previously applied creams and ointments from the wound allows for repeated assessment of the wound.

Superficial and partial-thickness wounds heal by regeneration of epithelium from existing basal cells at the wound surface.[89] Some mild contraction may be associated with the healing of superficial wounds, but seldom is there scarring. In contrast, deep wounds usually heal by a combination of reepithelialization and contraction.[89] Contraction serves to decrease the area of the wound. Wounds are then reepithelialized from the margins. Scarring and contraction of scar tissue are typically consequent problems to the healing of deep partial-thickness and full-thickness wounds.

The rate of reepithelialization may be enhanced by the application of bacitracin,[27,28] and polymyxin B and Neosporin in an ointment or TAB solution appear to either have no, or only a slight, inhibitory effect on keratinocyte proliferation.[29] In contrast, povidoneiodine,[38,39] silver sulfadiazine,[39,48,49] mafenide acetate,[39,48,49,59] nitrofurazone,[39] acetic acid,[29] and sodium hypochlorite[29,39] will likely inhibit reepithelialization.[47-90] A bland ointment (bacitracin, polymyxin B sulfate, neomycin, and their combinations) and possibly silver sulfadiazine are often the topical agents of choice for reepithelializing wounds. Bland ointments are also generally less expensive than the sulfa-based topical agents and therefore might be a more cost-effective choice for treatment of small, uncomplicated wounds.

Wound contraction is a natural process in which wounds heal by decreasing their size.[91] When a wound is located over or near a joint surface, however, excessive contraction may contribute to loss of joint motion. Further, when the wound encompasses a large surface area, contraction cannot successfully close the wound. Little is known about the effects of topical agents on the rate or amount of wound contraction. Bacitracin and silver sulfadiazine have been shown to retard wound contraction in a pig model,[28] but the direct clinical application of these findings is not yet understood. Additionally, the appropriate choices of topical treatment may speed wound coverage, thereby decreasing the risk of scarring and associated scar contracture. A hypertrophic scar, which results from a poorly treated wound or is the predictable result of a healed full-thickness wound, will continue to contract for several months, even following wound healing.

Conclusion

Because of the availability of several effective topical agents, wound care protocols may vary and still meet with success. Observation of the wound, along with the appropriate selection of a topical therapeutic agent, can improve the healing of wounds and lead to decreased patient morbidity. The physical therapist should be aware of the advantages and disadvantages of varying topical wound care agents. Collaboration with the physician in determining infective organisms at a wound site will assist with making acceptable decisions about the topical agents of choice. Future studies of importance to this clinical area should include controlled comparative clinical studies on the effects of various topical agents on different types of wounds, the interaction of various dressings with topical agents, the potential use of drug enhancers for these topical agents, the effect of different topical agents on wound and scar contraction, the rate of healing and its effect on scar formation, and the cost effectiveness of varying wound treatments.

References

1. Feedar JA. Clinical management of chronic wounds. In: McCulloch JM, Kloth IC, Feedar JA, eds. *Wound Healing: Alternatives in Management*. 2nd ed. Philadelphia, Pa: FA Davis Co; 1995:145-146, 150-156.

2. Ward RS. The rehabilitation of burn patients. Crit Rev Phys Med Rehabil. 1991;2:121-138.

3. Solem L. Classification. In: Fisher SV, Helm PA, eds. *Comprehensive Rehabilitation of Burns*. Baltimore, Md: Williams & Wilkins; 1984:9-15.

4. Goode PS, Allman RM. The prevention and management of pressure ulcers. *Med Clin North Am*. 1989;73:1511-1524.

5. Miller SF, Richard RL, Staley MJ. Triage and resuscitation of the burn patient. In: Richard SL, Staley MJ, eds. *Burn Care and Rehabilitation: Principles and Practice*. Philadelphia, Pa: FA Davis Co; 1994:109-110.

6. Holt MB, Matthews PJ. Pressure sore flowsheet. In: Carlson CE, ed. *Spinal Cord Injury: A Guide to Rehabilitation Nursing*. Rockville, Md: Aspen Publishers Inc; 1987:185.

7. Sande MA, Mandell GL. Antimicrobial agents: the aminoglycosides. In: Gilman AG, Goodman LS, Rall TW, Murad F, eds. *The Pharmacological Basis of Therapeutics*. New York, NY: Macmillan Publishing USA; 1985: 1161-1163, 1165-1166,

8. Lavelle KJ, Kleit SA, Forney RB. Iodine absorption in burn patients treated topically with povidone iodine. *Clin Pharmacol Ther*. 1975; 17:355-362.

9. Pietsch J, Meakins JL. Complications of povidone-iodine absorption in topically treated burn patients. *Lancet*. 1976;i:280-282.

10. Dela Cruz F, Brown DH, Leikien JB, et al. Iodine absorption after topical administration. *West J Med*. 1987;146:43-45.

11. Moncrief JA. Topical therapy for control of bacteria in the burn wound. *World J Surg*. 1978;2:151-165.

12. Harkess N. Bacteriology. In: Kloth IC, McCulloch JM, Feedar JA, eds. *Wound Healing: Alternatives in Management*. Philadelphia, Pa: FA Davis Co; 1990:60-61.

13. Hill MJ. Infections. In: Hill MJ, ed. *Skin Disorders*. St Louis, Mo: Mosby-Year Book Inc; 1994:89-93.

14. Brown CD, Zitelli JA, A review of topical agents for wounds and methods of wounding. *J Dermatol Surg Oncol*. 1993; 19:732-737.

15. Custer J, Edlich R. Studies in the management of the contaminated wound. *Am J Surg*. 1971;121:572-575.

16. Branemark PI, Ekholm R. Tissue injury caused by wound disinfectants. J Bone Joint Surg [Am]. 1967:49:48-62.

17. Tatnall FM, Leigh IM, Gibson JR. Comparative toxicity of antimicrobial agents on transformed human keratinocytes. J Invest Dermatol. 1987;89:316-317.

18. Viljanto J. Disinfection of surgical wounds without inhibition of normal healing. Arch Surg. 1980;115:253-256.

19. Lineaweaver W, Howard R, Soucy D. Topical antimicrobial toxicity. *Arch Surg*. 1985; 120:267-270.

20. Shelanski HA, Shelanski MV. PVP-iodine: History, toxicity and therapeutic uses. *J Int Coll Surg*. 1956;25:727-734.

21. Jacobs MR, Zanowiak P. Topical anti-infective products. In: Feldman EG, ed. *Handbook of Nonprescriptive Drugs*. 9th ed. Washington, DC: American Pharmaceutical Association; 1990:779, 781.

22. Gottardi W. Iodine and iodine compounds. In: Block SS, ed. *Disinfection, Sterilization, and Preservation*. Philadelphia, Pa: Lea & Febiger; 1983:183-196.

23. Craven DE, Moody B, Connolly MG, et al. Pseudobacteremia caused by povidone-iodine solution contaminated with Pseudomonas cepacia. *N Engl J Med*. 1981;305:621-623.

24. Polk H, Finn M. Chemoprophylaxis of wound infections, In: Simmon RI, Howard RJ, eds. *Surgical Infection Diseases*. New York, NY: Appleton Century Crofts; 1982:471.

25. Saffle JR, Schnebly WA. Burn wound care. In: Richard RL, Staley MJ, eds, *Burn Care and Rehabilitation: Principles and Practice*. Philadelphia, Pa: FA Davis Co; 1994:137-139, 174.

26. Arndt KA. Formulary, In: *Manual of Dermatologic Therapeutics*. 3rd ed. Boston, Mass: Little, Brown and Company Inc; 1983:299.

27. Eaglstein WH, Mertz PM, Alvarez OM. Effect of topically applied agents on healing wounds. *Clin Dermatol*. 1984;2: 112-115.

28. Watcher MA, Wheeland RG. The role of topical agents in the healing of full-thickness wounds. *J Dermatol Surg Oncol*. 1989;15:1188-1195.

29. Cooper ML, Boyce ST, Hansbrough JF, et al. Cytotoxicity to cultured human keratinocytes of topical antimicrobial agents. *J Surg Res*. 1990;48:190-195.

30. Saberwal G, Nagaraj R. Cell-lytic and antibacterial peptides that act by perturbing the barrier function of membranes: facets of their conformational features, structure-function correlations and membrane perturbing abilities. *Biochim Biophys Acta*. 1994; 1197:109-131,

31. Hansbrough JF, Zapata-Sirvent RL, Cooper ML. Effects of topical antimicrobial agents on the human neutrophil respiratory burst. *Arch Surg*. 1991;126:603-608.

32. Gette MT, Marks JG Jr, Maloney ME. Frequency of postoperative allergic contact dermatitis to topical antibiotics. *Arch Dermatol*. 1992;128:365-367.

33. Taddonio TE, Thomson PD, Smith DJ Jr, Prasad JK. A survey of wound monitoring and topical antimicrobial therapy practices in the treatment of burn injury. *J Burn Care Rebabil*. 1990; 11:423-427.

34. Sande MA, Mandell GL. Antimicrobial agents: tetracyclines, chloramphenicol, erythromycin, and miscellaneous antibacterial agents. In: Gillman AG, Goodman IS, Rall TW. Murad F, eds. *The Pharmacologic Basis of Therapeutics*. New York, NY: Macmillan Publishing USA: 1985:1191-1192.

35. Brown MRW, Wood SM. Relation between cation and lipid content of cell walls of *Pseudomonas aeruginosa, Proteus vulgaris*, and *Klebsiella aerogenes* and their sensitivity to polymyxin B and other antibacterial agents.

36. Kaiser W, von der Lieth H, Potel j Heymann H. Experimental study of the local application of silver sulfadiazine, cefsulodin and povidone-iodine to burns. *Infection*. 1984;12: 31-35.

37. Robin AL, MacArthur JD, O'Connor N. The influence of betadine ointment (povidone-iodine) on wound healing in rats. In: Georgiade NG, Boswick JA, MacMillan BG, eds. *Recent Antisepsis Techniques in the Management of burn Wound.* Norwalk, Conn: The Purdue Frederick Co; 1974:12-14.

38. Lineaweaver W, McMorris S, Soucy D, Howard R. Cellular and bacterial toxicities of topical antimicrobials. *Plast Reconstr Surg.* 1985;75:394-396.

39. Smoot EC, Kucan JO, Roth A, et al. In vitro toxicity testing for antibacterials against human keratinocytes. *Plast Reconstr Surg.* 1991; 87:917-924.

40. Mark JG. Allergic contact dermatitis to povidone-iodine. *J Am Acad Dermatol.* 1982; 6:473-475.

41. Steen M. Review of the use of povidone-iodine (PVP-1) in the treatment of burns. *Post-Grad Med J* 1993;69:S84-S92.

42. Monafo WW, West MA. Current treatment recommendations for topical burn therapy. *Drugs,* 1990;40:364-373.

43. Kucan JO, Robson MC, Heggers JP, et al. Comparison of silver sulfadiazine, povidone-iodine and physiologic saline in the treatment of chronic pressure ulcers. *J Am Geriatr Soc.* 1981:29:232-235.

44. Arndt KA, Mendenhall PV, Sloan KB, Perrin JH. The pharmacology of topical therapy. In: Fitzgerald TB, Eisen AZ, Wolff K, et al, eds. *Dermatology in General Medicine.* New York, NY: McGraw-Hill Inc; 1993:2838, 2839.

45. Arndt KA. Treatment principles. In: *Manual of Dermatologic Therapeutics* 3rd ed. Boston, Mass: Little, Brown and Company Inc; 1983:229.

46. Fox CL. Silver sulfadiazine: a new topical therapy. *Arch Surg.* 1968;96:184-188.

47. Monafo WW, Ayvazian VH. Topical therapy. *Surg Clin North Am.* 1978;58:1157-1171.

48. Cooper ML, Laxer JA, Hansbrough JF. The cytotoxic effects of commonly used topical antimicrobial agents on human fibroblasts and keratinocytes. *J Trauma.* 1991;31:775-784.

49. McCauley RL, Linares HA, Pelligrini V, et al. In vitro toxicity of topical antimicrobial agents to human fibroblasts, *J Surg Res*. 1989: 46:267-274.

50. Geronemus RG, Mertz PM, Eaglstein WH. Wound healing: the effects of topical antimicrobial agents. *Arch Dermatol*. 1979;115:1311-1314.

51. Zapata-Sirvent RL, Hansbrough JF. Cytotoxicity to human leukocytes by topical antimicrobial agents used for burn care. *J Burn Care Rehabil*. 1993;14:132-140.

52. Kiker RG, Carvajal JF, Mlcak RP, Larson DL. A controlled study of the effects of silver sulfadiazine on white blood cell counts in burned children. J Trauma. 1977;17:835-836.

53. Smith-Choban P, Marshall WJ. Leukopenia secondary to silver sulfadiazine: frequency, characteristics and clinical consequences. *Am Surg*. 1987;53:515-517.

54. Fuller FW, Engler PE. Leukopenia in nonspecific burn patients receiving topical 1 percent silver sulfadiazine cream therapy: a survey. *J Burn Care Rebabil*. 1988;9:606-609.

55. *Physicians' Desk Reference*. 49th ed. Montvale, NJ: Medical Economics Data Production Co; 1995:1143.

56. Lindberg RB, Moncrief JA, Mason AD Jr. Control of experimental and clinical burn wound sepsis by topical application of sulfamylon compounds. *Ann NY Acad Sci*. 1968; 150:950-960.

57. Shuck JM, Thorne AW, Cooper CG. Mafenide acetate solution dressings: an adjunct in burn wound care. *J Trauma*. 1975;15:595-599.

58. Mandell GL, Sande MA. Antimicrobial agents: sulfonamides, trimethoprimsulfamethoxazole, and agents for urinary tract infections. In: Gilman AG, Goodman LS, Rall TW, Murad F, eds. *The Pharmacological Basis of Therapeutics*. New York, NY: Macmillan Publishing USA; 1985:1101.

59. McCauley RL, Li YY, Poole B, et al. Differential inhibition of basal keratinocytes growth to silver sulfadiazine and mafenide acetate. *J Surg Res*. 1992;52:276-285.

60. White MG, Asch MJ. Acid base effects of topical manefide acetate in the burned patient, *N Engl J Med*. 1971;284:1281-1286.

61. Harrison HN, Shuck JM, Caldwell E. Studies of pain produced by mafenide acetate preparations in burns. *Arch Surg*. 1975;110: 1446-1449.

62. Kucan JO, Smoot EC. Five percent mafenide acetate solution in the treatment of thermal injuries. *J Burn Care Rehabil*. 1993; 14: 158-163.

63. Dube MP, Heseltine PN, Rinaidi MG, et al. Fungemia and colonization with nystatin-resistant *Candida rugosa* in a burn unit. *Clin Infect Dis*. 1994; 18:77-82.

64. Phillips I, Lobo AZ, Fernandes R, et al. Acetic acid in the treatment of superficial wounds infected by *Pseudomonas aeruginosa*. *Lancet*. 1968;1:11-12.

65. Sloss JM, Cumberland N, Milner SM, Acetic acid used for the elimination of *Pseudomonas aeruginosa* from burn and soft tissue wounds. *J R Army Med Corps*. 1993;139:49-51.

66. Gallico G, O'Conner N. Compton C, et al. Cultured epithelial autografts for giant congenital nevi. *Plast Reconstr Surg*. 1989;84:1-9.

67. Gruber RP, Vistnes L, Pardoc R. The effect of commonly used antiseptics on wound healing. *Plast Reconstr Surg*. 1975;55:472-476.

68. Heggers JP, Sazy JA, Stenberg BD, et al. Bactericidal and wound-healing properties of sodium hypochlorite solutions: the 1991 Lindberg Award. *J Burn Care Rebabil*. 1991;12:420-424.

69. Kozol RA, Gillies C, Eigebaly SA. Effects of sodium hypochlorite (Dakin's solution) on cells of the wound module. *Arch Surg*. 1988; 123:420-427.

70. Livingston DH, Cryer HG, Miller FB, et al. A randomized prospective study of topical agents on skin grafts after thermal injury. *Plast Reconstr Surg*. 1990;86:1059-1064.

71. Bellinger CG, Conway H. Effects of silver nitrate and sulfamylon on epithelial regeneration. *Plast Reconstr Surg*. 1970;45:582-585.

72. Bonder CC, Morris BJ, Wee T, et al. The metabolic effects of 0.5 percent silver nitrate in the treatment of major burns in children. *J Pediatr Surg.* 1967;2:22-31.

73. Moyer CA, Bretano L, Gravens DL, et al Treatment of human burns with 0.5 percent silver nitrate solution. *Arch Surg.* 1965;90:812-867.

74. Holder IA. Wet disc testing of mafenide hydrochloride, chlorhexidine gluconate, and triple antibiotic solution against bacteria isolated from burn wounds. *J Burn Care Rebabil.* 1990;11:301-304.

75. Harvey SC. Antiseptics and disinfectants; fungicides; ectoparasiticides. In: Gilman AG, Goodman LS, Rall TW, Murad F, eds. The *Pharmacological Basis of Therapeutics.* New York, NY: Macmillan Publishing USA; 1985: 963.

76. Andersen BL, Bradrup F. Contact dermatitis from chlorhexidine. *Contact Dermatitis.* 1985; 13:307-309.

77. Greener Y, McCartney M, Jordan L, et al. Assessment of the systemic effects, primary dermal irritation and ocular irritation of chlorhexidine acetate solutions. *J Am Coll Toxicol* 1985;6:309-319.

78. Laresen WG. Perfume dermatitis. J Am Acad Dermatol. 1985; 12:1-9.

79. Strock LL, Lee MM, Rutan RL, et al. Topical Bactroban (mupirocin): efficacy in treating burn wounds infected with methicillin-resistant staphylococci. *J Burn Care Rebabil,* 1990;11:454-459.

80. Maple PAC, Hamilton-Miller JMT, Brumfitt W. Comparison of the in-vitro activities of the topical antimicrobials azelaic acid, nitrofurazone, silver sulfadiazine and mupirocin against methicillin-resistant *Staphylococcus aureus. J Antimicrob Chemother.* 1992;29:661-608.

81. Smoot EC Jr, Kucan JO, Graham DR, et al. Susceptibility testing of topical antibacterials against methicillin-resistant *Staphylococcus aureus. Burn Care Rebabil.* 1992; 13:198-202.

82. Hunt TK. Physiology of wound healing. In: Clowes GHA, ed. *Trauma, Sepsis, and Shock: The Physiological Basis of Therapy.* New York, NY: Marcel Dekker Inc; 1988:443-471.

83. Knighton DR, Hunt TK, Scheuenstuhl H, et al. Oxygen tension regulates the expression of angiogenesis factor by macrophages. *Science*. 1983;221:1283-1285.

84. Knighton DR, Silver IA, Hunt TK. Regulation of wound healing angiogenesis: effect of oxygen gradients and inspired oxygen concentration. *Surgery*. 1981;90:262-270.

85. Hohn DC, MacKay RD, Halliday B, Hunt TK. The effect of O_2 tension on the microbial function of leukocytes in wounds and in vitro. *Surg Forum*. 1976;27:18-20.

86. Smith IM, Wilson AP, Hazard AC, et al. Death from staphylococci in mice. *J Infect Dis*. 1960;107:369-378.

87. Orgill D, Demling RH. Current concepts and approaches to wound healing. *Crit Care Med*. 1988; 16:899-908.

88. Levin ME. The diabetic foot. In: Jelinek JE, ed. *The Skin in Diabetes*, Philadelphia, Pa: Lea & Febiger; 1986:73--94.

89. Greenhalgh DG, Staley MJ. Burn wound healing, In: Richard RL, Staley MJ, eds. *Burn Care and Rehabilitation. Principles and Practice*. Philadelphia, Pa: FA Davis Co; 1994:81-85.

90. Monafo WW, Freedman B. Topical therapy for burns. *Surg Clin North Am*. 1987;67:133-145.

91. Peacock EE, Van Winkle W. Contraction. In: Peacock EE, Van Winkle eds. *Wound Repair*. Philadelphia, Pa: WB Saunders Co; 1976:54.

—by R Scott Ward and Jeffrey R Saffle

RS Ward, PhD, PT, is Staff Member, Intermountain Burn Center, and Assistant Professor and Co-Director, Division of Physical Therapy, University of Utah Health Sciences Center, Annex 1130, Salt Lake City, UT 84112 (USA).

JR Saffle, MD, FACS, is Director, Intermountain Burn Center, and Associate Professor, Department of Surgery, University of Utah Health Sciences Center, 50 N Medical Dr, Salt Lake City, UT 84132 (USA).

Chapter 24

Infectious Complications after a Burn Injury

Abstract

Since the inception of organized burn care nearly 50 years ago, infections complicating the care of thermally injured patients have been recognized as a major source of morbidity and mortality. The control of invasive infection and burn wound sepsis and improvements in the general care of these critically ill patients have resulted in unsurpassed survival; even so, infection remains the most frequent cause of death in these severely injured patients.

Introduction

Infectious complications continue to be the predominant determinant of outcome in thermally injured patients. Improvements in the general care of these critically ill patients and control of invasive infection and burn wound sepsis through the use of effective topical antimicrobial agents and timely excision and grafting have resulted in the survival of more patients who previously would have died soon after being burned.

Coincident with improvements in survival and prolongation of the hospital course of nonsurvivors, changes in the epidemiology of infection have occurred, resulting in a predominance of true fungi, yeast, and multiple antibiotic resistant bacteria as the causative agents of nosocomial infections. Control of the bacterial burn wound flora has been associated with a relative increase of infections in other sites, predominantly the lungs, as principal causes of morbidity and mortality.

Additionally, prolongation of the hospital course of nonsurvivors, most of whom die as a result of overwhelming infection or multiple system organ failure, has focused interest on the pathogenesis of the systemic inflammatory response syndrome and the role of systemic cytokine liberation, intestinal bacterial translocation, and polymorphonuclear leukocyte activation in the cause of multiple system organ failure.

Further characterization of the host response to thermal injury may identify potentially deleterious processes or pathways that contribute to an exaggerated systemic inflammatory response. Such information can be used to formulate selective pharmacologic interventions that ameliorate an uncontrolled inflammatory response or prevent its occurrence. This process recapitulates the events that led to the description of invasive bacterial burn wound infection and the development of effective topical antimicrobial agents, essentially eliminating bacterial burn wound infection as a clinical problem.

Epidemiology of Infection

During the past four decades, the prophylactic use of effective topical antimicrobial agents such as mafenide acetate burn cream, silver sulfadiazine burn cream, and dilute (0.5 percent) silver nitrate soaks has become routine, and prompt excision and early closure of the burn wound have become standard practice; at the same time, the occurrence of invasive burn wound infection and its related mortality have significantly diminished. Other factors that have contributed to the decrease in burn wound infections are listed in Table 24.1.

In a recent large series[1], in which the causes of mortality in thermally injured patients were reviewed, wound infection accounted for

Table 24.1. Factors Associated with Decreasing Incidence of Burn Wound Infection.

Effective topical antimicrobial therapy.
Timely excision of burn wounds.
Availability of effective biologic dressings.
Improved burn wound monitoring.
Cohort isolation techniques.
Improved general care.

only 5.1 percent of infection-related deaths between 1987 and 1991, compared with 25.5 percent in 1979. Additionally, the initiation of single-bed isolation of seriously burned patients was associated with an unchanged incidence of colonization of the burn wound by *Pseudomonas aeruginosa*; colonization was, however, significantly delayed, when compared with a historical cohort (25 days after the burn, compared with 15 days)[2]. *Pseudomonas pneumonia*, invasive burn wound infection, and bacteremia each occurred at a decreased frequency and longer after the burn when this isolation technique was used with a rigorous microbial surveillance program and strict environmental infection control practices.

Nonbacterial Infection

Longer survival of patients whose wounds remain open, either because of the extent of the burn or because of complications that necessitate the use of broad-spectrum antibiotics, increases the probability that organisms causing colonization or infection will be yeasts, fungi, or multiple antibiotic resistant bacteria. The moist, protein rich, avascular eschar of a burn wound creates an excellent microbial culture medium into which parenterally administered antibiotics penetrate poorly, if at all, and thus have no effect on the rapid bacterial colonization in the burn wound.

Topical agents effectively control the initially sparse, predominately Gram-positive burn wound flora; in patients in whom prompt wound closure cannot be accomplished, however, the colonizing flora not only of the burn wound but also of the respiratory, gastrointestinal, and urinary tracts are often replaced by nosocomial Gram-negative organisms and nonbacterial opportunists.

In a recent review of 2114 thermally injured patients admitted to our institution[3], fungal wound infection occurred in 141 patients, whereas bacterial wound infection was documented in only 68 patients. In patients in whom the causative organism could be identified by microscopic morphologic appearance or culture recovery from tissue samples, filamentous fungi and *Candida* species were present in 82 percent and 18 percent of specimens, respectively. *Aspergillus* and *Fusarium* species were recovered in 68 percent of specimens, whereas *Rhizopus* and *Mucor* species were detected in only 9.1 percent and *Microspora* and *Alternaria* species in fewer than 5 percent each. Thus, fungi have replaced bacteria as the most common microbes causing invasive burn wound infection in this series.

Histopathologic identification of fungal invasion of viable subeschar tissue in a wound biopsy specimen should mandate prompt local surgical debridement of all involved tissue. Parenteral administration of amphotericin B should be started in patients who exhibit spread of fungal infection beyond the confines of the burn wound or have evidence of microvascular or lymphatic invasion detected by wound biopsy. Parenteral treatment with fluconazole and topical antifungal therapy have not been proved to be effective in this setting.

The exact relationship of the administration of parenteral antibiotic therapy in burned patients to the emergence of fungi as the most common pathogens causing burn wound infection is unknown; these "opportunistic" infections of the burn wound, however, have been associated with the reduced incidence of Gram-negative burn wound infection brought about by the use of effective topical chemotherapeutic agents. To prevent or minimize the emergence of multiple antibiotic resistant bacteria and nonbacterial pathogens, strict criteria for parenteral antibiotic use should be followed, and empiric antibiotic therapy for "sepsis" in the absence of an identified source should be avoided.

Viral infections have also been recognized with increasing frequency in burned patients. At our institution, herpes simplex virus type 1, the most frequently identified virus causing infections, was identified as the cause of infection of the airway in nine patients and of the burn wound in five patients during a recent six year period[4••]. Cytomegalovirus infections of the airway were identified in six patients during the same period.

In a recent prospective study of cytomegalovirus sero-conversion in burned patients[5], cytomegalovirus antibody titer increased more than fourfold in 31 out of 87 patients but appeared to have no effect on outcome.

Clinical manifestations of indolent infection, such as persistent temperature elevation, hepatitis, and lymphocytosis, suggest a viral origin and, in the absence of an identifiable bacterial source of infection, speak for the withholding of antibacterial agents, which would be ineffectual. The administration of antiviral agents such as adenine arabinoside or ganciclovir is indicated in patients with systemic viral infection and progressive deterioration.

Methicillin-resistant Strains of Staphylococcus Aureus

Antibiotic-resistant bacteria of special note and of much controversy are the methicillin-resistant strains of S. *aureus*. The strains that are principally resistant to penicillinase-resistant penicillins and aminoglycosides are increasingly common nosocomial isolates. Since the 1960s, these strains have been treated and reported as if they were distinct pathogens with more virulence than other methicillin-sensitive *S. aureus* strains. Clearly, the emergence of antibiotic-resistant organisms is of concern, and reasonable efforts should be made to reduce this occurrence; the unique concern, however, about methicillin-resistant strains in particular, above and beyond concern for *S. aureus* infection in general, that has caused temporary closure of care facilities and restriction of patient movement among levels of care must be weighed against the clinical and economic value of these added control practices.

In a unique report[5••], the virulence and pathologic significance of methicillin-resistant *S. aureus* strains compared with methicillin-sensitive strains causing infections in burned patients were evaluated. Colonization with any *S. aureus* was identified in 658 burned patients, treated during a six year period. In 319 of the patients, colonization by methicillin-resistant *S. aureus* was identified. A total of 253 staphylococcal infections occurred in 178 patients. Fifty-eight per cent of the infections were pulmonary and 38 percent were bacteremic. In 58 of the 178 patients (32.6 percent), infections were caused by methicillin resistant *S. aureus*.

A severity index based on multiple logistic regression analysis of mortality in thermally injured patients was used to compare outcomes in patients infected by methicillin-resistant and methicillin-sensitive strains of *S. aureus*[6••]. In both groups, all patients were treated with vancomycin, and no differences in the observed and predicted mortality were found between groups. These results seriously questioned the need for unique precaution, isolation, or treatment in patients with methicillinresistant infection. Nevertheless, these concerns persist and continue to appear in the medical literature[7].

The availability of vancomycin in a generic formulation and its efficacy with twice-daily dosing regimens have increased its economic appeal in the treatment of staphylococcal infections. Additionally, the newer formulations appear to be associated with less ototoxicity and nephrotoxicity than previously reported. The main concern related to frequent use of vancomycin is the possible development of vancomycin-resistant *S. aureus*, prompted by the recent recognition of vancomycin-resistant strains of *Enterococcus* species. The clinical development of vancomycin-resistant staphylococcal strains, however, is yet to be reported. To avoid inappropriate prescription of this and other antibiotics, strict criteria for antibiotic use based on the prevalence of resistant organisms at individual institutions and for diagnosing specific infections in burned patients should be adopted at each burn center.

315

Pneumonia

The improved survival of patients with massive burns has been associated with a relative increase in infections in sites other than the burn wound as principal causes of morbidity and death[4••]. Pneumonia is now the most frequent septic complication after thermal injury, and, as the incidence of invasive burn wound infection has decreased, bronchopneumonia has surpassed hematogenous pneumonia as the predominant form. Other factors contributing to this epidemiologic change are listed in Table 24.2.

In a review encompassing a recent five year period at our burn center[8], pneumonia occurred in 169 out of 988 burned patients who were admitted. In 91 of the 166 fatally burned patients cared for during that period, pneumonia was present, and it was considered to be the primary cause of death in half of the patients who died.

The relative increase in the frequency of airborne pneumonia may also be, in part, attributed to improved survival in patients with severe smoke inhalation injury. Rue *et al.*[9••], using a logistic regression-derived mortality predictor based on patient age and extent of burn, recently compared the contemporary co-morbidity of inhalation injury and pneumonia with an historic cohort previously reported from the same institution[10]. Patients in the more recent period had a significantly lower mortality than predicted (29.4 percent compared with 41.4 percent). Patients with inhalation injury found on bronchoscopy, which was associated with a more severe injury, showed some improvement in outcome from that predicted (38.3 percent compared with 50.2 percent), but the rate of pneumonia was not different between cohorts.

A subset of 61 patients treated with high-frequency percussive ventilation was compared with patients treated with conventional

Table 24.2. Factors Associated with Emergence of Bronchopneumonia

Decreased incidence of burn wound infection.
Decreased incidence of suppurative thrombophlebitis.
Prolonged intubation of airway and gastrointestinal tract.
Perioperative antibiotic use.
Increased numbers of patients with inhalation injury.
Excessive fluid resuscitation.

volume-controlled ventilation[9**]. Despite similar age, burn size, and duration of intubation, the incidence of bronchopneumonia was markedly reduced, occurring in only 29.3 percent of the patients treated with percussive ventilation, compared with 52.3 percent of conventionally ventilated patients. Additionally, mortality was significantly less in patients treated with percussive ventilation than in the conventionally ventilated patients (16.4 percent compared with 42.7 percent) and significantly less than that predicted from the mortality predictor (16.4 percent compared with 40.9 percent).

In this study[9**], the combined effects of general improvement in care of all burned patients and the prevention of pneumonia by high-frequency percussive ventilation were shown to reduced mortality, compared with patients with pneumonia, and it significantly affected the survival of all patients with inhalation injury. This ventilatory mode appeared to have the beneficial therapeutic effect of facilitating the removal of endobronchial secretions and cellular debris while ventilating at airway pressures lower than those applied with conventional ventilation. Such effects interrupted the usual pathologic sequelae of severe inhalation injury and prevented or minimized small airway obstruction, distal atelectasis, progressive barotrauma, and pneumonia.

Hematogenous pneumonia is now encountered more rarely than bronchopneumonia and usually occurs later in the hospital course. Remote septic foci such as invasive wound infection, endocarditis, or suppurative thrombophlebitis are common causes. The radiographic hallmark is a solitary nodular pulmonary infiltrate, but progression to multiple nodular infiltrates throughout the lungs may occur. All possible sites of infection must be evaluated if a characteristic nodular pulmonary infiltrate appears, and the primary infection must be identified and treated. The pneumonic process is treated by systemic administration of antibiotics directed against the causative organism and ventilatory support as needed.

In addition to the relative change in frequency of pneumonia, the predominant organisms causing pneumonia in burned patients have changed markedly during the past decade. In 1982, *P aeruginosa* was considered the causative organism in 32 percent of the pneumonias occurring that year and S. *aureus* the causative organism of only 24 percent. In 1989, S. *aureus* was identified as the cause of 48 percent of pneumonias and *P aeruginosa* the cause of merely 16 percent after burn injury. A similar trend in the emergence of Gram-positive organisms as the predominant flora responsible for pneumonia and other infections after burns has been documented at other institutions [11, 12].

Infections at Other Sites

The control of invasive burn wound infection and the overall decrease in incidence of pneumonia have been associated with a relative increase in infections in other sites; the actual number of these infections, however, has decreased from previous years: suppurative thrombophlebitis is an example. At our institution, the incidence of suppurative thrombophlebitis decreased from 6.9 percent) of patients treated during 1969 and 1970 to 1.4 percent during 1977 and 1978. From the middle of 1982 to December 1990, only sixteen cases in 2268 burned patients were documented (0.71 percent)[4**]. Strict cannula discipline that limits cannula residence at a single site to a maximum of 72 hours and the current approach to wound care have contributed significantly to the marked decline of this infection. In recent years, much like colonization of the respiratory tract, staphylococci have replaced Gram-negative organisms as the predominant cause of suppurative thrombophlebitis, and nonbacterial pathogens have emerged as causative organisms. Early diagnosis and prompt surgical excision of the involved vein before hematogenous dissemination of the infecting organisms reduces the morbidity and mortality associated with this complication.

Acute infective endocarditis is an infrequent but well described site of infection in burned patients that has occurred in 1.3 percent of patients in recent years. Burn wound manipulation, prolonged intravenous cannulation, and septic thrombophlebitis are the most common sources of bacteria producing this complication. Preventive measures include effective topical antimicrobial therapy, timely excision and closure of the burn wound, and early discontinuation or frequent replacement of intravenous cannulae. *S. aureus* is the most common causative organism, and the right side of the heart is most frequently affected. Recurrent staphylococcal bacteremia in a burned patient with sepsis and no other apparent identifiable source of infection should suggest the diagnosis; heart murmurs are often difficult to diagnose in hyperdynamic, tachycardic patients. Transesophageal echocardiography is the preferred examination to detect valvular lesions. Systemic maximal-dose antibiotic therapy is directed against the causative organism and continued for six weeks after the last positive blood culture.

The occurrence of paranasal sinusitis and infections of the urinary tract are related to the presence of the foreign materials of the tubes, cannulae, and catheters placed to gain access to the alimentary tract, airway, or urinary bladder, respectively. The incidence of both of these infections increases with the duration of cannulation, arguing for prompt removal of the catheters for effective prevention of these infections.

In a study of sinusitis in transnasally intubated burned patients[13], 8 out of 22 patients who were intubated for more than seven days and underwent computed tomographic scan of all paranasal sinuses, with timing dictated by the patient's clinical condition, had findings consistent with sinusitis. Removal of all nasal tubes, application of topical nasal decongestants, and administration of culture-specific antibiotics were successful in treating the infection in all but one patient.

In association with the changes in burn wound care and patient management, the incidence of all infections, including bacteremia in burned patients, has also decreased. The increased mortality associated with Gram-negative bacteremia is not observed with Gram-positive bacteremia[14]. In addition, the present mortality associated with Gram-negative bacteremia usually caused by normal host flora is significantly less than that caused in the past by endemic infecting strains that were often resistant to multiple antibiotics[2].

The emergence of Gram-positive organisms as the predominant flora has contributed to a lessening in the impact of infection. The virulence of *S. aureus*, however, may be strain-specific. Bacteremia resulting from strains of *S. aureus* possessing the gene for the production of toxic shock syndrome toxin-1 has been associated with episodes of unexplained profound hemodynamic instability in several burned patients treated by us and described by others[15, 16]. This gene, however, has been identified in *S. aureus* strains recovered from patients with various infections, bacteremia, or wound colonization without evidence of profound physiologic alteration.

In burned patients with staphylococcal infections who manifest hemodynamic instability that responds poorly to treatment and that is out of proportion to that usually encountered in Gram-positive infections, the diagnosis of a variant of toxic shock syndrome should be considered. Acute management first requires aggressive intravenous fluid resuscitation to regain hemodynamic stability. Vancomycin should be administered intravenously unless the organism is known to be sensitive to methicillin, in which case a beta-lactamase-resistant antistaphylococcal antibiotic such as nafcillin may be given.

An antitoxin to the toxic shock syndrome toxin-1 is not clinically available. The prevalence of antibodies against the toxin is more than 90 percent in the general population, and nearly all patients with toxic shock syndrome related to menstruation have had undetectable antibodies at onset of the disease. Although this relationship has not been confirmed in burned patients with staphylococcal infections and clinical evidence of toxic shock syndrome, the isolation of a strain of *S. aureus* that produces the toxic shock syndrome toxin-1 and the absence of circulating antibodies to the toxin may establish the diagnosis.

Systemic Inflammatory Response

Prolongation of the time until death of nonsurviving burned patients and the overall reduction in the number of patients succumbing to infections have generated an increased awareness of the occurrence of multiple system organ failure and the systemic inflammatory response syndrome. Consequently, studies of the pathogenesis of systemic inflammation have markedly proliferated, with special emphasis on identifying important causal factors and mechanisms.

Cytokines

The cellular response to injury and infection has been associated with systemic liberation of cytokines such as tumor necrosis factor α, interleukin-1ß, and interleukin-6, and these cytokines have been extensively studied in various inflammatory diseases. The contributions of these cytokines to the initiation and perpetuation of the hypermetabolic state after burns and the host response to infection have recently been described[17, 18]. In serial plasma samples obtained from 27 thermally injured patients, interleukin-1ß, interleukin-6, and tumor necrosis factor α were measured by enzyme-linked immunosorbent assay, and correlations between core temperature and the presence or absence of infection were assessed. Interleukin-1ß responded modestly to injury alone but showed little response to infection, whereas interleukin-6 and tumor necrosis factor-α levels were increased in severely infected patients compared with patients who remained free of infection. Interleukin-6 and interleukin-1ß were also positively correlated with increases in core temperature. These results suggest that, in thermally injured patients, the observed alterations in cytokine concentrations may represent the effect rather than the cause of infection.

Bacterial Translocation

The concept that the gut plays a central role in the initiation and maintenance of a persistent catabolic state in severely injured patients has gained substantial popularity. Severe injury has been clearly associated with breakdown of gut mucosal integrity in animals and humans. Intestinal permeability has been shown to be increased shortly after injury [19] and increased before and during episodes of sepsis[20]. Endotoxin has been identified in the blood of burned patients within hours of injury, but no direct proof has been found that the endotoxin originates in the gut[21].

In a recent prospective, randomized clinical study of 76 burned patients[22]**, half of the patients were given intravenous polymyxin B for one week after the burn in doses designed to neutralize circulating endotoxin. The reduction in plasma endotoxin concentration compared with controls was statistically significant, although no reductions in interleukin-6 levels, Baltimore sepsis scores, or mortality were seen.

In recent clinical studies evaluating portal vein bacteremia[23] and the presence of bacteria in mesenteric lymph nodes[24] after mechanical trauma, investigators have also failed to substantiate the occurrence of significant bacterial translocation in humans. These recent studies seriously question whether alteration in intestinal permeability results in infection or represents only an epiphenomenon; the significance of bacterial translocation in the pathogenesis of clinical infection or systemic inflammation must also be questioned because of the lack of clinically significant bacteremia and endotoxemia in patients.

Granulocyte Response

Burn injury elicits a response from the immune system that is proportional to the extent of the burn and that causes impaired function in some cells while sensitizing other cells such that a second insult induces an exaggerated and prolonged response. The metabolic products of activated leukocytes such as cytokines and reactive oxygen species may act beneficially to enhance host resistance or deleteriously to depress remote organ function through an overwhelming systemic inflammatory response. Although the complexity of the leukocyte response to burn injury has not allowed formulation of a unifying hypothesis other than that of global immuno-suppression, recent studies have shown that, particularly in the case of granulocytes, certain characteristics once thought to represent hypofunction of polymorphonuclear leukocytes were actually due to systemic activation of these cells.

The classic observations documenting defects in chemotaxis, phagocytosis, bactericidal capacity, and superoxide and hydrogen peroxide production in granulocytes of thermally injured patients have been interpreted as evidence of dysfunction in these cells. Conversely, the concept of systemic activation of neutrophils after thermal injury has been supported in the recent literature. The historical development of the theories and evidence of polymorphonuclear leukocyte activation are thoroughly covered in a recent review by Cioffi et al.[25**].

In a recent study by the same authors[26], the effect of thermal injury on the oxidative potential of granulocytes serially collected from burned patients was evaluated by a fluorescent technique. Unstimulated granulocytes from burned patients showed a significantly higher baseline activity than did unstimulated cells from controls. The granulocytes from burned patients also displayed greater than normal oxidase activity after in-vitro stimulation by phorbal myristate acetate, suggesting in-vivo activation and priming for an exaggerated response to a second insult.

Other evidence for in-vivo neutrophil activation has been reported by Dobke *et al.*[27], who demonstrated that the resting oxygen uptake of neutrophils was significantly increased in burned patients, compared with controls.

The "second hit" concept, in which specific priming and activation sequences are postulated to result in significant in-vivo tissue injury, has recently been proposed on the basis of laboratory studies in a murine model[28]. In rats, low-dose lipopolysaccharide administration caused a priming of neutrophils that was partially mediated by platelet activating factor. Subsequent exposure of those cells to a non-injurious dose of f-met-leu-phe resulted in significant pulmonary injury. The organ injury was blocked by administration of a platelet activating factor antagonist before the challenge, suggesting that platelet activating factor was at least partially responsible for the neutrophil priming observed.

The function of neutrophils in a tissue matrix environment may also be very different from that of circulating cells. Various cell-surface receptors[29, 30, 31] are expressed after stimulation by various mediators, resulting in cell adherence and migration. Neutrophils adherent to extracellular matrix proteins such as fibronectin or laminin have been shown to be capable of a large respiratory burst in response to small quantities of cytokines compared with cells in aqueous suspension. The clinical importance of this observation remains undefined.

As a means of improving granulocyte function after burn injury, the administration of granulocyte-macrophage colony-stimulating factor to thermally injured patients has been studied[32]. In addition to stimulating proliferation of granulocyte and macrophage progenitor cells, this agent increases macrophage phagocytic and cytocidal activity, granulocyte RNA and protein synthesis, granulocyte oxidative metabolism, and antibody dependent cytotoxic killing in mature cells *in vitro.*

Treatment by Granulocyte-macrophage colony-stimulating factor in a small cohort of burned patients[32] increased granulocyte counts by 50 percent and reduced granulocyte cytosolic oxidative function and myeloperoxidase activity to control levels without changing superoxide production. After treatment was stopped, however, superoxide activity increased compared with untreated burned patients. These findings caution against clinical extrapolation of in-vitro results. A reduction in myeloperoxidase activity may actually be detrimental because bactericidal capability may be compromised, and increased superoxide production could potentiate endothelial cell damage, leading to increased capillary permeability and contributing to the systemic inflammatory response syndrome.

The inability of immunomodulatory drugs to alter significantly changes in immune function after burns may simply represent the inability of single agents to influence the complex and redundant cascade of pathophysiologic events occurring in extensively burned patients.

The clinical signs of infection or a systemic inflammatory response-like syndrome are often indistinguishable from those of uninfected hypermetabolic patients with extensive burns and include hyperthermia, tachycardia, tachypnea, glucose intolerance, and hyperdynamic circulation. Distinguishing between infection, hypermetabolism, and the "sepsis syndrome" is problematic both clinically with regard to initiating appropriate treatment and investigationally with regard to grouping patients according to the mechanism responsible for the altered physiology.

In an attempt to facilitate earlier identification of infected patients, serum neopterin, which is released by activated mononuclear leukocytes, was serially measured in burned patients and correlated with the development of infection[33]. Elevated levels correlated with the presence of infection and were sometimes elevated for up to ten days before treatment was started. Because of the similarity in clinical presentation of infections and inflammatory or hypermetabolic conditions, a laboratory tool that permits accurate and reliable separation of the entities would be extremely useful.

Conclusion

Despite significant improvement in the survival of thermally injured patients, infectious complications continue to be a significant source of morbidity and mortality. Control of invasive burn wound infection by effective topical antimicrobial agents and timely excision and skin grafting of the burn wound have been associated with changes in the predominant sites and types of infection. Strict isolation techniques and improved wound care have successfully controlled infections due to Gram-negative organisms. These infections have been supplanted by infections caused by true fungi, yeast, and multiple antibiotic resistant bacteria.

Improvements in fluid management, wound care, and nutritional support have markedly reduced early mortality from thermal injury and prolonged the hospital course of nonsurvivors. Thus, increased emphasis has been placed on elucidation of the systemic inflammatory response syndrome and multiple system organ failure as potential targets for future therapeutic interventions.

Despite a fervor of research activity, the complexity of the pathophysiologic events causing the systemic inflammatory response has limited the success of interventions intended to ameliorate cellular injury. Continued efforts to define the roles of the various immunologic cell populations and their cytokine mediators in the initiation and propagation of this response may eventually permit selective interruption of the deleterious effects of this redundant cascade.

References and Recommended Reading

papers of Particular Interest have been highlighted as:

- of special interest
- • of outstanding interest

1. Cioffi WG, Kim SH, Pruitt BA Jr: *Cause of Mortality in Thermally Injured Patients*. In Die Infektion beim Brandverletzten, Proceedings of the "Infektionsprophylaxe und infektionsbekampfung beim Brandverletzten" International Symposium. Edited by Lorenz S, Zellner PR. Darmstadt: Steinkopff Verlag; 1993:7-11.

2. McManus AT, Mason AD Jr, McManus WF, Pruitt BA Jr: Control of Pseudomonas aeruginosa infections in Burned Patients. *Surg Res Commun* 1992, 12:61-67.

3. Becker WK, Cioffi WG Jr, McManus AT, Kim SH, McManus WF, Mason AD, Pruitt BA Jr: Fungal Burn Wound Infection. *Arch Surg* 1991, 126:44-48.

4. •• Pruitt BA Jr, McManus AT. The Changing Epidemiology of infection in Burn Patients. *World J Surg* 1992, 16:57-67.

    A comprehensive review relating the evolution of burn care to the changing epidemiology of infection after thermal injury.

5. Bale JF Jr, Kealey GP, Massanari RM, Strauss RG: The Epidemiology of Cytomegalovirus Infection among Patients with Burns. *Control Hosp Epidemiol* 1990, 11:17.

6. •• McManus AT, Mason AD Jr, McManus WF, Pruitt BA Jr: What's in a Name? Is Methicillin-Resistant Staphylococcus aureus just Another S. aureus when Treated with Vancomycin? *Arch Surg* 1989, 124:1456-1459.

    The virulence and pathologic significance of methicillin-resistant strains of Staphylococcus aureus were compared with methicillin-sensitive strains isolated from burned patients. Vancomycin was used to treat all patients with S. *aureus* infections, and no difference in outcome was observed.

7. Pegg SP: Multiple Resistant Staphylococcus aureus. *Ann Acad Med* 1992, 21:664-666.

8. Pruitt BA Jr: Cadaverous Particles and Infection in Injured Man. *Eur J Surg* 1993, 159:515-520.

9. •• Rue LW III, Cioffi WG, Mason AD, McManus WF, Pruitt BA Jr: Improved Survival of Burned Patients with Inhalation Injury. *Arch Surg* 1993, 128:772-780.

    The improvements in the care of thermally injured patients and the use of high-frequency percussive ventilation in patients with smoke inhalation injury resulted in a decreased incidence of pneumonia and improved survival.

10. Shirani KZ, McManus AT, Vaughan GM, McManus WF, Pruitt BA Jr, Mason AD Jr: Effects of Environment on Infection in Burn Patients. *Arch Surg* 1986, 121:31-36.

11. Taylor GD, Kibsey P, Kirkland T, Burroughs E, Tredget E: Predominance of Staphylococcal organisms in Infections occurring in a Burns Intensive Care Unit. *Burns* 1992, 18:332-335.

12. Frame JD, Kangesu L, Malik WM: Changing Flora in Burn and Trauma Units: Experience in the United Kingdom. *J Burn Care Rehabil* 1992, 13:2816-286.

13. Bowers BL, Purdue GF, Hunt JL: Paranasal Sinusitis in Burn Patients following Nasotracheal Intubation. *Arch Surg* 1991, 126:1411-1412.

14. Mason AD Jr, McManus AT, Pruitt BA Jr: Association of Burn Mortality and Bacteremia. *Arch Surg* 1986, 121:1027-1031.

15. Frame JD, Eve MD, Hackett MEJ, Dowsett EG, Brain AN, Gault DT, Wilmshurst AD: The Toxic Shock Syndrome in Burned Children. *Burns* 1986, 11:234-241.

16. Egan WC, Clark WR: The Toxic Shock Syndrome in a Burned Victim. Burns 1988, 14:135.

17. Drost AC, Burleson DG, Cioffi WG Jr, Mason AD Jr, Pruitt BA Jr: Plasma Cytokines after Thermal Injury and their Relationship to Infection. *Ann Surg* 1993, 218:74-78.

18. Drost AC, Burleson DG, Cioffi WG Jr, Jordan BS, Mason AD Jr, Pruitt BA Jr: Plasma Cytokines following Thermal Injury and their Relationship with Patient Mortality, Burn Size and Time Postburn. *J Trauma* 1993, 35:335-339.

19. Deitch EA: Intestinal Permeability is Increased in Burn Patients Shortly after Injuries. *Arch Surg* 1990, 107:411-416.

20. LeVoyer T, Cioffi WG Jr, Pratt L, Shippee R, McManus WF, Mason AD Jr, Pruitt BA Jr: Alterations in Intestinal Permeability after Thermal injury. *Arch Surg* 1992, 127:26-30.

21. Winchurch RA, Thupari JN, Munster AM: Endotoxemia in Burn Patients: Levels of Circulating Endotoxins are Related to Burn Size. *Surgery* 1987, 102:808-812.

22. •• Munster AM, Smith-Meek M, Dickerson C, Winchurch RA: Translocation. Incidental Phenomenon or True Pathology? *Ann Surg* 1993, 218:321-327.

    A randomized, prospective clinical study of 76 burned patients, in which the impact of intravenous polymyxin B therapy on circulating endotoxin levels and outcome were evaluated. Plasma endotoxin levels significantly decreased, whereas interleukin-6 levels, Baltimore sepsis scores, and mortality were unaffected.

23. Moore FA, Moore EE, Poggetti R, McAnena Oj, Peterson VM, Abernathy CM, Parsons PE: Gut Bacterial Translocation via the Portal Vein: A Clinical Perspective with Major Torso Trauma. *J Trauma* 1991, 31:629-638.

24. Peitzman AB, Udekwu AO, Ochoa J, Smith S: Bacterial Translocation in Trauma Patients. *J Trauma* 1991, 31:1083-1087.

25. •• Cioffi WG, Burleson DG, Pruitt BA Jr: Leukocyte Responses to Injury. *Arch Surg* 1993, 128:1260-1267.

A current review of the literature, in which the pathophysiologic changes in leukocyte populations after burn injury were described. Evidence for leukocyte immunosuppression and activation was discussed.

26. Cioffi WG Jr, Burleson DG, Jordan BS, Mason AD Jr, Pruitt BA Jr: Granulocyte Oxidative Activity after Thermal Injury. *Surgery* 1992, 112:860-865.

27. Dobke MK, Deitch EA, Harner Tj, Baxter CR: Oxidative Activity of Polymorphonuclear Leukocytes after Thermal Injury. *Arch Surg* 1989, 124:856-859.

28. Anderson BO, Harken AH: Multiple Organ failure: Inflammatory Priming and Activation Sequences Promote Autologous Tissue Injury. *J Trauma* 1990, 30(suppl):44-49.

29. de la Ossa JC, Malago M, Gewertz BL: Neutrophil-Endothelial Cell Binding in Neutrophil-Mediated Tissue Injury. *J Surg Res* 1992, 53:103-107.

30. Mileski W, Borgstrom D, Lightfoot E, Rothlein R, Faanes R, Lipsky P, Baxter: Inhibition of Leukocyte-Endothelial Adherence following Thermal Injury. *J Surg Res* 1992, 52:334-339.

31. Bevilacqua MP, Nelson RM: Selectins. J Clin Invest 1993, 91:379-387.

32. Cioffi WG Jr, Burleson DG, Jordan BS, Becker WK, McManus WF, Mason AD Jr, Pruitt BA Jr: Effects of Granulocyte-Macrophage Colony-Stimulating Factor in Burn Patients. *Arch Surg* 1991, 126:74-79.

33. Burleson DG, Johnson A, Salin M, Mason AD Jr, Pruitt BA Jr:
     Identification of Neopterin as a Potential Indicator of Infec-
     tion in Burned Patients. *Proc Soc Exp Biol Med* 1992,
     199:305-310.

— by David W. Mozingo and Basil A. Pruitt Jr

David W Mozingo and Basil A. Pruitt Jr, US Army Institute of Surgical Research, 2322 Harney Road, Fort Sam Houston, TX 78234-6315,
USA.

Chapter 25

Nutrition in Patients with Severe Burns

Abstract

Postburn hypermetabolism can lead rapidly to deleterious consequences if adequate nutrition support is not provided. Several predictive formulas are used currently for estimation of the nutrition needs of both adult and pediatric patients with burn injuries. Adequacy of enteral or parenteral or both deliveries of nutrients must be interpreted in light of injury-induced effects on nutrition parameters. (J Burn Care, Rehabil 1996;17:62-70).

State of the Art

Severe burn injuries create an extreme state of physiologic stress. No other single insult results in such an accelerated rate of tissue catabolism, loss of lean body mass, and depletion of energy and protein reserves.[1,2] Multiple factors contribute to the postburn hypermetabolic response. After burn injury, metabolic rate reportedly is raised by increased levels of circulating catecholamines, glucagon, and cortisol; increased body temperatures; cool environmental temperatures; extent and depth of the burn wounds; evaporative losses from burn wounds; and infectious complications.[2,4] Occlusive dressings, warm ambient temperatures, and drug therapy such as ibuprofen can partially alleviate hypermetabolism.[3,5]

To prevent the detrimental consequences of postburn hypermetabolism, close attention to nutrition needs and aggressive nutrition support is essential. The purposes of this chapter are to summarize the methods of calculating and delivering nutrient requirements, and to review appropriate nutrition assessment parameters for patients with burn injuries.

Adult Nutritional Requirements

Calories. Patients with severe burn injuries require caloric deliveries elevated above basal requirements to meet increased energy expenditures.[6,8] The formulas that exist for predicting needs are flawed due to their inability to account for environmental temperatures and humidity, inhalation injury, dressing changes, skin grafting, pain, anxiety, use of sedatives, and varying activity levels. Values obtained from predictive formulas are approximate and should be used as guidelines only. Many burn-injury, dietetics professionals compare different formulas to determine ranges for estimated needs rather than absolute values.

Curreri[9]: 25 kcal/kg + 40 kcal/% TBSA burn

Long[1,13]: Basal energy expenditure (BEE) × activity × injury
  factors
  BEE for males–66.5 + (13.8 × wt) + (5 × ht) – (6.8 × age)
  BEE for females–655 + (9.6 × wt) + (1.9 × ht) – (4.7 × age)
    (Weight in kilograms, height in centimeters, age in years)
  Activity factor–1.2 (confined to bed)
              1.3 (out of bed)
  Injury factor for severe thermal burn–2.10

Ireton-Jones[7]:
  EEE (v) = 1925 – 10(A) + 5(W) + 281(S) + 292(T) + 851(B)
  EEE (sp) = 629 – 11(A) + 25(W) – 609(O)

EEE, Estimated Energy Expenditure kilocalories/day; *V*, ventilator dependent; *sp*, spontaneous breathing; *A*, age; *W*, weight in kilograms; *S*, sex (male 1, female 0); *T*, trauma; *B*, burns; *O*, obesity; (present 1, absent 0).

Figure 25.1. Adult formulas for calculating caloric requirements

According to a recent survey of burn units,[8] the most common methods of calculating adult energy needs are the Curreri formula and variations of the Harris-Benedict equation (BEE) (Figure 25.1). The Curreri formula, which uses only body weight and the percentage of total body surface area (TBSA) burned, is a regression equation that is predicated on the amount of calories needed for weight maintenance.[9] Investigators have found this formula to overestimate caloric requirements when compared to actual energy expenditures.[10,12] To modify the BEE for severe burns, an injury factor of 2.1, in addition to the activity factors of 1.2 to 1.3, has been suggested by Long.[13] However, allowances for different percentages of TBSA burned are not made with Long's formula. Others use the BEE with variable injury factors according to the percentage of TBSA burned as follows: 1.2 to 1.4 (<20 percent TBSA); 1.6 (20 percent to 25 percent TBSA); 1.7 (25 percent to 30 percent TBSA); 1.8 (30 percent to 35 percent TBSA); 1.9 (35 percent to 40 percent TBSA); 2.0 (40 percent to 45 percent TBSA); and 2.1 (>45 percent TBSA).[8]

Two alternative formulas, distinguished by ventilatory status, have been suggested by Ireton-Jones[7] (Figure 25.1). These formulas account for the presence of burn injuries, but not the extent or depth of the burns. The effect of the size of the burn wound on metabolic rate is a controversial issue.

Measured energy expenditure (MEE) by indirect calorimetry is the best method for determining caloric requirements.[10,12] Actual indirect calorimetry measurements have demonstrated the inaccuracies in predicting energy needs due to individual variations, daily fluctuations, operative procedures, and different stages of rehabilitation. A factor of 20 percent to 30 percent above the MEE is recommended to account for activity and stress of treatments.[12] Twice-weekly metabolic cart studies have been suggested because of changes in energy expenditures during a patient's clinical course.[6] Goals recommended for caloric distribution have been approximately 20 percent as protein, 50 percent as carbohydrate, and 30 percent as fat.[2,6,8.]

Protein. Because of the increased demand for protein for gluconeogenesis in the acute phase, for healing of extensive wounds, and for replacement of nitrogen losses from wounds and in the urine, more protein than the recommended daily allowances (RDA) is needed after severe burn injury. Current recommendations are based on 1.5 to 3.0 grams of protein per kilogram of ideal body weight (IBW), depending on the percentage of TBSA burn[14,18] or 20 percent of total kilocalories as protein.[6,8]

Specific amino acids have been under investigation to determine their roles in certain metabolic processes. In animals with 30 percent TBSA burns, arginine supplementation in the amount of 2 percent of the total calorie requirements appears to correlate with improved immunocompetence and survival.[16] A significant reduction in wound infection and in length of stay was demonstrated in patients with burn injuries with the use of a modular tube feeding that contains 9 percent of the protein source as arginine.[17] Other components of this tube feeding could also have contributed to these improved outcomes. The role of increased amounts of glutamine in patients with severe burns has not been established to this date. However, glutamine has a theoretic advantage in these patients because of its role in preserving the gut mucosa during stressed states. Branched-chain-amino-acid supplementation has not been shown to have beneficial effects on lean body mass preservation in patients with severe burns.[18] In comparison to free amino acids, intact protein has been associated with better weight maintenance, improved visceral protein status, and better survival after burn injury in animals.[19]

Carbohydrate. Glucose is an important energy source to promote sparing of lean body mass in patients with burns. However, there are limits to the amount of glucose that injured patients can metabolize. The optimal carbohydrate delivery of five mg of glucose per kilogram of body weight per minute has been established by Burke et al.[20] Excessive carbohydrate administration results in hyperglycemia and increased carbon dioxide production. Hepatic lipogenesis and liver function abnormalities can develop with excessive parenteral administration.

Fat. The fat distribution of 30 percent of total calories is commonly used by burn-injury dietetics professionals.[8] However, large amounts of fat, especially ω6 fatty acids, can have an immunosuppressive effect by stimulating the release of arachidonic acid. This precursor leads to the formation of prostaglandins that depress delayed cell-mediated hypersensitivity, lymphocyte proliferation, and natural killer-cell function.[6] ω3 Fatty acids, which are mainly found in fish oil and marine products, may have a beneficial effect on immunocompetence in patients with burn injuries.[7] Diets containing 15 percent to 20 percent of nonprotein calories as fat appear to be optimal.[21] Provision of adequate calories may be difficult, though, when fat intake is limited. The minimum amount of linoleic acid needed to prevent essential fatty acid deficiency is approximately 4 percent of total calories consumed.[18]

Occupational

615.8515

Burns-Rod

617.11

Critical Care

616.028

Micronutrients. Criteria for prescribing vitamins and minerals in individual patients include preburn nutritional status, dietary intakes, burn size, wound healing, and laboratory data.[18] Although specific vitamin and mineral requirements of patients with severe burns have not been established, provision of at least the RDA has been advocated.[15,22] For those micronutrients that are known to be beneficial in terms of wound healing—zinc, vitamins A and C, amounts in addition to the RDA should be given. Recommendations for micronutrient supplementation have been published by Gottschlich and Warden [22](Table 25.1).

Table 25.1. Vitamin and trace element recommendations[22,26]

IU, International unit.

> Minor burns (<10 percent-20 percent TBSA)
> > One multivitamin daily (all ages)
> Severe burns (>10 percent-20 percent TBSA)
> > One multivitamin daily (all ages)
> Ascorbic acid
> > 250 mg twice daily (<3 years of age)
> > 500 mg twice daily (all ages >3 years)
> Vitamin A
> > 5000 IU daily (<3 years of age)
> > 10,000 IU daily (all ages >3 years)
> Zinc sulfate
> > 100 mg daily (< 3 years of age)
> > 220 mg daily (all ages >3 years)

Pediatric Nutritional Requirements

More than 35 percent of burn victims in the United States are children. Infants and toddlers are at the greatest risk for major burn injuries, with scald burns comprising 72 percent of the total number.[23] Adolescent males are also at risk for burn injuries associated with attempts to increase the burning rates of existing fires, to clean with petroleum products, or to respond to peer-related dares. Pediatric patients with burn injuries present unique nutritional challenges due to their limited fat and lean body mass reserves, high basal metabolic requirements, increased body surface area (BSA) in relation to weight, and extra needs for growth and development, especially during infant and adolescent growth spurts.[24]

Calories. Unique determinants of caloric expenditures in pediatric patients include needs for growth and small caloric reserves. In addition, the larger BSA-to-weight ratio in children necessitates more calories per kilogram to meet basal metabolic needs than needed by adults.[24] Precise energy requirements for different age groups remain ill defined.

Various formulas for estimating caloric requirements of pediatric patients with burns have been suggested. Recently a questionnaire was mailed to 206 burn-injury dietetics professionals in the United States and Canada to determine actual burn nutrition practices. Forty-six burn-injury dietetics professionals responded and indicated that more than 23 different methods are being used for estimating caloric needs for pediatric patients.[8] The most commonly used formulas are listed in Table 25.2. Use of the RDA for age and the Davies method were indicated in the survey as the two most popular methods for calculating pediatric caloric needs.[8,25] Long's modifications of the BEE also have been used to estimate caloric needs of burned children.[26] Although this method is typically used for adult patients with a variety of different disease states, a factor for age is included in the BEE regression equation.

Estimates of caloric needs from the Wolfe and the RDA formulas are almost identical.[27,28] These two formulas suggest the lowest calorie requirements of any of the predictive formulas. Bell et al.[29] prospectively evaluated caloric delivery based on Wolfe's formula (Table 25.2) and associated weight loss.[29] Weight changes of 42 patients with burns, including 27 children, were evaluated by subtracting discharge weights from the corresponding premorbid weights. Adjustments in weight changes were made for escharotomies and for normal growth rates in children younger than 18 years of age. Results showed that 35 of the total patients experienced weight loss within 10 percent of their premorbid weight. Six of the remaining patients had weight loss within 20 percent of their premorbid weights. These authors concluded that the basal metabolic rate (BMR) x 2 was adequate to prevent significant weight loss in most patients.[29] For pediatric patients with burns, the Wolfe or RDA method is recommended as a starting point to provide adequate caloric intake.

Table 25.2. Pediatric formulas for calculating caloric requirements

Davies[25]: 60 kcal/kg/day + 35 kcal/% TBSA/day
Wolfe[27,28]: BMR × 2

Sex and Age range (yr)	BMR Equation (wt in kg)
Males	
Birth-3	
3-10	$(60.9 \times wt) - 54$
10-18	$(22.7 \times wt) + 495$
Females	$(17.5 \times wt) + 651$
Birth-3	
3-10	$(61.0 \times wt) - 51$
10-18	$(22.5 \times wt) + 499$
	$(12.2 \times wt) + 746$

RDA[28]

Age (yr)	Kcal/kg	Basal calories
Birth-0.5	108	320
0.5-1.0	98	500
1-3	102	740
4-6	90	950
7-10	70	1130
Males 11-14	55	1440
Males 15-18	45	1760
Females 11-14	47	1310
Females 15-18	40	1370

Solomon[28,30] RDA for age + added needs for % burn

Weight (kg)	Kcal/% burn
0-9	15
10-13	20
14-18 (burns >40%)	20
14 (all other burns)	30

Curreri junior[31]
Birth-1 year: basal kcal from RDA + (15 kcal/% burn)
1-3 year: basal kcal from RDA + (25 kcal/% burn)
4-15 year: basal kcal from RDA + (40 kcal/% burn)

Hildreth[32-36]
Less than 1 year old: 2100 kcal/m^2 BSA + 1000 kcal/m^2 BSA burned
Less than 12 years of age: 1800 kcal/m^2 BSA + 2200 kcal/m^2 BSA burned
Less than 12 years of age (revised): 1800 kcal/m^2 BSA + 1300 kcal/m^2 BSA burned
12-18 years of age: 1500 kcal/m^2 BSA + 1500 kcal/m^2 BSA burned

Although the RDA is designed for healthy children, investigators suggest that this is a rational method for determining energy needs in burned children.[26] The RDA, in addition to other factors, accounts for physical activity. It is suggested that increased calorie requirements for hypermetabolism are offset by reduced activity levels after burn injuries. Solomon's formula, which incorporates the RDA with a factor for percentage of BSA burned, has also been suggested to predict calorie requirements.[30]

The Curreri Junior[31] formula, which has been shown to overestimate actual requirements, predicts calorie needs by use of regression analyses of weight loss in 30 pediatric patients with burns of less than 50 percent BSA (mean 16 percent BSA burned). The modified Curreri

Junior formula is based on the RDA for basal needs in addition to kcal/percent TBSA burn for three different age groups.[27]

Hildreth and Carvajal[32] evaluated the efficacy of the Galveston formula (1800 kcal/m^2 BSA+ 2200 kcal/m^2 BSA burned) in estimating daily caloric needs. This predictive formula considers heat losses associated with predicted fluid losses from evaporation and exudation from burn wounds. Fifty-two children (infants aged two weeks to children aged fifteen years) with burns in excess of 20 percent of their BSA were evaluated for caloric needs according to this formula. With use of the weight on the fourteenth day after burn as baseline (dry weight), the children were divided into two groups. In group one, 40 patients received calories as estimated by the Galveston formula and gained weight. In group two, twelve patients received less than the recommended calories and lost weight. The authors concluded that the Galveston formula was accurate in estimating caloric requirements in burned children. Their conclusion is reasonable; however, their estimates were not compared to actual MEE.

A more recent study by Hildreth et al.[33] compared kilocalories estimated by the original Hildreth and Carvajal study[32] and the Curreri Junior formula to the actual consumed kilocalories needed to maintain weight in pediatric patients with burns >30 percent TBSA. The 121 patients were divided into three age groups—birth to one year; one to three years; and four to fifteen years—coinciding with those in the Curreri Junior formulas. Results of these comparisons indicated that the actual intakes required for weight maintenance in each group were significantly lower than the requirements estimated from either of the two predictive formulas. Calories were overestimated from 10 percent to 45 percent when these two formulas were used. Earlier excision and grafting may have partially explained the decreased caloric needs. A significant difference was also noted between the one- to three-year age group (1521 ± 104 cal/m^2 burn/day) and the 4- to 15-year age group (1136±87 cal/m^2 burn/day) in caloric requirements needed to maintain weights. It was concluded that overfeeding occurs with the Galveston and Curreri Junior formulas, and that a formula that uses m^2 BSA burn (Table 25.2) is appropriate for children because of the wide ranges in body size at different ages.[33]

To more accurately determine caloric requirements for weight maintenance, Hildreth et al.[34] studied 102 patients less than 12 years of age with greater than 30 percent BSA burned. Patients were divided into group one (maintained weight at ±5 percent, $n = 65$), group 2 (gained over 5 percent dry weight, $n = 34$) or group 3 (lost more than 5 percent of their dry weight, $n = 3$). From multivariate-regression analysis, it was determined that 1800 kcal was a valid estimate of calories per BSA. The multiplier for burned surface area was then estimated to be 1300 kcal/m² by regression analysis. The revised version of Hildreth's previously recommended formula is (1800 kcal/m² BSA+ 1300 kcal/m² BSA burned), for each day throughout the hospital admissions of children younger than twelve years of age.[2]

Although infants and adolescents were included in Hildreth's nutrition studies, growth and development needs in these two age groups are unique. Further research studies by Hildreth et al.[35,36] have addressed these needs. Thirty pediatric patients less than one year old who had burns over 25 percent TBSA were evaluated. Actual intakes required for weight maintenance were 11 percent lower than the amount published in the original Galveston formula[32] and 7 percent lower than the calories indicated in the revised Galveston formula.[34] The currently recommended formula suggested for infants is (2100 kcal/m² BSA + 1000 kcal m² BSA burned) per day.[35]

On the basis of their experiences with infants and children, Cunningham et al.[37] agreed that fewer calories are needed to support wound healing than popular burn formulas predict. These investigators compared actual caloric intakes of ten children <3 years of age who had burns >30 percent TBSA with estimates of caloric needs from four formulas—Wolfe's formula, the original Galveston formula, the Curreri formula, and the Curreri Junior formula (Table 25.2). Wolfe's formula, or the BMR x 2, predicted the lowest calorie target of all four formulas. Results showed that delivered calories did not meet targeted goals, but averaged 88 percent, 120 percent, 130 percent, and 175 percent of BMR during weeks one through four, respectively. Regardless, weight was maintained at 95 percent ± 7.6 percent IBW and wound healing was supported. The researchers concluded that caloric provision of 120 percent to 200 percent BMR is sufficient for infants and children with severe burn injuries.[37]

Adolescents (ages 11 to 20 years), including 21 males and 8 females with burns involving more than 35 percent TBSA, were studied by Hildreth et al. These investigators used the same methods as in their previous studies. All 30 patients maintained their weight at ±5 percent of their dry weight. MEE was obtained during the first two weeks after injury. Actual intakes of all patients were compared to caloric requirements, as calculated retrospectively, according to the original Galveston formula[32] and the Curreri junior formula.[31] Calorie intakes required for weight maintenance (resting energy expenditure x 1.6) and MEE were significantly lower (by 29 percent to 45 percent) than either formula estimated. A formula unique for adolescents was suggested to be (1500 kcal/m^2 BSA+ 1500 kcal/ m^2 BSA burn) per day.[36]

Use of indirect calorimetry is recommended in pediatric patients for accurate determination of calorie needs. MEE multiplied by a factor of 1.3 provides for weight maintenance in pediatric patients with burns.[38]

Protein. As with adults, protein needs are commonly based on IBW. When fluid retention is suspected and preburn weight is not known, the 50th percentile weight for length is used to calculate IBW for infants.[37] If an accurate length cannot be obtained for an infant, the 50th percentile weight for age is used. For children less than one year of age, 3 gm to 4 gm protein/kg IBW is recommended to ensure successful graft coverage and healing.[27,39] Excessive protein is not advised for infants because of their lack of ability to tolerate high renal solute loads. Cunningham et al.[37] concluded from their study that 3 gm protein/kg/day equals or exceeds the estimated protein losses in children 3 years of age who have >30 percent BSA burned.[37]

For older children and adolescents, 1.5 gm to 2.5 gm protein/kg of IBW has been recommended by Bell and Wyatt.[15] Another method for estimating protein needs is the modified Solomon formula (RDA for age+ 1 gm per percent BSA burned).[30] Hutsler[30] has suggested the following formula: [(24-hour urinary urea nitrogen (UUN) x 1.1) + (1 gm for stool losses) + (estimated wound losses of nitrogen)[40]] x 6.25 gm protein/gm of nitrogen. A factor of 1.1 is used to estimate nonurea urinary nitrogen losses. Wound losses of nitrogen (N) are estimated by body weight and percentage of open wounds (0.02 gm N/kg body weight for 10 percent open burn wounds; 0.05 gm N/kg body weight for 11 percent to 30 percent open burn wounds; 0.12 gm N/kg body weight for >30 percent open burn wounds).[40]

Aggressive protein feeding has had beneficial effect for some children with severe burns. Alexander et al.[41] prospectively randomized eighteen children (mean BSA burned, 60 percent) into two groups. The control group received a balanced diet providing 16 percent of calories as protein. The high-protein group received approximately 25 percent of their caloric intake as protein. At the end of six weeks, the investigators reported higher levels of serum proteins and amino acids, greater retention of administered protein, more positive nitrogen balances, fewer infections, and better neutrophil function in those randomized to receive the protein-enriched diets.[41] Improvement in mortality rates and morbidity was achieved with aggressive protein delivery in the amount of 20 percent to 22 percent in comparison to 16 percent of the total calorie intake.

Carbohydrate. Carbohydrates have been recommended to provide between 40 percent and 50 percent of the calories.[8,26] Carbohydrates are more effective than fat in promoting nitrogen retention. For infants, parenteral infusion of 5 percent dextrose in water can be initiated at a rate of 5 mg/kg/minute and advanced to 15 mg/kg/minute over a two day period.[26] In older infants and children, current guidelines restrict 5 percent dextrose in water to a maximum of 5 to 7 mg/kg/minute. Although these guidelines have been established for parenteral administration, it seems prudent to use the same guidelines when enteral nutrition support is indicated.[15]

Fat. Conservative delivery of fat, especially linoleic acid or ω-6 fatty acids, is also recommended in pediatric patients. A fat intake of 2 percent to 3 percent of total calories is necessary to prevent essential fatty acid deficiency.[26] When intravenous lipids are administered to infants, a maximum of 4 gm fat/kg of IBW daily is recommended as an energy source.[39]

Micronutrients. Gottschlich and Warden [22] have recommended vitamin and mineral supplementations for different age groups (Table 25.1).[26] Beyond the RDA for most micronutrients, additional amounts are recommended for vitamins A and C and for those that may have increased losses through the wounds or urine, such as phosphorus,[39] zinc,[42] and water-soluble vitamins.

Phosphorus supplementation needs special attention. Massive urinary losses of extracellular ions begin immediately after burn injury and continue during acute care.[39] Intravenous potassium phosphate in the amounts of 1.5 to 2 mmol/L phosphate/kg may be necessary for children with severe hypophosphatemia. For phosphorus levels less than 2.0 mg/dl, intravenous supplementation of phosphate is recommended due to uncertain absorption of oral phosphate supplements.[30] When serum levels are above 2.0 mg/dl, phosphorus supplements (Neutra Phos), can be given in daily enteral doses of six to twelve capsules (250 mg phosphate/capsule).[30]

Methods

Feeding Modalities

Adequate oral intakes can often be achieved by patients with burns less than 20 percent BSA if attention is given to their food preferences. Calorie counts can provide a picture of dietary intake adequacy.

However, children especially may not understand the rationale for adequate nutritional intakes and may exhibit negative eating behaviors that interfere with intake goals. Several suggestions for improving the feeding behaviors of children in the burn unit were outlined by White and Kamples[43]:

1   Provide meals at a consistent time and in a predictable environment,

2   Eliminate distractions during mealtimes, such as the television,

3   Encourage but do not force the child to eat adequately,

4   Give assertive directions and positive reinforcements to the child, but ignore negative behaviors, and

5   Educate staff and parents on feeding intervention plans.

When patients with burns are unable to meet dietary intake goals orally, and when total BSA burned is >20 percent, more aggressive nutrition support is warranted. Nocturnal tube feedings to supplement dietary intake during the day may be adequate to meet nutrition needs.

If full nutrition support is required, the enteral route is preferred in comparison to total parenteral nutrition (TPN) to increase gut blood flow,[44] preserve gut function, maintain mucosal integrity,[45] decrease the incidence of metabolic imbalances, eliminate the risk of infection at the TPN catheter site, and decrease the cost of nutrient delivery. Despite common concerns about postburn gastric ileus, immediate intragastric feeding after burn injury (within 6 to 24 hours) has been shown to be safe and effective.[46,47] Initiation of enteral feeding within 48 hours may significantly reduce length of stay.[48] A reduction in the hypermetabolic response also has been illustrated with early enteral feeding because of the prevention of excessive secretion of hormones.[48,49,50.] Enteral nutrition support is not always possible because of tube obstruction and dislodgment problems and frequent nothing-by-mouth status for surgical procedures.

Withholding continuous enteral feedings is a common practice due to frequent surgical procedures. The safety and feasibility of providing enteral nutrition throughout operative procedures has been investigated.[51] When duodenal feedings were delivered with conscientious monitoring of tube position and of gastric reflux, intraoperative feedings were reported to be well tolerated and resulted in increased caloric intake and decreased wound infections.

Special enteral formulas designed for patients with burns do not exist. Commercial infant formulas are utilized when more aggressive nutrition support is needed for patients less than one year of age. An infant formula with 20 calories/ounce can be increased with glucose polymers (Polycose) or (Modual) or a lipid emulsion, (Microlipid) to a 24-to-30 calorie/ounce product to meet an infant's estimated energy needs. For children aged nine months through six years, isotonic products (Pediasure or Kindercal) with higher caloric density (30 calorie/ounce) can be used. Formulas designed for adults, especially those with high-calorie, and protein density, are recommended for children more than six years of age, adolescents, and adults. Modular protein supplements (ProMod, Propac, or Casec) can be added to commercial formulas to increase the protein content.

Increased deaths have been associated with the use of TPN in patients with severe burn injuries.[52] Therefore, TPN should be limited to only those patients whose gut is not functioning. Extreme short bowel, enteric fistulas, severe pancreatitis, and prolonged ileus are examples of indications for TPN.

Nutrition Assessment Parameters

Although anthropometric measurements, plasma protein levels, and tests of immunocompetence typically are useful for nutrition assessment, injuryinduced changes in these parameters occur after thermal injury. These changes are independent of nutritional status. Recommended assessment measurements include body weight, laboratory analyses, nitrogen balances, and nutritional intake records. In interpreting these measures, one must consider factors unique to thermal injuries. Each of these parameters should be viewed as only one part of the overall assessment.

Weight. Preburn weights are difficult to assess. Fluid resuscitation performed in the first 48 to 72, hours results in a significant increase in body weight. Usual weight can be estimated by subtracting the amount of fluid received for resuscitation from the actual weight with the calculation: 1 L of fluid = 1 kg of body weight.[8] After hospital admission, daily weights without dressings and splints are recommended.[27] Records or graphs of these serial weights can be used to visualize weight patterns. Growth charts are appropriate for evaluating long-term weight changes. Loss of lean body mass cannot be accepted as a normal consequence of burn injury. Under normal circumstances, children gain weight and grow on a continual basis.

Weight maintenance is probably a more realistic goal during the acute postinjury phase in children.

Laboratory analyses. In the survey conducted by Williamson,[8] serum albumin in addition to body weight were listed as the most universal nutrition assessment parameters. The patient with burns may have fluid shifts and protein losses through wounds that may distort serum albumin values. Trends in albumin levels over time can show the adequacy of long-term nutrition support. The value of total protein as an index of nutritional status in patients with severe burn injuries is not known.[39]

Although prealbumin decreases initially after postburn injury, it is the most sensitive indicator of nutrition adequacy because of its short half-life of two to three days.[30] Prealbumin levels are not affected by intravenous albumin infusions. Measurements of serum prealbumin levels are recommended twice weekly during the acute phase after burn injury.

Nitrogen balance studies. Nitrogen balance [24-hour N intake — (24-hour UUN + 4)] is a common method of determining adequacy of nutrition support in many burn centers.[8] Accurate determinations of nitrogen intake and nitrogen losses are necessary for clinical decision making. Nitrogen losses account for both UUN and nonurea urinary nitrogen. In nonstressed patients, UUN multiplied by a factor of 1.25 accounts for nonurea urinary nitrogen and estimates total urea nitrogen (TUN) excretions. However, in hypermetabolic states, large discrepancies exist between this estimate and actual measurements of TUN.[53] When available, TUN is the most accurate method for determining urinary nitrogen losses.

Nitrogen balance studies are prone to considerable errors due to integumental losses through open, ungrafted wounds. Nitrogen balance calculations should be modified to include estimates of wound losses. Although work has been done to determine wound nitrogen losses in burned patients, these adjustments result in rough estimates at best.[40] Insensible nitrogen losses, according to pediatric age group, can also be added to the UUN as follows: UUN + 2 (birth to four years), UUN + 3 (four to ten years), UUN + 4 (>ten years).[27] Weekly measures of nitrogen balances have been suggested.[30]

Conclusion

Burn injuries have important ramifications from a nutritional perspective. No current consensus exists regarding which is the most appropriate or most accurate predictive formula for estimating calorie and protein needs. In any case, close attention to the increased needs for nutrients is warranted to ensure adequate nutritional intakes. When used in conjunction with each other, nutrition parameters can provide a reliable evaluation of nutritional status. The nutrition goals of weight maintenance in the acute postinjury phase, childhood growth in the rehabilitation phase, wound healing, and convalescence are realistic. Discovery of more precise methods for measuring nitrogen losses from wounds could facilitate more accurate evaluations of nitrogen balance. Future research is needed to determine more specific nutritional requirements, especially, of micronutrients.

References

1. Long CL, Schaffel N, Geiger JW, Schiller WR, Blakemore WS. Metabolic response to injury and illness: estimation of energy and protein needs from indirect calorimetry and nitrogen balance. *J Pen* 1979;3:452-7.

2. Muller MJ, Herndon DN. Hormonal interactions in burned patients. *Semin Nephrol* 1993;13:391-9.

3. Wallace BH, Caldwell FT, Cone JB. The interrelationships between wound management, thermal stress, energy metabolism, and temperature profiles of patients. *J Burn Care Rehabil* 1994;15:499-508.

4. Caldwell FT. Etiology and control of postburn Hypermetabolism. *J Burn Care Rehabil* 1991;12:385-401.

5. Wallace BH, Caldwell FT, Cone JB. Ibuprofen lowers temperature and metabolic rate of humans with burn injury. *J Trauma* 1992;32:154-7.

6. Waymack JP, Herndon DN. Nutritional support of the burned patient. *World J Surg* 1992;16:80-6.

7. Ireton-Jones C. Nutrition for adult burned patients: a review. *Nutr Clin Pract* 1991;6:3-7.

8. Williamson J. Actual burn nutrition care practices: a national survey (part II). *J Burn Care Rehabil* 1989;10(Pt 2):185-94.

9. Curreri PW, Richmond D, Marvin J, Baxter CR Dietary requirements of patients with major burns. *J Am Diet Assoc* 1974;65:415-7.

10. Turner WW, Ireton CS, Hunt JL, Baxter CR-Predicting energy expenditures in burned patients. *J Trauma* 1985;25:11-6.

11. Schane J, Goede M, Silverstein P. Comparison of energy expenditure measurement techniques in severely burned patients. *J Burn Care Rehabil* 1987;8:366-70.

12. Saffle JP, Medina E, Raymond J, Westenskow D, Kravitz M, Warden GD. Use of indirect calorimetry in the nutritional management of burned patients. *J Trauma* 1985;25:32-9.

13. Long C. Energy expenditure of major burns. *J Trauma* 1979;19:904-6.

14. Montegut WJ, Lowry SF. Nutrition in burn patients. *Semin Nephrol* 1993;13:400-8.

15. Bell SJ, Wyatt J. Nutrition guidelines for burned patients. *JADA* 1986;86:648-53.

16. Saito H, Trocki O, Wang S, Gonce SJ, Joffe GN, Alexander JW. Metabolic and immune effects of dietary arginine supplementation after burns. *Arch Surg* 1987;122:784-9.

17. Gottschlich MM, Jenkins M, Warden GD, et al. Differential effects of three enteral dietary regimens on selected outcome variables in burn patients. *JPEN* 1990;14:225-36.

18. Carlson DE, Jordan BS. Implementing nutritional therapy in the thermally injured patient. *Crit Care Nurs Clin North Am* 1991;3:221-35.

19. Trocki O, Mochizuki J, Dominioni L, Alexander JW. Intact protein versus free amino acids in the nutritional support of thermally injured animals. *JPEN* 1986;10:139-45.

20. Burke JF, Wolfe RR, Mullany CJ, Mathews DE, Bier DM. Glucose requirements following burn injury. *Ann Surg* 1979; 190:274-83.

21. Gottschlich MM, Alexander JW. Fat kinetics and recommended dietary intake in burns. *JPEN* 1987;11:80-5.

22. Gottschlich MM, Warden GD. Vitamin supplementation in the patient with burns. *J Burn Care Rehabil* 1990;11:275-9.

23. Heivig E. Pediatric burn injuries. *AACN Clin Issues* 1993: 433-42.

24. Harmel RP, Vane DW. Burn care in children:special considerations. *Clin Plast Surg* 1986:95-105.

25. Davies JWL, Liljedahl SL. Metabolic consequences of an extensive burn. In: Polk HC, Stone HH, eds. *Contemporary Burn Management*. Boston: Little Brown, 1971:151-69.

26. Gottschlich MM. Nutrition in the burned pediatric patient. In: Queen PM, Lang CE, eds. *Handbook of Pediatric Nutrition*. Gaithersburg, Md: Aspen Publishers, 1993:536-59.

27. O'Neil CE, Hutsler D, Hildreth MA. Basic nutritional guidelines for pediatric burn patients. *J Burn Care Rehabil* 1989; 10:278-83.

28. Food and Nutrition Board. Recommended dietary allowances. 10th ed. Washington DC: National Academy of Sciences, 1989.

29. Bell SJ, Molnar JA, Krasker WS, Burke JF. Weight maintenance in pediatric burned patients. *J Am Diet Assoc* 1986;86: 207-11.

30. Hutsler D. Nutritional monitoring of a pediatric burn patient. *Nutr Clin Pract* 1991:11-7.

31. Day T, Dean P, Adams MC, Luterman A, Ramenofsky ML, Curreri PW. Nutritional requirements of the burned child: the Curreri Junior formula. *Proc Am Burn Assoc* 1986;18:86.

32. Hildreth M, Carvajal HF. Caloric requirements in burned children: a simple formula to estimate daily caloric requirements. *J Burn Care Rehabil* 1982;3:78-80.

33. Hildreth MA, Herndon DN, Desai MH, Duke MA. Reassessing caloric requirements in pediatric burn patients. *J Burn Care Rehabil* 1988;9:616-8.

34. Hildreth MA, Herndon DN, Desai MH, Broemeling LD. Current treatment reduces calories required to maintain weight in pediatric patients with burns. *J Burn Care Rehabil* 1990;11:405-9.

35. Hildreth MA, Herndon DN, Desai MH, Broemeling LD. Caloric requirements of patients with burns under one year of age. *J Burn Care Rehabil* 1993;14:108-12.

36. Hildreth MA, Herndon DN, Desai MH, Duke MA. Calorie needs of adolescents with burns. *J Burn Care Rehabil.* 1989;10:523-6.

37. Cunningham JJ, Lydon MK, Russell WE. Calorie and protein provision for recovery from severe burns in infants and young children. *Am J Clin Nutr* 1990;51:553-7.

38. Gore DC, Rutan RL, Hildreth M, Desai M, Herndon DN. Comparison of resting energy expenditures and caloric intake in children with severe burns. *J Burn Care Rehabil* 1990-11: 400-4.

39. Cunningham JJ, Harris LJ, Briggs SE. Nutritional support of the severely burned infant. *Nutr Clin Pract* 1988;3:69-73.

40. Kien CL, Young VR, Rohrbaugh DK, Burke JF. Increased rates of whole body protein synthesis and breakdown in children recovering from burns. *Ann Surg* 1978;187:383-91.

41. Alexander JW, Macmillan BG, Stinnett JD, et al. Beneficial effects of aggressive protein feeding in severely burned children. *Ann Surg* 1980;192:505-17.

42. Cunningham JJ, Lydon MY, Briggs SE, DeCheke M. Zinc and copper status of severely burned children during TPN. *J Am Coll Nutr* 1991;10:57-62.

43. White S, Kamples G. Dietary noncompliance in pediatric patients in the burn unit. *J Burn Care Rehabil* 1990;11: 167-74.

44. Inoue S, Lukes S, Alexander JW, Trocki O, Silberstein EB. Increased gut blood flow with early enteral feeding in burned guinea pigs. *J Burn Care Rehabil* 1989;10:300-8.

45. Saito H, Trocki O, Alexander JW, Kopcha I, Heyd T, Joffe SN. The effect of route of nutrient administration on the nutritional state, catabolic hormone secretion, and gut mucosal integrity after burn injury. *JPEN* 1987; 11: 1-7.

46. McDonald WS, Sharp CW, Deitch EA. Immediate enteral feeding in burn patients is safe and effective. *Ann Surg* 1991; 213:177-83.

47. Hansbrough WB, Hansbrough JF. Success of immediate intragastric feeding of patients with burns. *J Burn Care Rehabil* 1993;14:512-6.

48. Garret DR, Davignon I, Lopez D. Length of care in patients with severe burns with or without early enteral nutritional support: a retrospective study. *J Burn Care Rehabil* 1991;12: 85-90.

49. McArdle AH, Palmason C, Brown RA, Brown HC, Williams HB. Early enteral feeding of patients with major burns: prevention of catabolism. *Ann Plast Surg* 1984;13:396-401.

50. Mochizuki H, Trocki O, Dominioni L, Brackett KA, Joffee SN, Alexander JW. Mechanism of prevention of postburn hypermetabolism and catabolism by early enteral feeding. *Ann Surg* 1984;200:297-310.

51. Jenkins ME, Gottschlich MM, Warden GD. Enteral feeding during operative procedures in thermal injuries. *J Burn Care Rehabil* 1994;15:199-205.

52. Herndon DN, Barrow RE, Stein M, et al. Increased mortality with intravenous supplemental feeding in severely burned patients. *J Burn Care Rehabil* 1989;10:309-13.

53. Konstantinides FN, Radmer WJ, Becker WK, et al. Inaccuracy of nitrogen balance determinations in thermal injury with calculated total urinary Nitrogen. *J Burn Care Rehabil*, 1992; 13:254-60.

— by Donna J. Rodriguez, RD, CNSD

Department of Surgery, University of New Mexico, School of Medicine. Albuquerque, New Mexico

Chapter 26

Second Skins

Last spring, a sixty-eight year old Northern California man suffered deep, third-degree burns when he dropped a cigarette and his pants leg caught fire. Unfortunately, such injuries are all too common. What's unusual is that this man became the first patient treated outside clinical trials with a new artificial skin that the Food and Drug Administration had just approved for marketing the month before.

A serious burn is one of the most horrendous traumas the body can suffer. Every year, about 51,000 Americans are hospitalized for burn treatment, according to the American Burn Association, and 5,500 die. The good news is that the incidence and severity of burn injuries have declined significantly over the past twenty years. And patient survival keeps improving.

"This is a very exciting area," says Charles Durfor, Ph.D., in FDA's division of general and restorative devices. "Thirty to forty years ago, many burn patients didn't live. Advances in treatment have created a whole new patient population that not only lives, but has an improving quality of life."

The first great strides were in getting patients through the initial shock, and preventing fluid loss. Controlling infection, a serious threat to burn patients, also improved. Specialized nutritional support has helped. Another leap occurred when doctors began surgically removing, or excising, all burned tissue from the wound as soon as possible.

1997 January/February *FDA Consumer*.

After stabilizing the patient and cleaning out the wound, the next step is to cover it.

"The sooner you close the wound, the sooner the patient gets better," says Robert Klein, M.D., medical director of the regional burn center at Children's Hospital Medical Center of Akron, Ohio.

"The problem is, we've never had an optimal way to do it," says Jerold Kaplan, M.D., director of the burn centers at Alta Bates Hospital in Berkeley, Calif., and at Children's Hospital in nearby Oakland. The need to cover wounds as quickly as possible while minimizing scarring and additional trauma has driven development of advanced wound dressings and skin substitutes. Kaplan treated the sixty-eight year old California man's wounds with Integra Artificial Skin Dermal Regeneration Template, from Integra LifeSciences Corp., Plainsboro, N.J. "Integra is a significant addition to the armamentarium of the burn surgeon," Kaplan says, and other surgeons agree.

Skin Deep

Surgeons also agree that no single product or technique is right for every burn situation. And so far, there's no true replacement for healthy, intact skin, which is the body's largest organ, and one of the most complex. It's the first line of defense against infection and dehydration, but it's more than just a physical barrier. Skin also helps control temperature, through adjustments of blood flow and evaporation of sweat. It's an important sensory organ, too.

Skin thickness varies with age and body location, but averages only 1 to 2 millimeters (0.04 to 0.08 inches) thick. Thick or thin, it has two layers. The thin outer epidermis is nourished from the thicker, more sensitive dermis below. The outermost surface is a tough, protective coating of dead, flat cells resembling paving stones. As these cells wear away, they're replaced from beneath. The innermost part of the epidermis consists of rapidly dividing cells, called keratinocytes, which produce keratin, a tough protein. Epidermis also contains a unique fatty substance that makes skin waterproof.

The skin's blood vessels, lymph vessels, and nerves are in the dermis. Hair follicles, sweat glands, and oil glands also reside deep in this layer, which is mainly connective tissue. A network of collagen, the most common protein in the body, gives flexibility and structural support to the skin. Fibroblasts are the dominant cell type. Dermis plays a role in preventing wound contraction and scarring.

Treatment of burns depends on how deep and extensive they are, and the overall health of the patient. First-degree burns (such as sunburns) affect only the epidermis; they may peel but generally heal quickly. Second-degree burns damage the skin more deeply, causing blisters but sparing some of the dermal layer. Unless they're extensive, these burns usually heal without serious scarring. Third-degree burns destroy the full skin thickness, sometimes exposing muscle or bone, and require specialized treatment and skin grafts to obtain complete wound healing and reduce scarring. Left alone, the body tries to close wounds quickly by contraction, which results in serious scarring that is not only disfiguring, but can also be disabling.

Currently, the best wound covering most often is the patient's own skin. Healthy skin from another body site can be transplanted, which is called an autograft (autos means self). Sometimes little slits are cut so the resulting meshed graft can be stretched to cover more area. A split-thickness graft takes only the upper skin layer, and the donor site usually heals within several days. The thinner the graft, the faster the donor site heals. Surgeons may even take additional thin grafts from healed sites. Full-thickness grafts usually give a better-looking final result, but sometimes they don't adhere and survive. Donor sites are limited and autografting isn't always possible.

"People with great big burns don't have enough of their own skin, so you have to have some other way of covering them," says David M. Heimbach, M.D., director of the University of Washington Burn Center at Harborview, Seattle. Some patients can't withstand the additional trauma of a donor site wound. Older patients heal slowly and have thinner skin to begin with. And grafting creates another scar.

Doctors often use temporary coverings while patients get stronger, or while donor sites heal for additional harvesting. Two traditional possibilities are an allograft (allos means other) of human skin, usually cadaver skin, or a xenograft (xenos means stranger, in this case from another species) of pig skin. Cadaver skin is preferable, but as with other donated organs, sometimes it's in short supply and transmission of infectious agents is a concern. Human skin is regulated under FDA's Human Tissue Program, which requires donor screening for HIV (the AIDS virus) and hepatitis. In any case, the immune system rejects allo- and xenografts in a matter of days or weeks, and they must be removed and replaced. To avoid such problems, researchers and manufacturers are developing better wound dressings.

Advanced Dressings

FDA recognizes two broad categories of wound dressings interactive and noninteractive. A variety of noninteractive dressings are available for covering first- and second-degree burns and other wounds. An interactive dressing is intended to actively promote wound healing by interacting directly with body tissues. Manufacturers must submit safety and effectiveness data to FDA in a premarket approval application. FDA has approved two interactive wound dressings for use on third-degree burns: Integra Artificial Skin and Original BioBrane (Blue Label), marketed by Dow B. Hickam, Inc., New York.

BioBrane is a knitted nylon fabric bonded to an ultra-thin silicone rubber membrane coated with a protein (gelatin) derived from pig tissue. Clotting factors in the wound interact with the gelatin in the dressing, causing it to adhere to the wound within a day or so. The dressing remains in place until autografting becomes possible.

Integra is a two-layer membrane a dermal layer that's a porous lattice of cross-linked collagen fibers, and a synthetic epidermal layer. The dermal layer acts as a biodegradable template that helps organize dermal tissue regeneration. Fibroblasts and other cells migrate into the lattice from surrounding healthy tissue, as do blood and lymph vessels. The fibroblasts degrade the temporary scaffold and recreate their own collagen matrix.

"The dermal part of the product is a permanent cover which the body converts into something which looks more like dermis than it looks like scar tissue," Heimbach says.

The outer synthetic layer provides the barrier functions of epidermis for two to three weeks; then the surgeon replaces it with a very thin autograft. "The ability to have the donor site be very thin and heal in just a few days is the big benefit," says Kaplan. "You're actually adding a procedure, but the end result is positive."

"It's a neat concept and it appears to work," says Heimbach, who has used Integra on more than 100 patients during clinical trials. He says the final results look much better than the alternative, meshed autografts. "We're excited about the new composite skin substitutes," he says.

Cultured Skin

Doctors prefer a thin graft to a thick one, but eliminating the donor site wound and scar altogether would be even better. That's done by growing the patient's skin in the lab, under special tissue culture conditions. Lab-grown skin products also have other potential uses for wounds other than burns, and for laboratory testing. From a postage stamp-sized piece of skin, technicians can grow enough skin in about three weeks to nearly cover the body. Some medical centers are equipped for this sort of cell culture, and Genzyme Tissue Repair, Cambridge, Mass., does it as a commercial service. Cultured skin has been available for treating burns for about a decade, and in certain circumstances it can work well.

"The problem here is you're putting on epidermis and not dermis," Kaplan says.

"Without both parts, you don't really have skin," Heimbach says. "You're grafting on scar tissue and that's not a satisfactory skin covering."

Less than ten cells thick, it's also tricky to handle. "It's like gossamer," Kaplan says. And something has to cover the wound in the meantime. That's where Kaplan and others see a potentially useful combination. The patient's epidermis could be cultured during the two to three weeks while Integra's dermal layer becomes a suitable bed for grafting. "They're complementary," says Kaplan.

"You would have the best of both worlds. You don't have any donor sites, and you have a good, durable, cosmetically acceptable cover," says Heimbach.

"Another approach we're actively working on is the one-step procedure," says Frederick Cahn, Ph.D., senior vice president, technology, Integra LifeSciences. The patient's own epidermal cells are isolated, as they would be for culturing, then seeded onto the dermal layer of Integra before it is applied to the wound. Both skin layers regenerate in place simultaneously, and only one surgical procedure is required. This procedure has worked well in animals, but hasn't been tried in humans yet.

Although physicians welcome new ways to help their patients, they're leery of "scar in a jar" products that might solve some problems while creating others. Last year, FDA held hearings on using the patient's own cells for structural repair in therapy, and heard a strong call for measures of efficacy. Based on the testimony presented, FDA has decided to regulate such therapy and is developing guidance documents to assist manufacturers in completing the premarket review process.

"FDA recognizes that the area of tissue substitutes is a rapidly evolving area and that medical and biochemical practice are also growing rapidly and it's working aggressively to make sure it doesn't stifle development while continuing to ensure patient safety," says FDA's Durfor.

Investigators have developed other variations on cultured skin in the hope of providing off-the-shelf, living, temporary or permanent dressings. Clinical trials are under way testing them on burns and other wounds. For example, Advanced Tissue Sciences, La Jolla, Calif., developed its Dermagraft-TC skin replacement to be used as an alternative to cadaver skin for burns.

Treatment for burns keeps improving, but burn surgeons still have another important concern. "I think 95 percent of the burns we see are completely preventable," says Heimbach. He credits smoke detectors for a huge drop in the number of burns and deaths from house fires, but he hasn't seen much change in the number of accidents caused by carelessness or ignorance.

"The answer to the burn problem is prevention. Once it happens, it's too late," Klein says. "Be careful so you never need us."

Skin under Glass

In addition to its potential as an advanced wound dressing, cultured skin may also prove useful in laboratory testing. Many cosmetic, household product, pharmaceutical, and petrochemical companies are experimenting with cultured skin in the hope that in vitro (in glass, meaning in lab vessels) assays can replace or reduce animal testing for evaluating raw materials and final product formulations. FDA has long supported development of such methods, but the state of the science hasn't progressed yet to where it can fully replace animal testing, according to FDA's John Bailey, who heads the Office of Cosmetics and Colors in the agency's Center for Food Safety and Applied Nutrition.

Scientists can use isolated skin tissue to test skin penetration, irritation, toxicity, and other effects of various substances. Although cadaver skin works for some purposes, its uses are limited because the cells are dead. Cultured skin contains live, metabolizing cells that can better mimic how skin responds to various stimuli.

One example is the EpiDerm System, a model of human epidermis marketed by MatTek Corp., Ashland, Mass. Human-derived epidermal cells are grown under culture conditions that encourage formation of the characteristic cell subtypes and layers of epidermis. Another example is Skin^2, developed by Advanced Tissue Sciences, Inc., La Jolla, Calif. Some versions of Skin^2 contain dermis as well as epidermis. These products are intended to be used for testing, not as dressings.

Lab-grown skin is used in two general ways. As a membrane to measure skin absorption, it doesn't work very well because it's much more permeable than skin, according to Robert L. Bronaugh, Ph.D., chief of the skin absorption and metabolism section in FDA's Office of Cosmetics and Colors. "A lot more work needs to be done before it can be used to simulate accurately the barrier properties of human skin," he says.

However, as an alternate test to measure irritation, cultured skin looks encouraging, according to Bronaugh. The U.S. Department of Transportation has approved the use of a Skin² in vitro test kit as an alternative to animal testing of potentially corrosive materials. Although FDA wouldn't accept final safety data acquired from these in vitro assays, companies can use cultured skin in early screenings, and that saves animals, as well as money.

Hope for Wounds That Won't Go Away

It may be hard for a healthy person to imagine having a wound that just won't heal, but that problem plagues millions of Americans. Non-healing wounds not only take an emotional toll, but also leave patients, their families, and society with a serious economic burden, ranging into billions of dollars.

The incidence of chronic wounds is far greater than burns and is expected to continue to increase as the population ages. Some of the treatment concerns are similar because the barrier function of skin is lost, putting the patient at risk for infection, and chronic wounds can be life threatening.

There are three general types of chronic wounds: pressure ulcers (bedsores or decubitus ulcers), venous ulcers, and diabetic ulcers. They have different causes, but the result is the same localized tissue death. The factors that cause an ulcer to develop in the first place also interfere with healing. The cost per healed ulcer when they heal at all can climb into the tens of thousands of dollars, and as many as half recur within a year. Roughly three-quarters of a million American diabetics suffer with foot ulcers, which are responsible for more than 50,000 amputations a year.

Recent research efforts in pursuit of various growth factors to promote wound healing have been disappointing. Figuring out which growth factors to put in a wound and when and at what dose is a daunting, perhaps impossible, task. Some investigators have turned to cultured skin, arguing that applying cultured skin to wounds makes more sense than using growth factors because living cells already know how to produce growth factors at the right time and in the right amount.

Organogenesis Inc., of Canton, Mass., has developed Apligraf (formerly Graftskin), a two-layer living skin substitute derived from infant foreskins. The upper layer contains keratinocytes, the dominant cell type in the epidermis. The lower layer contains collagen and fibroblasts, the main constituents of dermis. Other cell types that trigger immunological response are absent, and, as a result, this engineered tissue is not rejected. Human trials of Apligraf for treating burns, diabetic ulcers, and for use in other skin surgeries are under way.

Cultured skin offers new hope for chronic wounds, but, as with burns, prevention is the best bet.

—by Carolyn J. Strange

Carolyn J. Strange is a science and medical writer living in Northern California.

Chapter 27

The Evolutionary Development of Biologic Dressings and Skin Substitutes

The outlook for patients with burns has significantly improved over the last four decades so that today the LA_{50}, the size of burn that is fatal to half the people with that size burn, in all young adult patients with burns admitted to the U. S. Army Institute of Surgical Research is 75.6 percent of the total body surface; if you eliminate patients with inhalation injury, it is approximately 83 percent.[1] In the case of burned children younger than 15 years, the LA, approaches 90 percent.[2] Consequently, today we are faced with the challenge of dealing with an increasing number of patients with massive burns and a paucity of donor sites. As early as 1556 Gasparo Becerra depicted the fact that you can remove all the skin from any patient, but we now know that there has to be a second procedure to resurface that wound. When donor sites are scarce, the resulting therapeutic void has historically been filled by biologic dressings (Table 27.1).

The Ebers Papyrus, dated 1500 BC, is the first reference of which I am aware that describes the use of a biologic dressing.[3] That document recommended that one treat a burn by rubbing a frog that had been dipped in warm oil on the burn wound. That is not how we usually apply biologic dressings today, but it certainly established a precedent. There are also biblical references to the importance of skin. In the book of Job it is stated, "Skin for skin yea, all that a man hath will he give for his life." However, a problem arises when a man has no donor sites from which skin can be given. Naturally occurring tissues consisting of cutaneous allografts, xenografts, and amniotic membranes have been used for many years to provide temporary coverage in such a situation.

The transplantation of human tissues apparently began in the third century AD when Saints Cosmos and Damian transplanted a lower limb to Deacon Justiniano. That operation has been depicted by many artists who have shown the leg of a Moor transplanted to the chorister. Persistence of that transplant remains unconfirmed to this day. Even so, of the available naturally occurring materials, cutaneous allograft is considered the gold standard for coverage of open wounds when there are no available donor sites. The properties of viable cutaneous allograft considered beneficial are enumerated in Table 27.2, and all synthetic dressings need to possess those properties to some degree to function effectively. There are also specific limitations of allograft skin ranging from limited supply to the transmission of viral disease. The risk of human immunodeficiency virus transmission by allograft skin is the same as for blood, as is the risk of transmission of hepatitis. Other forms of cutaneous allograft, lyophilized, formalinized, and glycerol-preserved, are available. Those forms have less risk of transmitting disease and have essentially an indefinite shelf life. However, they adhere less well to the wound bed than does viable cutaneous allograft, and there is often dermal-epidermal separation followed by prompt desiccation of the exposed dermal surface.[4]

Canaday[5] was among the first to use xenograft tissue; in 1692 he reported the use of water lizard skin for wound care. The modern analog of that early work may be the use of frog skin as recently proposed by physicians in Brazil.[5] In the United States Haldor Sneve[6] was an early proponent of the use of xenograft skin in burn treatment. In 1906 he proposed using guinea pig, chicken, or rabbit skin and favored the last. In modern times Bromberg et al.[7] popularized the use of porcine xenografts, and canine xenografts were used extensively by others.[8] Cutaneous xenografts have been used, as have the other naturally occurring dressings, to fill the therapeutic void that exists when all available donor sites have been used and "mesh" expansion of the skin grafts does not close the wound. The disadvantage of xenograft is that because it does not establish vessel-to-vessel connection, it is not rejected as is allograft and undergoes avascular necrosis and sloughs.[9] Consequently, even though xenograft skin is more easily available, it is less effective as a biologic dressing as manifested by a greater number of subgraft bacteria compared with viable allograft skin. Amniotic membranes, which are said to have been first used in 1913 by Sabella, just like xenograft skin, are not vascularized by the process of inosculation and like allograft skin have the potential for disease transmission.[10]

The limitations of the naturally occurring biologic dressings have focused attention on the development of skin substitutes consisting entirely of synthetic materials or a combination of synthetic material and collagen. One of the earliest synthetic materials used in the United States was the plastic spray developed by Choy[11] in 1954. However, the first skin substitute to be used by more than a few investigators was the Ivalon sponge developed by Chardack et al.[12] in the early 1960s. Desiccation and inspissation of wound exudate in the interstices of the Ivalon sponge permitted extensive accumulation of suppurative material beneath the membrane. The Ivalon also fragmented on removal and left behind foreign bodies that initiated granuloma formation.[3] A variety of amino acid films have also been evaluated, and they characteristically showed no bio logic union with attachment to the wound by the serous crust that formed at the margin of the graft. Even in unilamellar membranes with porosity that facilitated water vapor transmission, inspissation of wound exudate reduced water vapor transmission, which resulted in submembrane accumulation of fluid.[9]

Studies at many laboratories have repeatedly demonstrated that a bilaminate structure that mimics the morphologic characteristics of skin is critically important for an effective biologic dressing.[9] An epidermal analog must be present to serve a barrier function, and a dermal analog is required to allow biologic union by the ingrowth of fibrovascular tissue to attach the membrane to the host. However, studies by Levine et al.[13] with formalinized allograft in laboratory models of burn wound excision have demonstrated that viability is not an essential characteristic of a biologic dressing. Those investigators developed a totally synthetic bilaminate. The epidermal analog consisted of a finely porous sheet of polytetrafluoroethylene, and the dermal analog consisted of six to eight layers of micromesh knit into which fibrovascular tissue could grow.[9] The membrane allowed secretion "strike through," but the appearance of such served as a clinical index of the need to change the membrane. When applied to a freshly excised burn wound, the totally synthetic skin substitute protected the wound and allowed the formation of uniformly vascularized granulation tissue that was easily graftable. The material had sufficient tensile strength to prevent fragmentation on removal and thereby avoid foreign body granuloma formation. Submembrane suppuration was common when the material was applied to other than a freshly excised burn wound.

There are now a variety of what are termed collagen-based bilaminate skin substitutes. Biobrane consists of an epidermal analog composed of a thin sheet of Silastic and a dermal analog composed of type I porcine collagen gel.[14] This skin substitute is translucent so that one can observe suppuration beneath the membrane and has sufficient strength so that it does not fragment on removal. As is the case with other composite membranes, this one functions best when applied to a freshly excised surgical wound.

All of the biologic dressings can be graded in terms of various desirable properties. Biobrane has been compared with xenograft skin

Table 27.1. Biologic dressings

Naturally occurring tissues

 Cutaneous allografts
 Cutaneous xenografts
 Amniotic membranes

Skin substitutes

 Synthetic bilaminate
 Collagen-based composites
  • Biobrane
  • Integra
  • Dermagraft-TC
 Collagen-based dermal analogs
  • Deepithelized allograft
  • Alloderm

Culture-derived tissue

 Cultured autologous keratinocytes
 Fibroblast seeded dermal analogs
  • Collagen-glycosaminoglycan membrane
  • Polyglycolic or polyglactin acid mesh

in terms of granulation tissue formation, suppuration, adherence, confirmation, and pliability. A wound dressing index can be calculated by adding the individual gradings for each of those five characteristics.[15] Biobrane was found to function as well as porcine xenograft, with the quality of granulation tissue being moderate to good under each dressing and suppuration rare under both.

The recently approved bilaminate skin substitute, Integra, was developed by Burke et al.[16] The epidermal analog of this membrane is a Silastic film, and the dermal analog consists of a mat of collagen fibrils enriched with chondroitin-6-sulfate. After it is applied to an excised burn wound, the dermal analog becomes vascularized. When adequate vascularization is visible through the thin outer Silastic film, the Silastic can be removed and the vascularized "neodermis" covered with ultrathin cutaneous autografts. The limitations of this material are its susceptibility to infection and the potential for greater scar formation as mentioned by some investigators. In a multiinstitutional evaluation the investigators reported that because thinner epidermal grafts could be used, there was more rapid healing of the donor sites, and reharvesting could be accomplished with greater rapidity.[17] In that study less hypertrophic scarring was claimed, as was greater patient preference compared with each institution's customary biologic dressing.

This several-decade experience with various skin substitutes permits us to define the essential properties of an effective skin substitute (Table 27.3). A bilaminate structure with both an epidermal and a dermal analog is critical. A skin substitute should have sufficient drapability to conform intimately to the wound surface, and it should be nontoxic with low antigenicity. There are desirable value- added properties, principal among which is that it be non inflammatory so that it will not induce a systemic inflammatory response when applied to the wound. It should possess adequate resistance to linear and shear stress and should be bacteriostatic so that there is no unbridled microbial proliferation below the membrane. In today's cost-conscious milieu of managed care, a low cost is ever more desirable.

The ultimate limitation of any biologic dressing is that it is only temporary. Consequently, one has to have a means of effecting definitive wound closure, and that need has focused attention on culture-derived tissues. The first such material and that which has been most extensively evaluated, consists of sheets of cultured keratinocytes, also called cultured epidermal autografts (CEA). At the U. S. Army Institute of Surgical Research Rue et al.[18] conducted a clinical evaluation of cultured epidermal autografts. Sheets of culture-derived keratinocytes were

Table 27.2. Beneficial properties of viable cutaneous allograft

1. Prevents desiccation of wound surface
2. Promotes development of granulation tissue
3. Decreases evaporative water loss
4. Decreases heat loss
5. Limits bacterial proliferation
6. Prevents exudative protein and red cell loss
7. Decreases wound pain
8. Facilitates movement of involved joints
9. Protects exposed tendons, vessels, and nerves
10. Enhances healing of partial-thickness burns

Table 27.3 Properties of Skin Substances

Essential
   Bilaminate structure: epidermal analog, dermal analog
   Drapability: absence of toxicity, low antigenicity

"Value-added": Noninflammatory, resistance to linear and shear stress, bacteriostatic activity, low cost.

applied on thirty-one occasions to nineteen patients whose burns involved an average of 71.9 percent of the total body surface (range 42 percent to 89 percent). The average area covered was 10.8 percent of the body surface, with the largest area covered being 24.5 percent. At the first dressing change, ten days after application, 47.8 percent of the grafted tissue was adherent. At the end of the study period (twenty-one to twenty-eight days) only 30.6 percent of the grafts were adherent, but the average surface area closed was only 2.8 percent, which one would anticipate to exert at best only a modest adjunctive effect. Most discouraging was the fact that engraftment of the CEA was inversely proportional to the extent of the burn. In patients with burns of 50 percent or less of the total body surface, adherence was generally good; that is, less than 20 percent of the CEA was lost. However, as the size of the burn increased, the amount of rejection increased proportionally.

The character of the wound bed also appears to influence the take of the CEA. CEA shows the least adherence on granulation tissue and similarly better adherence when applied to dermis exposed by excision or to subdermal tissue after excision of a full-thickness burn. The extent of coverage achieved was greatest for the intradermal wounds. The flora on the wound also influenced the take of CEA and subsequent wound coverage, which were decreased on wounds from which gram-negative organisms and fungi were recovered. In addition to early CEA loss, variable later loss has been attributed to mechanical (defective anchoring fibrils) and immunologic (reaction to xenogeneic proteins) factors.[19,20]

Cultured keratinocytes, both autogenous and allogeneic, have also been used as overlay grafts placed on widely expanded mesh autografts. The effectiveness of CEA used in this fashion and whether it is superior to a split-thickness cutaneous allograft used in similar fashion remain undefined.

The modest results achieved by using sheets of culture-derived keratinocytes have prompted the development of new variants of such tissues. Several investigators have reported favorably on the engraftment and persistence of CEA applied to previously placed cutaneous allografts from which the epidermal cells have been removed.[21] Allogeneic dermis that has been treated to remove antigenic determinants has been used in a similar fashion.[22] Cultured keratinocytes can apparently be applied to this "nonimmunogenic" allodermis after it has become attached and vascularized by host tissue. Attempts have also been made to delete the Langerhans cells from cultured keratinocytes to reduce antigenicity and allow the use of allogeneic tissue. An exciting initiative in this area is the use of what has been termed "chimeric" allogeneic tissue produced by culturing as little as 6.25 percent and up to 25 percent of autologous cells with allogeneic cells.[23,24] Applications of sheets of such "chimeric" tissue have been reported to achieve permanent wound closure. Presumably the allogeneic tissue is imperceptibly replaced by host tissue. Other preparations of cultured-derived tissue being evaluated include keratinocyte suspensions. The cells in such suspensions appear to adhere well to flat surfaces, but the effects of gravity may compromise their application to lateral and posterior body surfaces.

There is also a physical means to improve the acceptance and apparent persistence of foreign tissue, which is the application of low-amperage direct current. A current density of 0.6 $\mu A/cm^2$ with a silver-impregnated nylon cloth as an anode exerts an antibacterial effect, modifies vascular permeability, maintains dermal blood flow, increases the number of grafts that can be harvested from a given donor site, and reduces the antigenicity of allodermis.[25] In a murine model of a dorsal surface, full-thickness, excised wound to which allogeneic dermis was applied and covered with widely meshed autoepidermis, application of the low- amperage direct current was associated with minimal wound contraction (comparable to that of wounds covered with only autogenous tissue) and statistically less than that associated with wounds covered with only autogenous tissue) and statistically less than that associated with wounds covered with allogeneic tissue alone. The heated wound demonstrated pliability comparable to that of wounds covered with only autogenous tissue. Whether the allogeneic dermis persists or is gradually replaced by host tissue has not been determined.

Other cultured-derived tissues that have been evaluated to variable extent include a collagen gel seeded with autologous fibroblasts to effect in vitro contraction of the gel before application as a replacement for dermis.[26] A composite graft studied by Hansbrough et al.[27] in the late 1980s consisted of a collagen mat seeded with neonatal fibroblasts upon which cultured keratinocytes could be layered. The results of laboratory studies of that material have not been confirmed in the clinic.

As a variant of cultured tissue used for "permanent" engraftment, Dermagraft-TC (Advanced Tissue Sciences, Inc.) is a newly developed bilaminate skin substitute de signed to provide temporary coverage of open wounds. This membrane consists of a dermal analog containing collagen produced by human dermal fibroblasts cultured on nylon mesh and a silicone "epidermis."[28] At the time of removal of engrafted vascularized Dermagraft-TC, satisfactory adherence and take of subsequently applied cutaneous autografts have been customary. In a multiinstitutional clinical study Dermagraft-TC has been compared with cryopreserved allograft skin.[29] The only disadvantage attributed to Dermagraft-TC was a statistically greater sub membrane fluid accumulation, although the mean accumulation of fluid beneath both dressings was considered "minimal." There were numerous comparabilities of the two materials ranging from adherence to the wound bed to the incidence of wound infection. More important, there were definite advantages associated with Dermagraft-TC such as easier removability, less bleeding at the time of removal, no laminar separation, and of course no possibility of disease transmission. Those advantages assume particular importance in today's milieu of cost-conscious managed care and may promote ready acceptance and wide use of Dermagraft-TC for the temporary coverage of excised burn wounds.

References

1. Pruitt BA Jr, Mason AD Jr. Epidemiological, demographic and outcome characteristics of burn injury. In: Herndon DN, editor. *Total burn care*. Philadelphia: WB Saunders; 1995:5-15.

2. Herndon DN, Gore D, Cole M, Desai MH, Linares H, Abston S, et al. Determinants of mortality in pediatric patients with greater than 70 percent full-thickness total body surface area thermal injury treated by early total excision and grafting. *J Trauma* 1987;27:208-12.

3. Pruitt BA Jr, Silverstein P. Methods of resurfacing denuded skin areas. *Transplant Proc* 1971;3:1537-45.

4. Pruitt BA Jr, Sell K, O'Neill JA Jr, Lindberg RB, Moncrief JA. Clinical evaluation of freeze-dried and fresh frozen homograft in burned patients. *Annual Research Progress Report*, US Army Surgical Research Unit, Fort Sam Houston, Texas, Section 10, June 30, 1967.

5. Piccolo N, Piccolo-Lobo M, Piccolo-Daher M, Cardoso V, Silveira F. Use of frog skin as a temporary biological dressing [abstract]. *Proc Am Burn Assoc* 1992;24: abstract #39.

6. Sneve H. The treatment of burns and skin grafting. *JAMA* 1905;45:1-8.

7. Bromberg BE, Song JC, Mohn MP. The use of pig skin as a temporary biologic dressing. *Plast Reconstr Surg* 1965;36:80-90.

8. Switzer WE, Moncrief JA, Mills W Jr, Order SE, Lindberg RB. The use of canine heterografts in the therapy of thermal injury. *J Trauma* 1966;6:391-5.

9. Pruitt BA Jr, Levine NS. Characteristics and uses of biologic dressings and skin substitutes. *Arch Surg* 1984;119:312-22.

10. Colocho G, Graham WP III, Greene AE, Matheson DW, Lynch D. Human amniotic membrane as a physiologic wound dressing. *Arch Surg* 1974;109:370-3.

11. Choy DSJ. Clinical trials of a new plastic dressing for burns and surgical wounds. *Arch Surg* 1954;68:33-43.

12. Chardack WM, Brueske DA, Santomauro AP, Fazekas G. Experimental studies on synthetic substitutes for skin and their use in the treatment of burns. *Ann Surg* 1962;155:127-39.

13. Levine NS, Salisbury RE, Mason AD Jr. The effect of early surgical excision and homografting on survival of burned rats and of interperitoncally-infected rats. *Plast Reconstr Surg* 1975;56:423-9.

14. Frank DH, Wachtel T, Frank HA, Sanders R. Comparison of Biobrane, porcine, and human allograft as biologic dressings for burn wounds. *J Burn Care Rehabil* 1983;4:186-90.

15. Roberts LW, McManus WF, Shirani KZ, Mason AD Jr, Pruitt BA Jr. Evaluation of burn wound care in troops with burn injury: synthetic burn wound dressing—a comparative study. *Annual Research Progress Report*, US Army Institute of Surgical Research, Fort Sam Houston, Texas, 88-102, Sept 30, 1985.

16. Burke JF, Yannas IV, Quinby WC, Bondoc CC, Jung WK. Successful use of a physiologically acceptable artificial skin in the treatment of extensive burn injury. *Ann Surg* 1981;194: 413-28.

17. Heimbach D, Luterman A, Burke JF, Cram A, Herndon D, Hunt J, et al. Artificial dermis for major burns: a multi-center randomized clinical trial. *Ann Surg* 1988;208:313-20.

18. Rue LW, Cioffi WG, McManus WF, Pruitt BA Jr. Wound closure and outcome in extensively burned patients treated with cultured autologous keratinocytes. *J Trauma* 1993;34;662-7.

19. Woodley DT, Peterson HD, Herzog SR, Stricklin GP, Burge son RE, Briggaman RA, et al. Burn wounds resurfaced by cultured epidermal autografts show abnormal reconstitution of anchoring fibrils. *JAMA* 1988;259:2566-71.

20. Meyer AA, Manktelow A, Johnson M, et al. Antibody response to xenogeneic proteins in burned patients receiving cultured keratinocyte grafts. *J Trauma* 1988;28:1054-9.

21. Compton CC, Hickerson W, Nadire K, et al. Acceleration of skin regeneration from cultured epithelial autografts by trans plantation to homograft dermis. *J Burn Care Rehabil* 1993; 14:653-62.

22. Wainwright DJ. Use of an acellular allograft dermal matrix (Alloderm) in the management of full-thickness burns. *Burns* 1995;21:243-8.

23. Rouabhia M, Germain L, Bergeron J, Auger FA. Allogeneic-syngeneic cultured epithelia. *Transplantation* 1995;59:1229- 35.

24. Suzuki T, Ui K, Shioya N, Ihara S. Mixed cultures comprising syngeneic and allogeneic mouse keratinocytes as a graftable skin substitute. *Transplantation* 1995;59:1236-41.

25. Chu CS, McManus AT, Matylevich NP, et al. Enhanced survival of autoepidermal-allodermal composite grafts in allosensitized animals by use of silver-nylon dressings and direct current. *J Trauma* 1995;39:273-8.

26. Bell E, Ehrlich HP, Sher S, et al. Development and use of a living skin equivalent. *Plast Reconstr Surg* 1981;67:386-92.

27. Hansbrough JF, Boyce ST, Cooper MI, et al. Burn wound closure with cultured autologous keratinocytes and fibroblasts attached to a collagen-glycosaminoglycin substrate. *JAMA* 1989;262:2125-30.

28. Hansbrough JF, Morgan J, Greenleaf BS, et al. Development of a temporary living skin replacement composed of human neonatal fibroblasts cultured in Biobrane, a synthetic dressing material. *Surgery* 1994;115:633-44.

29. Hansbrough JF, Mozingo DW, Kealey GP, et al. Clinical trials of a biosynthetic temporary skin replacement. Dermagraft—Transitional Covering, compared to cryopreserved human cadaver skin for temporary coverage of excised burn wounds. *J Burn Care Rehabil* 1996;18:43-51.

—by Basil A. Pruitt, Jr, MD, FACS
San Antonio, Texas

Chapter 28

Burn Scars

One of the inevitable outcomes of deep thermal injury is the scarring of the body. And, in spite of the pain and suffering, the guilt, the many losses, perhaps even disability with which the burn survivor must cope, it is the scarring that may be the most difficult aspect of the recovery and adjustment to the new body image. Even those who are able to conceal their scars with clothing or hair often have great difficulty in accepting their new body image. We have designated this the Hidden Burn Syndrome.

Here are some things you should know about scars. For more detailed information, consult your physician or therapist. Beneath the skin is a fibrous connective tissue known as subcutaneous tissue composed of cells called fibroblasts. After injury these cells are stimulated to grow into granulation tissue, which knits the wound together if the wound is small enough. If the wound is too large to close spontaneously, skin grafting is required. Dense masses of granulation tissue create scars. Sometimes excessive collagen forms in the layer of the skin called the dermis during this connective tissue repair, resulting in sharply raised, progressively enlarging and discolored scar tissue. These are keloid scars, and are actually benign tumors that are generally considered harmless and non-cancerous. They may increase contractures of the tissue and may be more prone to occasional itching sensation.

Some people heal with less noticeable scars than others. Keloids are more common in some ethnic groups and in certain types of burns. Surgical removal is usually not effective because there is a high rate of recurrence. However, injection of steroids directly into the scar, cryotherapy, which freezes and destroys the tissue, and x-ray therapy may all offer substantial help. X-ray therapy presents some risk to surrounding tissue.

Scar removal using tissue expansion surgery or flap surgery may be a final resort and may be successful although new scars are created elsewhere.

Although scars are forever, as they become more mature (over a period of years) they become less and less noticeable. We also react differently psychologically and emotionally to this disfigurement to our bodies. To some it may seem like the end of the world. To others, particularly in males, scars are considered macho.

What can you do to help reduce the scarring? Not very much. Some people believe that vitamin E, the gel from the Aloe vera plant or cocoa butter will make a difference. Unfortunately there is no consistent scientific evidence that these will have any beneficial results on the scar's long-term appearance. Since scars usually improve just with the passage of time, people may mistakenly attribute improvement to the treatments they were applying.

The use of pressure therapy, in which custom-manufactured garments are used to apply uniform pressure to the healing area (approximately 25 mm of mercury), is generally thought to result in a more successful outcome. However, some recent research does not confirm this in all cases and there is some indication that pressure may only be beneficial with keloid scars. When these garments are prescribed, they must be worn twenty-three hours a day allowing only enough time to shower and change sets of garments.

Often, instead of a fabric face mask for facial burn scars, a hard plastic mask, molded to the facial features, may be more effective. Hard plastics may also be lined with various synthetic gel sheets, such as silicone, for even better effect and comfort. The hard mask is generally able to apply more uniform pressure over the entire structure of the face.

Sun can cause the scars to become more pigmented and is generally avoided during the period of healing. Sunscreen is recommended during this time. However, obsessive concern regarding sun exposure after full healing should be avoided. There appears to be a slight increase in skin cancer in burn survivors. Overexposure to sun is not healthy for anyone and protective creams should always be used.

In addition to surgical removal of scars and steroid injections, dermabrasion may be an option for some scars. This is a process of sanding down the scar to the level of the surrounding skin. It is usually only effective with small irregularities.

When all else fails, the final solution may be to conceal the scars with the use of camouflage cosmetics. These are very effective in concealing discolorations but have a lesser effect on texture, especially if the scars are raised significantly. But even smoothing out the color will prove very satisfactory. There are many excellent cosmetic products and practitioners of the art of Paramedical Cosmetology. Many of them will provide their services free of charge to burn survivors.

Sometimes, if a scar is lighter in color than the surrounding tissue, permanent pigmentation, which is a form of tattooing, can be used to match the scar color with the surrounding skin.

But when all is said and done, the most important step toward a full and good recovery is the survivor's acceptance of the new body image. Although our culture stresses perfection in our appearance, only a rare few ever attain it, either through great effort and sacrifice or by camouflage techniques.

Scars are an anathema because we are upset by people staring at us because of them. This appears to be an almost universal concern. How we cope with this is something we at The Phoenix Society may be able to help you with. It may be the most difficult but important part of your recovery.

If you are concerned about your scars, discuss them with your physician and therapists. If you want help in learning to accept your new body image, please contact us. We may be able to help.

For more information, contact.

Phoenix Society for Burn Survivors, Inc.
National Headquarters
33 Main Street, Suite 403
Nashua, New Hampshire   03060
(603) 889-3000* (603) 889-4688 Fax
888-BURN (2876) (toll free for burn survivors)
email: information@burns-phoenix-society.org
web page: www.burns-phoenix-society.org

371

Chapter 29

Prevention and Correction of Burn Scar Contracture

Introduction

Contractures and hypertrophic scars are two of the most frustrating sequelae of thermal injury. Frequently the burned patient has a satisfactory appearance upon discharge; however, three to four weeks later hypertrophy of the scar begins and progresses to severe deformity. Hypertrophic scars occur in any area of the body except those areas in which the skin is splinted by its attachment to underlying structures.

Joint contractures are not only a problem during healing, but also are a constant threat throughout the post-recovery period for a minimum of six months. The development of hypertrophic scars and the formation of contractures are so common, especially in children, that they are frequently accepted by many physicians as the natural course of events following thermal injury.

Our experience in treating approximately 800 acute and reconstructive burned patients yearly has resulted in the conclusion that those sequelae can be significantly altered and controlled with special techniques. The application of continuous and controlled pressure through the use of custom-formed splints and custom made anti-burn-scar elastic supports has yielded a high degree of both non-surgical control of scar contracture and hypertrophic scar formation.

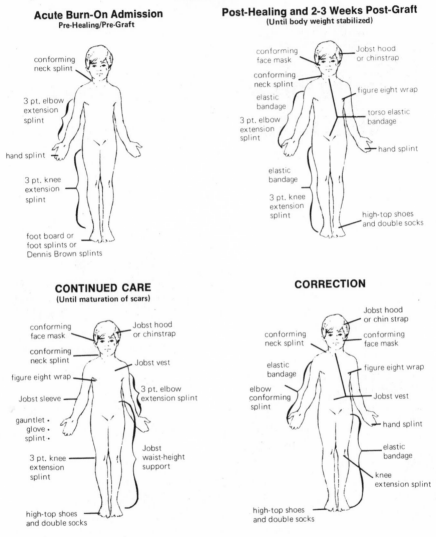

Figure 29.1. Non-Surgical Control of Burn Scar Hypertrophy and Contracture

"The Position of Comfort Is the Position of Contracture."

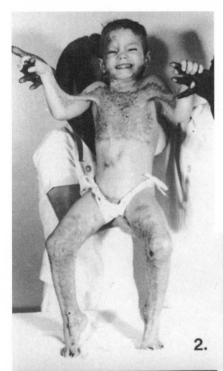

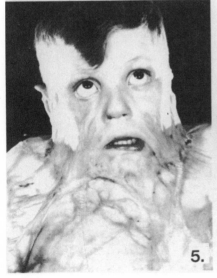

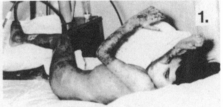

1-2. Because the healing process begins from the time of injury, the "Position of Comfort" preferred by the patient (1) facilitates and predisposes the development of contractures (2).

3. The radial wrinkle lines, sunburst effect, indicate the centripetal direction of contracture which is thought to be due to the contractile force of the fibroblasts.

4. The hypertrophic scar will form a bridge across crease lines of the body. The severity of the contracture is directly related to the severity of the scarring.

5. Thus, when the scar is anterior to a flexor surface, severe contractures may result. (six and one-half months post burn)

Post Healing Problems: Hypertrophic Scars and Contractures

1. This patient, having suffered deep second-degree burns to the face, healed spontaneously one month post burn. The logical expectation for this patient is an acceptable cosmetic result.

2. This the same patient four months later. The continued fibroblastic activity of the deep second-degree burn resulted in hypertrophy with distortion of facial features, betraying the original expectation.

3. Spontaneously healed and grafted second-and third-degree burns of the dorsum of the hand demonstrates an apparently excellent cosmetic result two months post burn.

4. The same hand seen six months later showing severe hypertrophy.

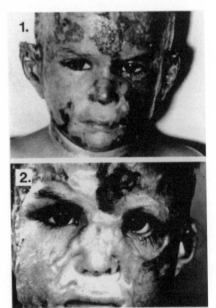

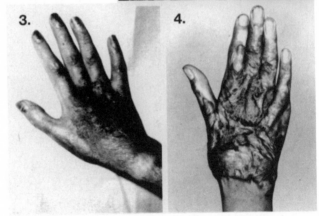

Morphology and Pathophysiology of Hypertrophic Scarring

1. Gross appearance of typical hypertrophic scarring.

2. Normal skin. Reticularis layer of the dermis showing the tridimensional arrangement of the collagen fibers. (L.M. Masson's stain orig. magn. x 156.25).

3. Collagen bundles in the dermis of normal skin The major fiber bundles are composed of finer, parallel, close-packed fibrillar subunits. (S.E.M.* x 7,500).

4. Hypertrophic scar. Reticularis layer of the dermis showing predominant whorl-like and nodular patterns of the collagen fibers. (L.M. Masson's stain orig. magn. x 156.25).

5. Upper: Collagen bundles in a hypertrophic scar are very tortuous and twisted as are the fibers making up the bundles, when the wound is allowed to heal in a shortened position by the unopposed centripetal force of the fibroblast or the voluntary flexion position of the patient. The wound is thus held in a contracted position. (S.E.M. x 7,500). Lower: The whorls and twisting can result in nodules, a characteristic sign of hypertrophic scar. (S.E.M. x 5,400).

6. Non-hypertrophic scar. Reticularis layer of the dermis showing the predominant parallel orientation of the collagen fibers (L.M. Masson's stain orig. magn. x 156.25).

7. Dermis from mature scar. Areas of previous hypertrophy demonstrate a loosening of the compact collagen. "Holey" pattern is characteristic for mature scar. (S.E.M. x 7,500).

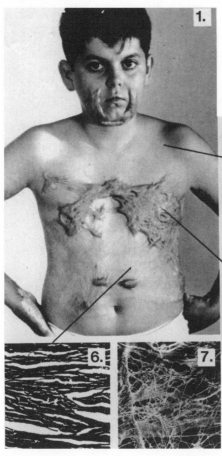

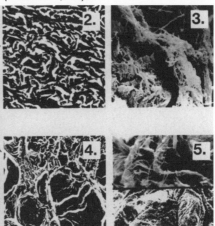

*Scanning Electron Microscope donated by Houston Endowment, Inc.

Morphology According to the Diameter of Collagen Filaments

1. A. Normal skin—round shape, largest size, few interstitial materials. Note sheath about many filaments. (E.M. x 250,000). B. Mature scar—ovoid to round shape, near normal size, amorphous interstitial material, no sheaths. (E.M. x 250,000). C. Hypertrophic scar—irregular to ovoid shape, half size of normal, prominent interstitial material, no sheaths. (E.M. x 250,000). D. Granulation tissue—angular and irregular shape, smallest size, prominent interstitial material, no sheaths. (E.M. x 250,000).

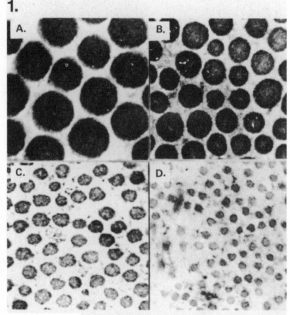

2. Nodules can be seen on gross examination of a section of hypertrophic scar. The majority occur in the deeper, reticularis layer of the dermis.

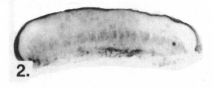

MUCOPOLYSACCHARIDE DISTRIBUTION

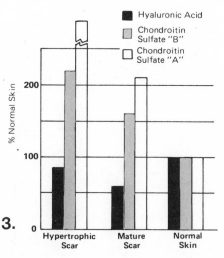

3. By measurement of percent of total mucopolysaccharides, Chondroitin Sulphate A is increased markedly in hypertrophic scar. This decreases with the application of constant pressure. Note: Normal dermis has small amount of Chondroitin Sulfate A.

Prevention—Positioning and Splinting

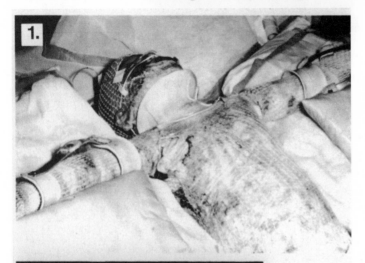

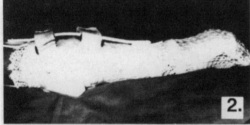

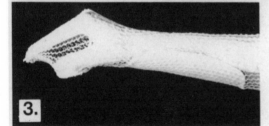

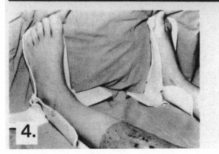

1. *The prevention of contracture deformities should begin as early as possible post burn. Positioning of joints in a neutral, non-fetal position is absolutely necessary. Splints may be used to facilitate positioning.*

2. *A basic three-point extension positioning splint is used for both upper and lower extremities.*

3. *Custom-made positioning hand splints ensure complete extension of the interphalangeal joints, while maintaining optimal wrist, metacarpophalangeal and thumb position.*

4. *Positioning of both involved and non-involved joints is necessary to prevent tendon shortening. Custom-made foot splints may be used instead of the standard footboard as positioning.*

Prevention—Grafting

1. Skin grafts decrease hypertrophic scar formation Note the scarring between the grafts.

2. Diagrammatic demonstration of hypertrophic scar piling up between grafts and covered by thin epidermis.

3. Verhoeff's stain reveals elastic fibers (black strings) in dermis of graft overlying scar. (L.M. orig. magn. x 43.75).

4. The graft limits the excessive proliferation of the connective tissue of the underlying wound and by its natural pressure acts to avoid to some extent the formation of the whorl-like or nodular arrangement of the collagen fibers. Thus in this picture it is possible to see a more regular pattern in the scar tissue under the graft. (L.M. Masson's stain orig. magn. x 43.75).

5. Thin epidermis covering scarred dermis is vulnerable to trauma. Note absence of elastic fibers (compare with Fig. 3). (L.M. Verhoeff's stain x 25).

6. The borders of the graft, where an open space is left between the grafts or between graft and normal skin, the collagen fibers of the dermis, through spontaneous healing, adopt a predominant whorl-like or nodular arrangement to form a hypertrophic scar. This evolution will result in the peculiar hypertrophic scarring shown in Fig. 1. (L.M. Masson's stain orig. magn. x 43.75).

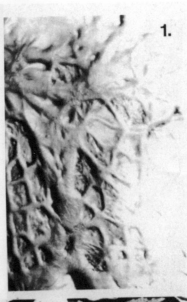

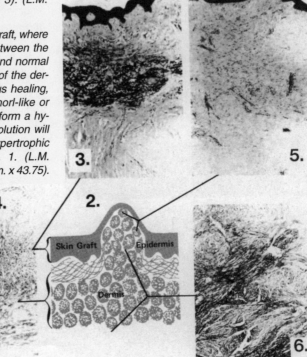

380

Prevention—Pressure and Splinting

1. To prevent facial scar hypertrophy, a custom made silicone foam conforming face mask is applied and held in place under moderate pressure with a Jobst hood of elasticized material.

2. The effect of eight days of pressure is shown sixty-five days post burn. A ridge is evident in front of the ear, curving toward the chin. Pressure to this area was reduced by tenting of the Jobst hood over the outer and lower borders of the face mask.

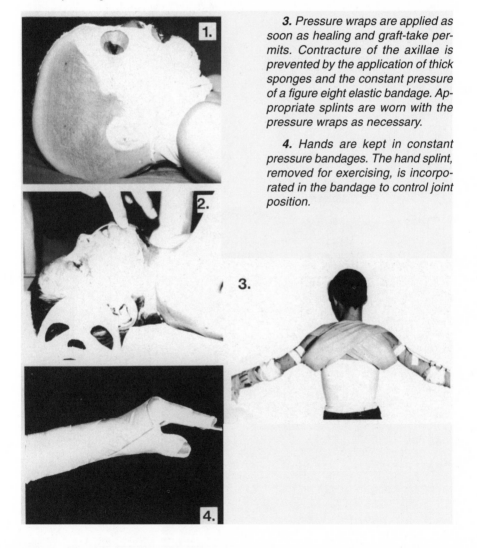

3. Pressure wraps are applied as soon as healing and graft-take permits. Contracture of the axillae is prevented by the application of thick sponges and the constant pressure of a figure eight elastic bandage. Appropriate splints are worn with the pressure wraps as necessary.

4. Hands are kept in constant pressure bandages. The hand splint, removed for exercising, is incorporated in the bandage to control joint position.

Prevention—Pressure

1. Burns covering large areas of the body, three months post burn.

2. Custom-made Jobst anti-burn-scar supports* replace wraps to facilitate and control pressure application. Light topical dressings can be continued as shown here to areas of skin breakdown or slow healing. Zippers to sleeves and hose permit application of the supports without shearing of vulnerable skin. The hood was worn with a facial splint.

3. Result after four months of continuous and controlled pressure.

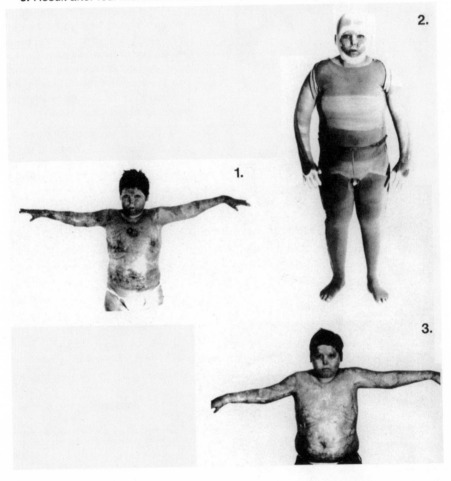

*Made to order by the Jobst Institute, Inc. 653 Miami Street, Toledo, Ohio 43694.

4. Spontaneously healed deep second-degree burns, two months post burn.

5. Custom-fitted Jobst glove worn continuously night and day.

6. Result shown after five months of pressure.

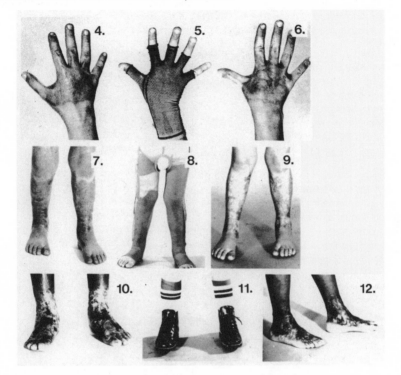

7. Mixed second-and third-degree burns three months post burn.

8. Jobst anti-burn-scar waist-height support applied to facilitate and control pressure. Zippers ankle to waist permit easy application without skin damage.

9. Result after four months of continuous pressure.

10. Burns to the dorsum of the feet result in dorsal tightness and inability to flex the toes, forty-seven days post burn.

11. High top shoes, laced toes to top, the tongue padded with 1/2 inch orthopedic felt and with a metatarsal bar under the sole and possibly a steel shank, are fitted as soon as skin condition permits and worn continuously night and day. To reduce friction and subsequent shearing of the skin, vulnerable areas of the foot are painted with tincture of Benzoin. A thin nylon sock is worn next to the skin. A second, thick cotton sock is worn over this. The result is a transfer of the shearing action to between the two layers of socks.

12. Soft pliable scar with absence of contracture at ten months post burn.

Prevention—Pressure

1. Constant pressure with elastic bandages decreases scar formation. Proximal portion of the upper arm (right) had no pressure. Note flattening of scars on distal portion (left) where pressure was applied. Long biopsy includes areas of pressure and no-pressure. Both areas healed spontaneously.

2. Hypertrophic scar showing the considerable amount of mucopolysaccharides (dark areas) within the nodules. (L.M. colloidal iron's stain orig. magn. x 156.25).

3. Portion of specimen not under pressure reveals increased amounts of compact collagen. (S.E.M. x 5,000).

4. Hypertrophic scar under pressure. This section shows a moderate amount of mucopolysaccharides. The collagen fibers are in a predominantly parallel orientation (contrast the white background with the grey background of Fig. 4). (L.M. colloidal iron's stain orig. magn. x 156.25).

5. Portion of specimen under pressure reveals less collagen and individual fibers are visible. (S.E.M. x 5,000).

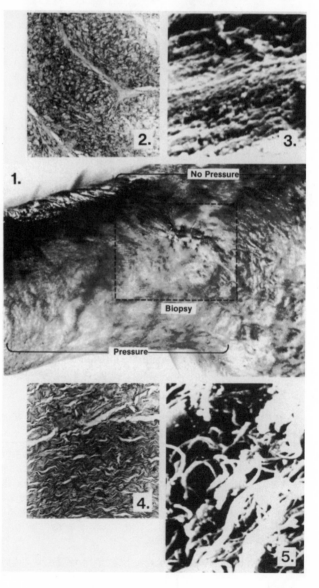

Correction: Traction

1. Severe contracture of the elbow, four months post burn.

2. Before traction: (patient shown—Fig. 1) Section of the skin demonstrates the epithelium with rete ridges and the collagen fibers of the reticularis layer of the dermis, showing a predominant whorl-like pattern. (L.M. Masson's stain orig. magn. x 43.75).

3. One day of constant traction with radial pin.

4. Three days of constant traction with radial pin.

5. Five days of constant traction with radial pin. Note the elbow is almost straight and the scar appears flat and comparatively soft. The wound is the biopsy site, shown in Fig. 6.

6. After fourteen days traction: Similar area to Fig. 2, showing the absence of rete ridges. Collagen fibers now have a predominant parallel orientation. (L.M. Masson's stain orig. magn. x 43.75).

7. Result achieved without surgical correction. Constant elastic bandage support and an elbow extension splint were used after traction, to maintain the correction. [Serial splinting together with constant pressure is preferred to traction for correction of contractures.]

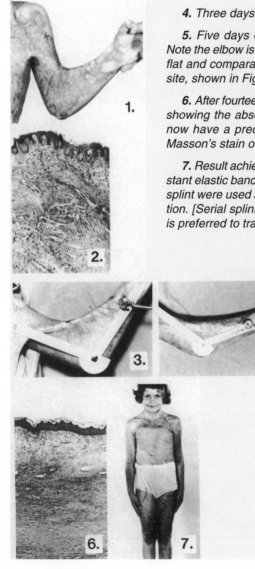

Correction—Splinting

- Avoids Surgery
- Does Not Require Hospitalization
- Treated on Outpatient Basis

1. Severe contracture deformity of the elbow, wrist, and hand with axillary involvement three months post burn, mixed second-and third-degree burns. Mesh grafts were used and hypertrophy of the interstices is evident.

2. Biopsy of scar of patient, Fig. 1, before pressure, shows increased, compact collagen. (S.E.M. x 6.000).

3. Elastic bandages and splints were applied and worn continuously without primary traction. The splints were modified daily as the scar tissue softened and permitted more range of motion.

4. After three to four weeks of treatment.

5. After three to four weeks: compact collagen beginning to loosen. (S.E.M. x 6.000).

6. After six weeks of treatment.

7. After six weeks of pressure and splinting, the collagen is less compact, and individual fibers are now visible. (S.E.M. x 6.000).

8. After three months of treatment. There is marked smoothing and fading of the scar with return of contour without surgery.

9. After three months pressure and splinting, fibroblasts are seen in a loose collagen network. (S.E.M. x 6.000).

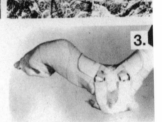

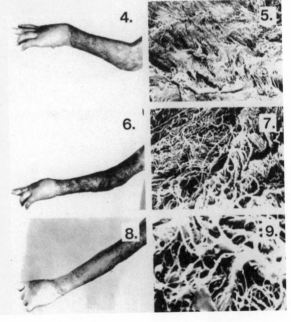

1. A closeup of the radial aspect of the hand three months post burn before treatment.

2. A custom-made hand splint is applied with elastic bandage pressure and worn continuously. As pressure softens the scar tissue, daily correction of the wrist and finger-positioning splint is possible.

3. One week of pressure and splinting.

4. Three weeks of pressure and splinting.

5. Six weeks of pressure and splinting.

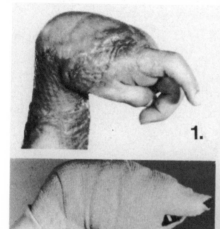

1.

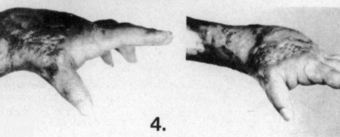

2.

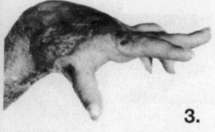

3.

4.

5.

6. The result achieved with eleven weeks of pressure and splinting on an outpatient basis, without surgery.

6.

Correction—Splinting

Special Problems—Skin Breakdown

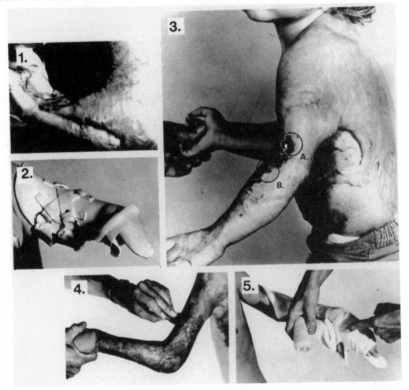

1. *Pressure should be applied as soon as possible for most effective results, but may be implemented as long as the scar remains hyperemic. This scar, one year post burn, is the result of a spontaneously healed second-degree scald.*

2. *Elastic bandages and splints were applied and worn continuously. The splints were modified daily during the first two weeks as the scar tissue softened and permitted more range of motion.*

3. *The remodeling and correction of the hypertrophic scar contracture is the result of six months continuous pressure and splinting, without surgery. Continuous application of pressure can cause breakdown of vulnerable skin (note open area upper arm "A") either by the shearing action or the inconsistency of the elastic bandage pressure wraps.*

4. *To prevent shearing action, tincture of Benzoin is applied to vulnerable skin.*

5. *Two layers of coarse mesh gauze are laid over the Benzoin. Elastic bandages and splints are then applied as usual. The shearing action is thereby transferred from between skin and bandage to between gauze and bandage. Benzoin is reapplied daily, as necessary, and permitted to build up a protective layer (see upper forearm Fig. 3B). Half-inch foam padding is inserted under the bandage over specific pressure areas to permit natural resolution of hematomas that may occur from undue pressure.*

Correction—Splinting and Pressure

1. Contracture of the fifth finger three months post burn.

2. A custom-made splint was molded to fit the contracture anteriorly and applied with an elastic bandage. The splint was modified daily as softening of scar tissue permitted increasing extension.

3. Full correction of the contracture was achieved within five weeks. The result is shown here, eighty-four days post splinting. All splinting adjustments were made by the parents at home. The total hospital attendance was only two days.

4. Hyperextension contracture of the wrist with loss of palmar arch, five months post burn.

5-6-7. Five weeks post splinting. Serial, anterior, conforming hand splints were applied with elastic bandage wraps. As the scar softened, correction of the wrist and thumb position increased and the modification of the splint was possible till a neutral splinting position was obtained. (5). Pressure was continuous during correction and continued until scar maturation was evident. The splint was removed for short periods during the day for exercise and activity (6). At this time wrist flexion was possible with fair opposition of the thumb (7).

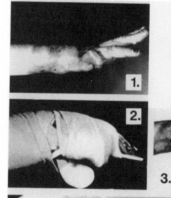

8. Before pressure: (Patient shown in Fig. 4) The collagen fibers of the dermis run in a predominant whorl-like arrangement as seen in hypertrophic scar. (L.M. Masson's stain orig. magn. x 43.75) The hole is an artifact caused by forceps during biopsy excision.

9. After pressure: (Patient shown in Figs. 5, 6, 7).Note the predominant parallel orientation of the collagen fibers of the dermis. Thickness of the scar reduced from 10 mm. to 3 mm. (L.M. Masson's stain orig. magn. x 43.75) Compare with Fig. 8.

Correction—Splinting

1. Hypertrophic scar contracture of the neck, four months post burn.

2. Correction of the contracture achieved by the application of five neck conformers, fitted serially over a period of eight weeks.

3. The result achieved after eight weeks continuous wear of the neck conformers. Although the contracture had been corrected, the scar was still hyperemic and showed signs of activity. Splinting was therefore continued to maintain the correction until there was evidence of scar maturation.

4. This is the result after one year continuous splinting, at which time the splint was discontinued.

5. Follow-up three months after discontinuation of splinting shows no recurrence of contracture or hypertrophy.

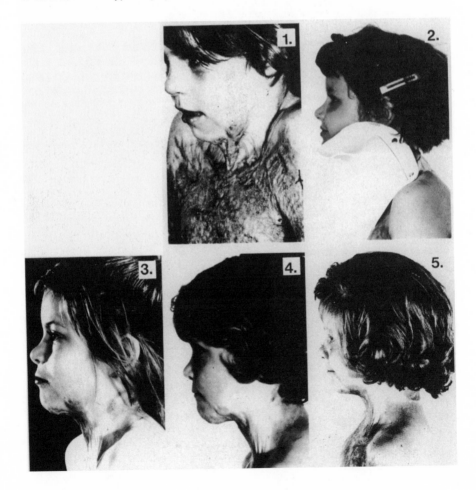

Correction—Pressure

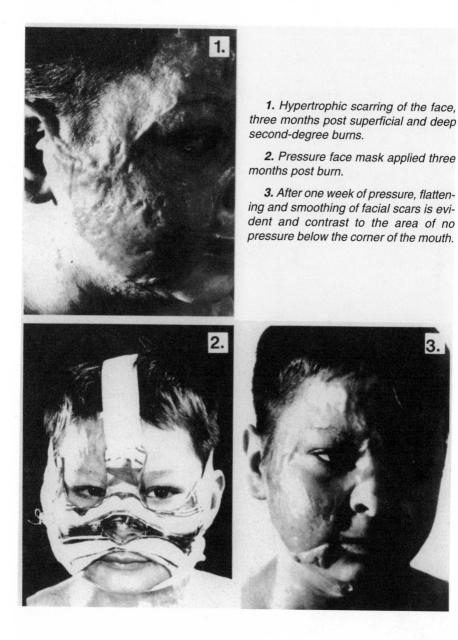

1. Hypertrophic scarring of the face, three months post superficial and deep second-degree burns.

2. Pressure face mask applied three months post burn.

3. After one week of pressure, flattening and smoothing of facial scars is evident and contrast to the area of no pressure below the corner of the mouth.

Correction—Pressure

1. Mesh grafts to the scalp and a mixture of grafted and spontaneously healed areas to the right side of the face, four months post burn.

2. A custom-made Jobst anti-burn-scar hood was applied and worn continuously. A nasal conformer was fitted to apply pressure to the scar on the right side of the nose.

3. Smoothed and softened result achieved after one month pressure.

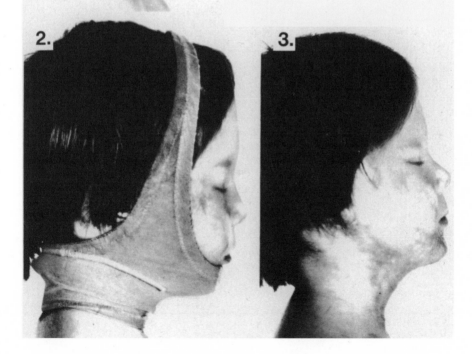

1. Facial scarring ten months post burn.

2. A Jobst custom-made chin strap was applied and worn continuously night and day.

3. This is the result achieved after five months of continuous pressure.

Summary

Non-surgical control of scar contracture and hypertrophic scar formation.

Method: Continuous splinting and pressure.
Duration: Until the scar tissue has matured (average time: six to twelve months).

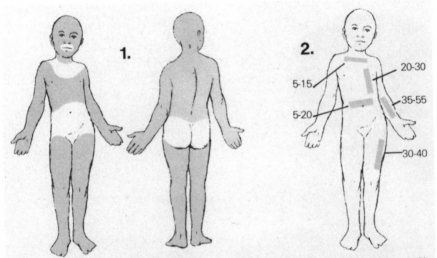

Shaded areas most consistently responsive to pressure.　Average pressure reading mm Hg

1. Evaluation of patients during the initial period of our use of pressure techniques indicated there were certain body areas which were consistently responsive to pressure. These areas are shaded in the diagram.

2. Pressure readings in the mm Hg taken with patients wearing Jobst anti-burn-scar supports during the initial period indicate high readings on the extremities and thorax. The lower readings obtained on the upper chest and abdomen are due to anatomical contour and unresistive underlying structures. Additional padding to these areas of difficulty will increase pressure to effective levels of 20 mm Hg or over.

References

Evans, E.B.; Larson, D.L.; Abston, S.; and Willis, B.; Prevention and Correction of Deformity After Severe Burns, *Surgical Clinics of North America* 50:1361-1375, 1970.

Larson, D.L.; Abston, S.; Evans, E.B.; Dobrkovsky, M.; and Linares, H.A.: Techniques for Decreasing Scar Formation and Contractures in the Burned Patient, *The Journal of Trauma* 11:807-823, 1971.

Larson, D.L., Abston, S.; Evans, E.B.; Dobrkovsky, M.; Willis, B.; and Linares, H.A.: Development and Correction of Burn Scar Contracture, *Transactions of the Third International Congress on Research in Burns*, Prague, 1970. Edited by P. Matter, Hans-Huber Publishers, Vienna.

Linares, H.A.; Kischer, C.W.; Dobrkovsky, M.; and Larson D.L.: The Histiotypic Organization of the Hypertrophic Scar in Humans, *J Invest Derm* 59:323-331, 1972.

Linares, H.A.; Kischer, C.W.; Dobrkovsky, M.; and Larson, D.L.: On_the Origin of the Hypertrophic Scar, *Journal of Trauma* 13:70-75, 1973.

Linares, H.A.: Granulation Tissue and Hypertrophic Scars, International Symposium and work shop on the relation of the ultrastructure of collagen to the healing of wounds and to the Surgical Management of hypertrophic scar, Cincinnati, Ohio, 1973 in press.

Shetlar, M.E.; Larson, D.L.; Shetlar, C.L.; Dobrkovsky, M.; Linares, H.A.; and Villarante, R.: The Hypertrophic Scar, Glycoprotein and Collagen Components of Burn Scars, *Proceedings of the Soc. for Exp. Biol. and Med.* 138:298-300, 1971.

Shetlar, M.E.; Shetiar, C.L.; Su-Fang Chien; Linares, H.A.; Dobrkrovsky, M.; and Larson, D.L.: The Hypertrophic Scar, Hexosamine Containing Components of Burn Scars, *Proc. Soc. Exp. Biol. and Med.* 139:544-547, 1972.

Willis, B.: The Use of Orthoplast Isoprene in the Treatment of the Acutely Burned Child: Preliminary Report, *American Journal of Occupational Therapy* 23:57-61, 1969.

Willis, B.: The Use of Orthoplast Isoprene in the Treatment of the Acutely Burned Child: A Follow-Up, *American Journal of Occupational Therapy* 24:187-191, 1970.

Willis, B.: Splinting the Burn Patient, Shriners Burns Institute, Galveston (Texas) Unit, UTMB Galveston, 1971.

Willis, B.: Burn Scar Hypertrophy—A Treatment Method, Shriners Burns Institute, Galveston (Texas) Unit and Jobst Institute, Inc. Toledo, Ohio, 1973.

Willis, B.: Custom Splinting the Burned Patient, Symposium on the treatment of burns, Lynch, J.B.; and Lewis, S.R. (Edit.), C.V. Mosby Co., Saint Louis, 1973, pp. 93-97.

Willis, B.; Larson, D.L.; and Abston, S.: Positioning and Splinting the Burned Patients, Heart and Lung: *The Journal of Critical Care*, Sept./Oct. 1973. pp. 696700.

—by Duane L. Larson M.D.

Part Four

Rehabilitation and Coping

Chapter 30

Burn Rehabilitation

"I'm told I'm lucky to be alive—that only five years ago a person burned as severely as I would have died. Maybe that would have been best." Shortly after his injury and months before his initial hospitalization ended, the young man quoted above was trying desperately to answer the question: *What about the quality of my life as a survivor of a severe burn injury?*

Survival rates for severely burned people have increased dramatically during the past twenty years, so this question deserves careful deliberation. The improvements have been attributed to the application of basic principles of medicine and systematic research into physiological and metabolic problems. For instance, less than ten years ago, it was learned that burn patients were dying of malnutrition because a severely burned body requires an enormous number of calories to maintain body temperature. Now careful attention is given to adequate calorie intake.

The medical aspects of treating burns have improved significantly. By contrast, the systematic application of rehabilitation principles and practices has not kept pace with acute treatment advances, according to Dr. Irving Feller. Concerned about this lag, Dr. Feller of the University of Michigan Burn Center and his colleagues at the National

NIHR Publication No. 0732-2623 *Rehab Brief* . Vol. VI No.5 May 1983. Although relatively old, this document is currently circulated by the National Institute of Handicapped Research and offers a useful framework for understanding burn rehabilitation.

Table 30.1. Personal and Environmental Factors Affecting the Occurrence of a Burn.

PERSON

Age

Sex

Premorbid Psychopathology
—Behavior problems
—Psychiatric diagnosis/ hospitalization
—Alcoholism-drug abuse
—Suicide
—self-destructive behaviors

Previous Physical Disability
—Neurological disorders
—Cardiovascular disease
—Obesity

Pre-existing Behavior Patterns
—Presence of accident behavior
—Absence or lack of protective behavior

ENVIRONMENT

Socio-Economic Factors
—Unskilled or semi-skilled wage earner
—Crowded housing
—Poor housing

Family Behaviors
—Lack of information about safety, danger, protection
—Presence of accident-prone behaviors

Family Stress
—Poor physical/emotional health
—Pregnancy
—Marital problems
—Conflict with immediate or extended family members

New Environments
—Frequent moves
—Migrants/immigrants
—Isolation

Institute for Burn Medicine (NIBM) began a program of research into burn rehabilitation in 1959. In 1977, the Rehabilitation Services Administration awarded a grant to NIBM. The project was later continued by the National Institute of Handicapped Research. *A Comprehensive Rehabilitation Program for Severe Burns: Final Report* summarizes the project work carried out by Dr. Feller and colleagues at NIBM. The report forms the basis of this BRIEF and answers some basic questions for the rehabilitation practitioner who becomes involved only upon referral late in the rehabilitation process.

Who Gets Burned?

Each year approximately two million people who are burned require medical attention. Seventy thousand require hospitalization and nine thousand die of their injuries. The comprehensive literature review and the three studies done by Dr. Feller and colleagues helped to identify and describe the burn population. While burn patients comprise a heterogeneous group with diverse needs, some generalizations about factors that make the occurrence of a burn more likely can be made. More males than females are burned, except for the population over sixty-five. Of adults, those in their twenties are more likely to be burned. The presence of other significant personal and environmental factors likely to contribute to a burn are summarized in Table 30.1. The reader is reminded that only a limited amount of research has been published and summaries and conclusions are only suggestive, not definitive.

What Is a Severe Burn?

The depth of the burn wound and the percentage of the body surface burned determine the severity of the burn. The depth of the wound is commonly classified in three degrees, but it is measured more precisely in terms of the thickness of the burn. A first-degree or superficial burn involves only the epidermis (top layer of the skin). A second-degree or partial thickness burn involves the dermis as well as the epidermis. A third-degree or full-thickness burn involves both layers of skin and the skin appendages—the hair follicles, sweat glands, and sebaceous glands. Generally, anyone with partial and full-thickness burns over twenty percent of the body is considered to be severely burned. Other factors such as age, pre-existing health problems, and body parts burned are considered also.

What Is the Rehabilitation Process for People Who Have Been Burned?

Successful rehabilitation requires the simultaneous management of all problems—especially medical and psychological—according to an individualized plan. To help the practitioner understand the complicated process, Dr. Feller and colleagues have divided it into three phases (described later). The medical aspects can more reliably be assigned to phases than the psychological aspects. Psychological reactions to a severe burn, like reactions to any disablement, depend on the nature of the disability and many variables relating to the person and the environment. The nature of the disability is influenced by many factors, too, including the resulting functional impairments, visibility of the scars, number of readmissions for corrective surgery, secondary complications, and cause of the burn (suicide attempt, accident, or inflicted burn). Personal characteristics that influence reactions to burns include sex, activities affected, lifestyle, and personality. The immediate environment is especially influential in determining the outcome or adjustment to a severe burn. Family acceptance and support, income, community resources, and hospital capabilities (burn center vs. general hospital) are a few of the environmental factors. Bearing all of these factors in mind and allowing for individual reactions, the practitioner can nevertheless recognize common reactions in each phase.

The Emergent Phase

From the scene of the accident, the severely burned person is rushed to the hospital where the burns are bathed and assessed. The first objective is to stabilize the body's fluids. Damaged capillaries allow fluids to escape to the surrounding tissues and since the skin no longer can control evaporation, the patient becomes dehydrated and goes into shock. Large volumes of fluids are pumped back into the body during the first twenty-four hours after injury. A great deal of swelling occurs and large incisions are sometimes made to release the pressure caused by the swelling. A second objective is to maintain the body temperature since there may be little skin to regulate heat loss. The body uses excessive calories to maintain the temperature and these must be replaced to prevent malnutrition. A weight loss of one pound per day is common. Debridement, or cutting away loose, dead skin begins. This is a painful process—despite injections of morphine. The burns are then coated with solutions to destroy bacteria and antibiotics are also injected. A range of behaviors from passivity and numbness to extreme agitation may be observed as the individual attempts to assimilate what has happened. This phase lasts from one to five days.

The Acute Phase

As the patient slowly understands what has happened, s/he may begin to feel the isolation required to subdue the possibility of infection. The person may realize that s/he has caught the last glimpse of a human face until this phase of rehabilitation is over. Every visitor—family, friend, or medical staff—must wear cap, gown, gloves, and mask. Only the eyes can be seen, but much can be read from them by a person who may be looking for signs of rejection. Having "things" done to one's body without full understanding of the planned outcome can create confusion and fear. Support and acceptance from staff and family are critical during this phase. Daily visits to the hydrotherapy tank continue where the burned, dead flesh is cut away with small, sharp scalpels designed to lessen the blood loss. The loss is so great that only a small area can be cleaned at any one time. Since the person's own skin will be needed for grafting, the muscle and fat are initially covered by pig skin or the skin of cadavers to allow those tissues to heal before grafting.

The pain increases, and although that is a sign of improvement (the pain receptors in full thickness burns are rejuvenating), it only complicates the emotions of the patient. S/he may be asking, "If getting better means adding pain to an already intolerable amount, then why get better?" Depression and anxiety are common and the person most likely wants to withdraw from all interaction. Still the physical therapist visits daily to manipulate joints to prevent loss of range of motion. Once a healthy base of tissue develops in the partial and full thickness burns, grafting can proceed. A donor site is chosen from an unburned area of the body and the skin taken can be stretched up to six (rarely, even to ten) times its original size to cover the wounds. Slowly, the grafts can be expected to cover the body and lower the risks of infection.

The Rehabilitation Phase

This phase begins when the burn wound is decreased to less than 20 percent of the total body surface. It is geared toward preventing cosmetic and functional deformities and returning the person to a place in society. The work done by NIBM indicates that social support from family, friends, peers, and personnel in community agencies facilitates the rehabilitation process independent of the severity of the burn injury.

This support network is challenged by the transition from hospital to home. If the burn happened in the home, fear and anxiety of returning to that environment may occur. Nightmares of being on fire are common for those who have been burned by flames. Unresolved issues about the accident and pre-existing disabilities or personal and family problems which may have been factors in causing burn injuries may surface as complications. Discipline is tested when energy levels are low and physical demands are high. Skin care is essential and physical therapy must be continued. Splints and elastic pressure garments to reduce contractures or scarring must be worn twenty-four hours a day by some people. Financial hardship may increase the strain of new procedures and experiences. The result may be frustration and anger. Gradually the medical condition improves and the person can be expected to assume preburn roles and responsibilities. Then, just as progress is being made, it may be interrupted. Twenty to 30 percent of all survivors require at least one readmission to the hospital and sometimes many more. Most surgeries to correct cosmetic deformities and functional limitations are performed within the first several years after injury, but some people will undergo recurrent surgeries for as many as twenty years. This is especially true for children who require release of scar contractures around developing breasts or growing joints.

As a person begins to realize that s/he will never look or be the same as before the injury, anger, remorse, and despair may surface. Some people reminisce with old photographs about "the way things used to be." They may try to believe that surgery will restore them completely. Yet, they know it is not true. Grief and emotional withdrawal are common as the individuals vacillate between reality and false hope. One young man, a year after injury and several corrective surgeries, realized that his appearance had not improved as much as he had hoped. He angrily tore to shreds every picture of himself taken before the injury. After several more months of depression and grieving, he decided to have only enough additional surgeries to correct contractures, and to forego surgeries intended only to improve appearance. He decided the pain was not worth the improvement he could realistically expect. Practitioners should be careful not to hold out false hopes about what the person can expect from surgery. The significance of the injury should be discussed openly and grief should be respected, but the person is usually helped most if encouraged to resume preburn roles, responsibilities, and activities as soon as possible. Slowly, s/he must be helped to accept a life that has been unalterably changed, but also must be helped to recognize that the quality of a changed life is not necessarily lessened. It is encouraging to note that severely burned people often emerge from the whole process with higher self-esteem than before injury. Sometimes, the support found during the rehabilitation process not only helps them accept the results of being burned, but also helps them learn to master other problems.

What Are the Vocational Implications?

Feller and his colleagues found that the majority of those employed pre-burn resume employment and that a quick return to employment is related to successful rehabilitation. Size of full-thickness burns was found to be an important variable in determining time it took to return to work, but other factors also played a role. Employees who did not return to the same jobs took significantly longer than those who did. Married people returned to work faster than single people. Those who had an adequate to good adjustment preburn returned faster. Litigation almost doubled the time it took to return. Skilled workers were more likely to return to previous jobs than laborers. Coverage by Worker's Compensation did not seem to be a factor. For those who were injured at work, fear of objects or situations (e.g., ovens, torches, carburetors), and physical impairments led to job change. Inability to work as long or as hard as before injury also caused job change. On-the-job complaints were most often related to hand, feet, and leg functioning.

Additional common problems that interfere with work or education are:

- **Contractures**. Contractures result when scar tissue forms over or adjacent to a joint or skin fold. The shortened skin causes a loss of range of motion. These may be corrected through continued physical therapy, but may often require surgery.

- **Hypertrophic scars**. This ropey, thick formation of skin is an abnormal configuration of collagen fibers. The scars may be corrected with elastic pressure garments, steroid injection, or partial removal of scar and regrafting. (Keloid formation is a special kind of scarring and is common to dark pigmented skin.)

- **Eye Injuries.** Inability to close the eyes due to badly burned eyelids can be corrected with grafting. Scarring of the corneas often responds to medication, but a corneal transplant may be helpful.

- **Body part loss**. Amputations may be required if burns involve muscle and bone. The loss of the nose and ears is a fairly frequent complication and requires plastic surgery.

- **Neuromuscular problems**. Peripheral neuromuscular problems are evidenced by numbness, tingling, peripheral weakness, impaired hearing, or other nerve deficit signs. Hemiplegia, seizure disorders, aphasia, encephalitis, and meningitis have been found.

- **Loss of sweat glands**. The person must avoid overheating.

- **Hair loss**. A full-thickness burn involves the hair follicles and thus the grafted areas will not grow hair. If the scalp is involved, hair transplants may be desired, if the person works with the public.

- **Loss of sebaceous glands**. Daily lubrication is needed to maintain pliable skin.

- **Delicate skin**. During the first year after grafting, even scratching can break the skin and the skin will sunburn easily.

- **Itching**. Itching is a common complaint.

- **Lack of sensation.** Grafted areas lack the sensation of normal skin.

- **Drug dependency**. Whether a problem before or after injury, drug dependency complicates vocational planning.

Other serious complications are total loss of hearing and brain damage. Electrical burns merit special consideration. All electrical burns are full-thickness burns and usually occur at work. They often appear to involve only small areas where the current entered and exited, but the tissue beneath the skin may be severely damaged. This can lead to amputation and/or serious neuromuscular problems.

While a person with many physical complications may present a challenge to the rehabilitation practitioner, severity of the injury may not be the major factor influencing return to preburn activities. Often a person with relatively few complications will take a long time to return to work and other activities. Evidence exists to show that young adults with no previous work experience represent a supreme challenge regardless of the severity of physical limitations or complications.

What Are the Components of a Model Program for Burn Care?

One of the most important tasks of the project undertaken by NIBM was to identify the components of a model rehabilitation program. Outlined in depth in the Final Report to the National Institute of Handicapped Research, the six components are listed below:

1. The planning and organization of a regionalized burn care system.

2. The development of a program designed to meet the needs of the burn patient population it serves.

3. The process of rehabilitation for the burn patient.

4. The burn rehabilitation team.

5. Education and involvement of the patient, family, and community.

6. Rehabilitation research.

How Can Information Be Shared?

The National Burn Information Exchange (NBIE) was started by NIBM to provide a method to define the natural course of burn trauma by collecting and disseminating information from burn centers throughout the world that can be used to more knowledgeably plan for rehab needs. Presently, over 65,000 cases are on file from over 100 hospitals.

Conclusions

NIBM studies indicate that a person who is treated at a major burn center and is provided with a supportive environment during the rehabilitation process can be expected to achieve social, emotional, and vocational adjustment. Indeed, some report higher self-esteem and life satisfaction than before injury. Thus, the practices demonstrated to be effective in such a supportive environment should be systematically applied to all settings providing burn-related services.

Rehabilitation professionals' roles and responsibilities must be clearly defined. The literature defines the roles of practitioners on the primary care team-surgeon, psychologist, psychiatrist, nurse, social worker, occupational therapist, and physical therapist—but not the roles of professionals in community agencies to which referrals are made. The rehabilitation counselor is particularly important in that return to productive work is recognized as a major factor contributing to overall adjustment. Yet, of the 325 people studied, only 16 per cent could remember being referred to a state vocational rehabilitation agency and only 11 percent reported contact with an agency. The results of that small study are not definitive, but raise questions as to why rehabilitation counselors are not more involved in the rehabilitation of people who are burned. Improvements may have been made since 1977, but counselors might ask themselves if greater efforts could be made to service this population. Assigning liaison counselors to burn units and burn centers would be one step in the right direction.

Counselors should recognize that while medical and physical facts may differ from other populations, the human reactions are similar to those they've observed with other disabilities. Therefore, the roles and responsibilities of the rehabilitation counselor are not new. They include:

1. Facilitating independence;
2. providing support and counseling;
3. providing vocational guidance and placement;
4. involving and educating the family; and
5. recognizing the long-term implications and providing follow-up when possible.

Counselors can contribute to the management of psychological stresses during the medical treatment and provide counseling and guidance aimed toward a quick return to preburn activities. The most outstanding medical treatment can be negated by lack of appropriate counseling and guidance. State rehabilitation agencies must see that this doesn't happen.

Sources

Three books developed during the grant are appended to, but not included in the Final Report:

Bowden, M.L. and Feller, Irving, M.D. *Progress in Burn Rehabilitation: A Report of Three Studies*, Ann Arbor, Michigan: NIBM, 1982.

Bowden, M.L.; Jones, Claudelia A.; and Feller, Irving, M.D. *Psycho*-Social *Aspects of a Severe Burn: A Review of the Literature*. Ann Arbor, Michigan: NIBM, 1979.

Feller, Irving, M.D. et al. *Reconstruction and Rehabilitation of the Burned Patient*. Ann Arbor, Michigan: NIBM, 1979.

Chapter 31

Aquatic Access for
the Disabled

Abstract

Innovations in rehabilitation engineering can now provide aquatic access for the disabled. In the regional burn center, the Bodi-Gard cart shower system (Hospital Therapy Products, Inc., Wood Dale, Ill.) uses three flexible hoses to provide precise hydrotherapy and debridement. Its main mixing valve controls temperature and pressure and is easily disinfected by an in-line chamber. This shower system is complemented by the foldable Bodi-Gard Mobile seat shower system (Hospital Therapy Products, Inc.). This system, which is covered by a disposable liner, surrounds the patient with eight water jets that empty into any floor drain. The Bather 2001 (Silcraft Corp., Traverse City, Mich.) is a fiberglass hydrotherapy bathtub with a unique Aqua-Seal door (Silcraft Corp.) that can be raised to provide patient access. Its unique closed-loop disinfection system prevents contamination of its internal components. The Nolan Tublift (Aquatic Access, Louisville, Ky.) is a lightweight, removable lift that uses water power to gently raise and lower its seat. It can be manually swiveled to allow access from a wheelchair. Transfer benches span the tub wall to provide access to the shower and bathtub. Although they are a less expensive alternative to the Tublift, they allow water to spill outside the tub, which may create a slippery bathroom floor. The Nolan Poolift (Guardian Products, Arleta, Calif.) is a water-powered pool lift that automatically rotates as it descends. It can lift up to 135-kg with a home water pressure of 55 psi. In contrast, the water-powered Aquatic Access Poolift is a less expensive pool lift that rotates manually with assistance. Because no part of any of these pool lifts is underwater except during use, the lifts are portable and not susceptible to corrosion by pool water. (J Burn Care Rehabil 1992;13:356-63).

Whether it be for recreation, therapy, or hygiene, access to water is a necessary and important part of our lives. When the disabled cannot gain access to water, they become frustrated with personal hygiene and cannot enjoy the celebration of aquatic exercise. With the advents of rehabilitation engineering, technologic advances have been made that allow the disabled to gain access easily and safely to water. In burn centers, hydrotherapy systems have been designed to allow wound cleansing with reduced risks of auto-and cross-contamination. In addition, showers and bathtubs that are easily accessible to the disabled have been designed. These adaptive modes of access can easily be incorporated into devices in the home. With the development

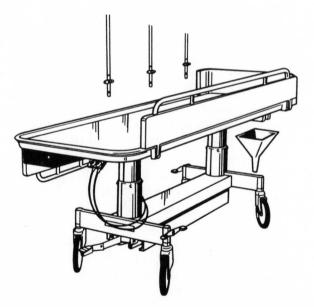

Figure 31.1. *The Bodi-Gard cart shower system (Hospital Therapy Products, Inc.) has three overhead retractable spray reels to provide precise hydrotherapy and a stainless steel cart that can transport and weigh a patient.*

of pool lifts, the disabled can now enjoy the benefits of aquatic exercise. It is the purpose of this chapter to describe the most recent advances in rehabilitation engineering that provide aquatic access for the disabled.

Aquatic Access Systems

Table Shower System. In many burn centers, patients receive daily hydrotherapy. This procedure offers many practical advantages:

1. It appears to facilitate dressing changes by loosening adherent dressings;

2. It encourages removal of the antimicrobial cream in preparation for reapplication;

3. It softens the eschar, which allows it to separate from underlying tissue during daily debridement and thus permits the patient to independently initiate range-of-motion activities.[1]

Control of infection in the burn wound may be another benefit of hydrotherapy. When the patient with burns undergoes hydrotherapy in a tank or tub, the water becomes heavily contaminated by viable bacteria. These bacteria originate either from the endogenous microflora of the patient (e.g., skin, stool) or from the burn wound. Because this contamination not only poses a threat to the patient but is a potential source of cross-contamination for other patients, disinfection of the hydrotherapy tank or tub is mandatory after each treatment.[1]

However, the addition of antiseptic agents to the water in the hydrotherapy tank is viewed by the patients and staff as a double-edged sword. Whenever the dilute solution of the antiseptic agent comes in contact with the patients burned skin, it elicits more discomfort than does tank water without the antiseptic agent. Furthermore, agitation of the water that contains the antiseptic agent releases vapors that are irritating to the conjunctival and nasal mucosa of personnel. The problems encountered with hydrotherapy tanks or tubs have been eliminated by the development of the Bodi-Gard cart shower system (Hospital Therapy Products, Inc., Wood Dale, Ill.), which was specially designed for regional burn centers (Figure 31.1). This system reduces autocontamination from the patient and cross-contamination from other patients. In addition, this system simplifies transfer of the patient from the bed to the treatment room. The patient is transferred to the cart and then taken to the hydrotherapy room for treatment.

413

The patient remains on the same cart for treatment and dressing changes. The cart is used to return the patient to his or her bedside and to transfer the patient to his or her bed. At the appropriate time during treatment, the patient is weighed with the built-in electronic scale.

The cart tray itself is made of stainless steel with coved corners and minimum seams for ease in cleaning. Long side rails offer maximum freedom of access for the patient, including a lowered height of 0.66 M, which allows ambulatory patients the ability to sit on the cart and then be raised to a working level by the staff. The cart is approximately 0.81 M wide by 2.13 M long and has a height range from 0.66 M to 0.86 M. The controls for raising and lowering the cart and the operation of the weighing scale is located at the head of the cart. The cart is rated for a 225-kg capacity with self-locking side rails to support lateral pressures from the patient. The casters have brakes that may be operated from either end with a swivel-lock function to aid in steering.

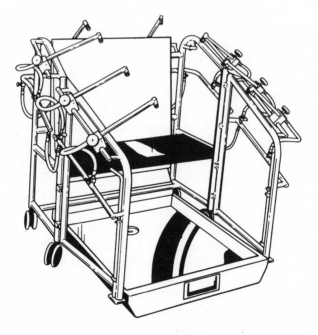

Figure 31.2. *The foldable Bodi-Gard Mobile seat shower system (Hospital Therapy Products, Inc.) surrounds the patient with eight water jets and can be placed over any floor drain.*

Three retractable overhead spray reels provide for hands-free soaking of the patient and wound-specific cleaning. Special stainless steel nozzles have a full cone spray pattern designed for full coverage of the patient from the neck to the ankles. A drip-free shutoff valve offers individual control of pattern and pressure on each nozzle. The main mixing valve assembly controls the water flow to the overhead spray reels. This assembly incorporates a thermostatic valve to control the temperature and a pressure-balancing unit to equalize the hot and cold incoming pressures. Together this assembly allows for control of output temperatures to within 2° F. of the set-point temperature. Overall pressures may be adjusted with the main input regulators on both the hot and cold water supplies. For safety, the system will automatically shut down if there is a loss of pressure on one side of the supply line or an uncontrolled increase in temperature.

Bodi-Gard disposable liners (Hospital Therapy Products, Inc.) reduce the possibility of cross-contamination between patients. Each individually packaged liner acts as a barrier between the patient and the cart. After each treatment, the liner is removed and replaced by a new liner in preparation for the next patient. Mounted in series with the main mixing valve is a sterilizing chamber to allow cleaning of the inside of the water lines from the chamber to the tip of the nozzles. The disinfectant solution in our burn center is Hibiclens (Stuart Pharmaceuticals, Wilmington, Del.).

Seat Shower System. The Bodi-Gard seat shower system (Hospital Therapy Products) was designed to complement the cart shower and allow ambulatory patients to be treated more quickly and with little handling by the nursing staff. Constructed of stainless steel and reinforced polycarbonate materials, the seat shower system measures approximately 1.1 M^2, is 0.81 M high at the front, and slopes to a height of 1.1 M at the rear. A low tip at the entrance of the shower allows most patients to walk easily into the shower and sit down on the wide bench seat. Surrounded by eight adjustable, fine-spray nozzles, the patient may clean himself or herself and even shave, if permitted.

One of the ideal functions of the seat shower is that the nursing staff may treat the patient without climbing into the shower and getting wet. The low height of the shower allows access to the patient from all four sides, and even the feet may be washed while the nurse remains outside the shower. For those patients with perineal wounds, it is common to remove the bench seat and have them stand or stoop in the shower for cleansing. The seat shower uses the BodiGard disposable liner system (Hospital Therapy Products) to reduce the possibility of infection and minimize equipment cleaning between patients. The polypropylene liners cover the shower's side walls, seat, and top opening and can be tucked around the patient's neck. The overhead spray reel and mixing valve assemblies used in the cart shower system are also incorporated into the seat shower system.

The Bodi-Gard seat shower is also available in a mobile design constructed of stainless steel with the same controls and spray nozzles (Figure 31.2). An important feature of the mobile shower is that it folds up to approximately 0.89 M x 1.27 M for storage or movement to another treatment room. Tepid water is supplied through a quick-disconnect assembly, and the base fits over a 15 cm flush floor drain, which eliminates the need for fixed plumbing assemblies.

Prefabricated Bath System. The Bather 2001 (Silcraft Corp., Traverse City, Mich.) is a compact patient bathing and hydromassage system with a unique Aqua-Seal side-opening door (Silcraft Corp.) that minimizes the need for lifting devices (Figure 31.3). It is a complete patient hygiene system that offers sit-down showering, deep soaking,

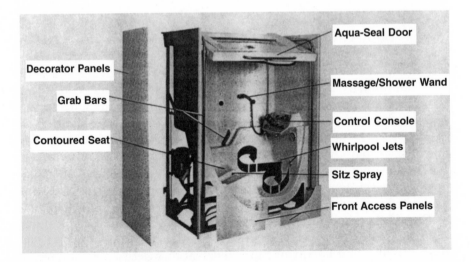

Figure 31.3. The Bather 2001 (Silcraft Corp.) is a hydrotherapy bathtub with a unique side opening door and closed-loop disinfecting system. Arrows show direction of circulation of water.

416

sitz spray, and hydrotherapeutic whirlpool massage. The tub is made of a one-piece fiberglass shell bonded to an inner aluminum tube frame and has the following inner dimensions: 0.79 M deep, 0.53 M wide at the tub floor, and 1.2 M long. The interior features a semireclined contoured seat with a perineal cutout to allow thorough cleaning. The unique side-opening door is raised manually on two glide rails to provide access for nonambulatory patients. In the down position, an Aqua-Seal Mechanism prevents any leakage. The tub is 2 M high and has outer dimensions of 1.6 M x 0.88 M. The movable door measures 0.79 M x 1.3 M, and when raised, its top is 0.10 M above the tub wall. When filled, the tub holds approximately 209 L of water, which is circulated by a 3/4 hp pump through a filtered inlet at a maximum rate of 258 L/Min. The filtered inlet provides 46 cm^2 of filtrate surface area.

Water enters the tub through two adjustable whirlpool jets in the front. A single water intake is located near the place for the patient's left foot. An adjustable body sprayer is located in front of the tub above the water line. An adjustable sitz sprayer is located in the seat's cutout and can direct water to the perineal area. A shower spray can be mounted on the tub wall in two different positions or can be handheld. Water temperature and pressure are selected and regulated by the control panel at the front of the tub. Also controlled here are the Aqua-Seal door lock, whirlpool intensity, drain, sitz spray, and body spray. A temperature-sensitive coil constantly monitors water temperature and shuts down water flow in less than five seconds when water temperature exceeds 38° C. A 5 cm drain empties the tub at a rate of 114 L/ Min., which usually takes about 1 1/2 minutes. Although the external surface of the tub can be cleaned with chemical disinfectants, a unique closed-loop disinfecting system is used to clean the internal components (pump, impeller, tubing, exit jets) and uses very little disinfecting solution. The jets are first turned and closed off and a small amount of disinfectant solution is then introduced into the system through, a reservoir at the front of the tub. After ten minutes of contact time, the jets are reopened and the solution is purged.

In many hospitals and homes, the disabled do not have the luxury of either a portable shower system or a prefabricated bath system. Most hospitals and homes have tubs that are not accessible to the handicapped. With the advent of the Nolan Tublift (Aquatic Access, Louisville, Ky.) and the Guardian transfer bench (Guardian Products, Arleta, Calif.) the handicapped can now safely enjoy a relaxing bath or shower.

Tublift. The Nolan Tubfift is a major technologic advance that provides the handicapped easy access to a tub or shower (Figure 31.4).

The entirely waterpowered lift is composed of an anodized aluminum frame and a polypropylene seat. The seat height in the raised position is either 43.2 cm or 53.3 cm from the tub floor, depending on the model. These two different models allow for variation in bathtub height. The seat is also available with or without arms. The H-frame base is 45.7 x 35.6 cm and attaches to the bottom of the tub with suction cups. The seat manually swivels to allow wheelchair access in the raised position. The seat is 40.6 x 38.1 cm, with a back that is 38.1 cm high. In the lowered position, the seat rests 5.1 cm from the tub bottom. The Tublift weighs 8.5-kg and can be removed for normal tub use.

The lift is totally water-powered and can lift up to 108-kg with 20 psi. A valve on the seat controls the flow of water into and out of the system for seat raising and lowering. On the models with arms, the control valve is on the arm. The water connection is made through a hose connected to a diverter on the shower head or to a special replacement spout with its own built-in diverter. Adult and child seat belts are available as optional

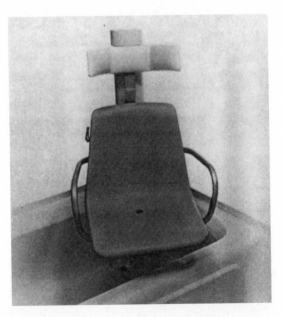

Figure 31.4. The water-powered Nolan Tubfift (Aquatic Access) raises, lowers, and swivels its seat to provide bathtub access. An optional water sprayer can be attached to the Tublift to facilitate bathing.

accessories. A hand-held shower that allows push-button water control can also be added, which eliminates the need to reach for faucets during the bath.

Transfer Bench. Less expensive alternatives to the Nolan Tublift are transfer benches. Although they provide the handicapped access to the tub and shower, their design does not prevent splashover, which allows spillage of water over the tub wall, an invitation to slipping on the wet bathroom floor. Transfer benches (Guardian Products) have two legs in the tub and two legs on the bathroom floor, thereby extending over the tub wall (Figure 31.5). They are designed to support the individual in the shower as well as during transfer to and from

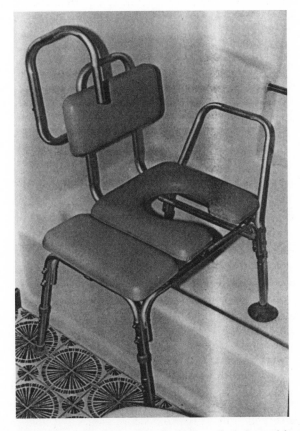

Figure 31.5. Transfer benches span the tub wall and provide support during transfer to and from the bathtub or shower.

419

it. Each transfer bench is made of an aluminum tube frame and polypropylene seat. Different models offer padded seats and backs, commode seats, suction-cup feet, and tub clamps.

The Deluxe padded transfer bench (Model 98017, Guardian Products) has two legs attached by suction cups to the tub floor; two other legs remain outside the tub, creating a supporting bridge into the shower. The bench measures 0.65 M x 0.52 M at its base and has a seat height that is adjustable from 0.46 M to 0.53 M. The padded seat measures 0.40 M square and has a commode opening. The seat's back is 0.34 M high. The transfer bench has an aluminum tube frame and vinyl-coated foam padding. Side arms on each side of the seat can be raised to allow access. A handrail on the seat's back provides another grasping site.

Pool Lifts. A variety of hydrotherapy pools have been specially designed for rehabilitation.[2] Many hydrotherapy pools are prefabricated, which facilitates their installation in the hospital setting. Most of these prefabricated pools rest fully above the floor, although one is an in-ground pool with its sides inset into the floor. An alternative to these prefabricated pools is a custom-designed in-ground hydrotherapy pool. In all cases, the handicapped must gain access to the pool with either a self-operated or manual-use pool lift.

Self-Operated Pool Lift. The Nolan Poolift (Guardian Products) is a water-powered lift that has a stainless steel tube frame and polypropylene seat. Wheelchair-bound individuals transfer to the seat in its upright position over the deck and automatically rotate 90 degrees as it descends into the pool (Figure 31.6, A and B). Seat travel is 1.1 M, the main vertical support is 2.4 M, and the distance between the main vertical support and the stanchion is adjustable from 12.7 cm to 43.2 cm. Self-operated use is achieved with call/send control levers at both the deck and water levels. The Nolan Poolift weighs approximately 38.2-kg and is installed by insertion into either an in-deck recessed or above-deck socket. The main vertical support rests against the side of the pool. This configuration eliminates the need for any underwater attachment and allows removal and storage of the unit.

The lift operates exclusively on water power and can be connected to a standard garden hose. It lifts up to 45-kg with 30 psi and up to 135-kg with 55 psi (normal city water psi ranges from 35 to 70 psi). The lift is raised with less than 7.6 L of water, which is then drained into the pool when the seat is lowered (Figure 31.6, C). The seat can

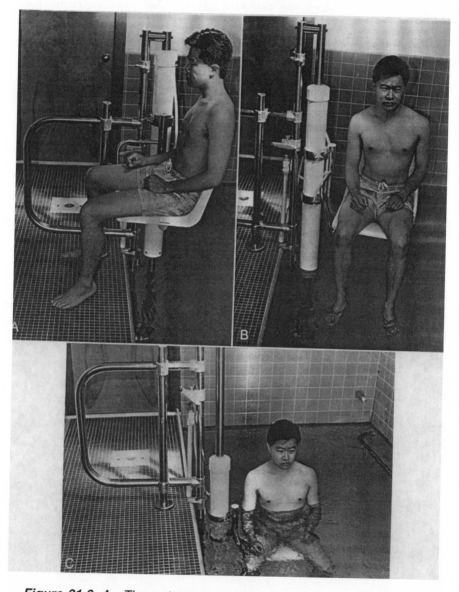

Figure 31.6. *A—The water-powered Nolan Poolift (Guardian Products) mounts into an in-ground or above-ground socket and has a vertical support that rests against the side of the pool. B—The Nolan Poolift automatically rotates 90 degrees as it ascends or descends, allowing an above-deck transfer for ambmbulatory and nonambulatory patients. C—The Nolan Poolift descends 1.1 M into the pool and can then be returned to the surface with the use of an additional water-level control valve.*

be locked to keep it in the raised position when water pressure is turned off. Optional accessories include a seat belt and a wheel assembly to ease transport and storage. A water sprayer can also be added to help rinse chlorinated pool water from the body.

Manual-Use Poolift. The Aquatic Access pool lift is less expensive than the self-operated pool lift but must be manually operated by an assistant (Figure 31.7). The pool lift is installed into a flush mounted bronze socket 25.4 cm to 35.6 cm from the edge of the pool. It is boarded completely over the deck and then manually rotated 180

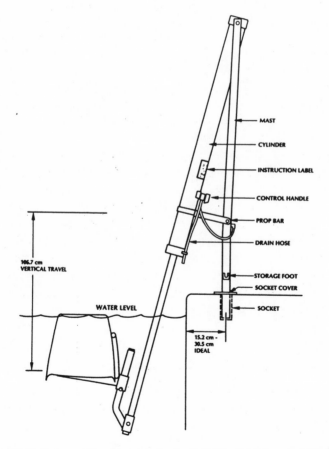

Figure 31.7. Schematic of manual-use Aquatic Access pool lift. The main vertical support of the Aquatic Access pool lift is never submerged, which reduces the chances of corrosion from pool water.

degrees over the water by an assistant. The control valve is then turned to lower the lift into the water. The seat travels 1.1 M. The Aquatic Access pool lift is constructed of polypropylene, polyvinyl chloride, and stainless steel; it is 1.8 M tall and weighs 30.6-kg. When not in use, no part of the pool lift is in the pool, and it can be easily folded or removed for storage. Normal city or household water pressure is adequate to lift up to 112.5-kg. Adult and child seat belts are available as options.

Discussion

Hydrotherapy is an essential component of burn care from the time of hospitalization until rehabilitation is complete. After burn injury, daily hydrotherapy facilitates dressing changes, encourages removal of the antimicrobial cream, and prepares the wound for debridement.[1] Hydrotherapy also offers the opportunity for personal hygiene and cleansing of the unburned skin. Hydrotherapy is also commonly used in the rehabilitation of patients with burns to promote physical fitness.[3] Aquatic exercise results in muscle strengthening, increased musculoskeletal extensibility, and cardiac conditioning, which have favorable psychologic benefits.

The design of aquatic access systems for patients with burns is based on three fundamental principles. First, the patient with burns must achieve access to water easily, without being fatigued. Second, the patient must receive hydrotherapy with reduced risks of cross- and autocontamination. Finally, health professionals must operate aquatic access systems without risk of occupational injury caused by musculoskeletal injury or hospital-acquired infection. As the patient with burns benefits from these unique aquatic access systems, both patient and health professional will appreciate the importance of medical engineering to burn care and rehabilitation.

References

1. Cardany CF, Rodeheaver GT, Horowitz JH, Kenney, JG, Edlich RF. Influence of hydrotherapy and antiseptic agents on burn wound bacterial contamination. J Burn Care Rehabil 1985;6:230-2.

2. Edlich RF, Abidin MR, Becker DG, Pavlovich LJ Jr, Dang MT. Design of hydrotherapy exercise pools. J Burn Care Rehabil 1988;9:505-9.

3. Edlich RF, Towler MA, Goitz RJ, et al. Bioengineering principles of hydrotherapy. J Burn Care Rehabil 1987;8: 580-7.

—by Richard F. Edlich, MD, PhD.

Ira W. DeCamp Burn Center, University of Virginia School of Medicine, Charlottesville, Virginia.

Chapter 32

Itching: What Helps

One of the major irritants during the healing process after burn injury is severe itching. In a survey of our burn members, 79 per cent of them complained of severe itching as a source of great discomfort during their recovery period. Vitale, *et al.*, found 87 percent of the patients they studied reported problems with itching.[1]

Itching, or pruritus, as it is medically termed, is a poorly localized cutaneous sensation induced by a wide variety of physical, systemic and dermatological stimuli. Pruritus, induces inflammatory changes in the burn wound and increases scarring. Patients are prone to scratching or rubbing newly grafted or healing burn wounds, often causing damage. Scratching may work to relieve the itching sensation at least temporarily because it acts as a competing stimulus that tends to block the itch. That may explain why itching is greater during sleep and relaxation.[2]

Itching interferes with daily living, sleep and therapy routines. The patient's concentration may be impaired due to the itching. In a large study done at Royal Adelaide Hospital, Australia, the incidence of severe itching in patients with healed burn scars was significantly higher than patients with severe surgical scars. There was no significant difference between burn scars that resulted from tangential excision when compared with burn scars that healed spontaneously.[3] Partial thickness burns appear to itch more than grafted areas.

Ambulatory patients seem to experience less itching than those who were bedfast.[4] *No succinctly defined method of treatment is found in the literature.*[4]

Itching is caused by the release of histamine which is synthesized in connective-tissue cells, called mast cells, and released locally, not only during injury or inflammation but also by large proteins and polypeptides and by drugs such as morphine alkaloids, thiamine and atropine. Morphine most likely promotes itching through action on the central nervous system.[2]

Itching after a burn may result from the formation of new nerve attachments during the healing process but also to dry, dehydrated skin. In burned tissue, lubricating and sweat glands may be damaged or eradicated by grafting and/or scarring. A good moisturizer should be used to compensate for this dysfunction.[6]

Generally, anti-itching agents are effective only for a few days, and then the patient will develop a tolerance to the medication.

What Helps

Here are some remedies that have been tried to relieve the effects:

Antihistamines, such as **Benadryl (diphenylhydramine)** (Park-Davis, Morris Plains, NJ)in pill or ointment form, **Atarax (piperazine)** (Roerig Div., Pfizer, Inc., New York, NY) and **Polyhist Forte** (blend of agents from **ethylenediamine** and **alcole-amine** families), usually give some transient relief, but they are often associated with an undesirable level of drowsiness. They are the most commonly recommended treatment.[3]

Moisturizing agents, such as **Nivea Cream** or **Lotion** (Beiersdorf Inc., Norwalk, CT), **baby oil**, **Tylox** and **Tylenol with codeine** (McNeil Pharmaceuticals Inc., Farmington, MI). **Vaseline Intensive Care Lotion** (Chesebrough-Pond's) also have been used with some effect.[9]

In my own case, **Temaril pills** (2.5 gm) were prescribed with little beneficial effect. **Cold packs** sometimes were effective as was a gentle slapping of the area. **Massage** with **Cocoa Butter** seemed partially effective.

Area Coordinator Delmar Scott tells us that cool showers helped and advises the use of white *Dial* soap. His dermatologist, Dr. E. Hozelrigg, recommended **Seldane**, **Hydroxyzine**, **Valisone Cream** and **Kenalog injections**.[7]

Our colleagues in New Zealand also highly recommend a **synthetic detergent soap**, *Rescue*.[8]

Area Coordinator Ellin Tolchin reported that **Benadryl** prescribed for her, did not work at all, but her psychiatrist put her on **Xanax**, an anxiolytic, and that did the trick for her.[8]

A blind, elderly, burned woman, also told us that Benadryl was not too good for her, but **Temaril** worked, as did **Aloe Vera** (99 percent liquid) and **Cocoa Butter**.[9]

Burn survivor Sean Harrison was burned in an explosion of spray lubricant. Severe itching set in within ten days of the event along all perimeters of the burns on his arms and legs. The itching awakened him during the night and "infuriated" him during the day. **Benadryl** caused side effects for him: disorientation, nausea, dehydration and the need for ever-increasing doses. Instead, he turned to Homeopathic remedies. **Homeopathic remedies** stimulate the body's immune system by introducing microdosages of elements that are similar to the cause of the disease. They are natural medicines derived from plants and minerals and administered as small tablets that dissolve under the tongue.

The greatest benefits from these remedies are the lack of side effects and their compatibility with many traditional medications. Sean was prescribed **Apis Mellifica** (30c) and **Sulphur** (30c). "My condition was drastically reduced using these cures," wrote Sean. **Topical ointments** and **olive oil** also increased his comfort and healing.[10]

Gary Crystal, a burn survivor from Tarzana, California, suffered constant frustration and irritation from itching for two and a half years following his burn injury. He tried an assortment of medications and topical creams, all of which either had no effect or provided only moderate relief. He finally found that **Neutrogena Norwegian Formula Hand Cream** gave him "tremendous relief," in his own words. Although it is expensive, only a small amount need be used in each application.[6]

Catherine McHugh, of Prince Edward Island, Canada, reports that **Cyclocort Ointment** combined with **Serax**, worked wonders for her. It is possible, she says, that the Serax may not be necessary.[7]

Also recommended is **Dr. Watson's Burn Cream**, an over-the-counter medication.

The Phoenix Society does not recommend any of these treatment methods. What worked for one survivor may not work for another. The good news is that itching generally subsides with time for most burn survivors and becomes only a distant memory.

References

1. Vitale M, Fields-Blach C, Luterman A Severe itching in the patient with burns *J Bn Care Rehab* 12(4):330-333 Jul/Aug 1991.

2. Lynch JB *Pain Management in the Burn Patient—A Workshop Review* The Medicine Group USA, Yardley, PA 1992.

3. Leitch IOW Itching in healed burn scars: a comparative review *ANZBA Bull* (8):7 1992

4. "Itching and Scratching," *New York Times, Science Times* 7/31/90

5. Bell L, McAdams T, Morgan R, Parshley PF., Pike RC Riggs P, Carpenter JE Pruritus in burns: a descriptive study *J Bn. Care Rehab* 9(3):305-311 May/Jun. 1988.

6. Henderson, PP. Private communication.

7. Private communication.

8. Manufactured in New Zealand by Love Your Skin (International) Ltd. P.O. Box 8283, Auckland, NZ Marketed by Marketing Brokers Australasia, 66 Model Farms Rd., Winston Hills, NSW 2153, Aust.

9. Private communication.

10. Private communication. For more information contact **National Institute of Homeopathy**, 801 N. Fairfax Suite 306, Alexandria, Virginia 22314,(703) 548-7790, or the **International Foundation for Homeopathy**, 2366 Eastlake Avenue East, Seattle, Washington 98102, (206) 324-8230. Both are non-profit organizations.

—by Alan J Breslau

Alan Breslau is Executive Director of The Phoenix Society for Burn Survivors. In 1963 he was burned over 45 percent of his body deep full thickness, in a crash of a commercial airliner In Rochester, New York.

Chapter 33

The Trauma of Hidden Burns

It was, until recent years, generally accepted that psychosocial adjustment varied directly with size of burn injury or extent of disfigurement.

Later studies contradicted this belief and now it has been well-established that no correlation exists between degree of burn and/or disfigurement with psychosocial adjustment.

Indeed, we and others have found that the correlation could be an inverse one: those suffering with relatively small burns, particularly when the scars can be concealed by clothing, suffer far more deeply and extensively than the massively and visibly disfigured burn survivor. This discovery came about when our organization received its first national media exposure that identified our support group for burn survivors.

We noticed that the influx of mail included a large number of letters from young women who had suffered essentially small burns as children who had never come to terms with the marring of their bodies. They were often not married, and they never (or rarely) exposed their residual scars by wearing bathing suits, shorts, or sleeveless blouses. Many expressed their unhappiness and a few mentioned thoughts of suicide.

The existence of this group, which we labeled "the hidden burn," was further confirmed when a series of national television talk shows displayed our toll-free telephone number. Again, the hidden burn population leaped from the incoming data. The calls received included women of all ages, some of whom were in the seventh decade of their lives, still unmarried and concerned about their childhood scars.

At the time, it seemed that this population was almost totally female. Most were burned as children, both pre-and post-adolescent (although pre-adolescent seem to predominate), and were able to conceal their scars with clothing.

We did not often encounter male burn survivors that matched this pattern; we assumed it was essentially a female problem. When we explored with some of these patients the root cause of their problem, we found in many cases, that the parent (more usually the mother) encouraged the child to conceal the scars from classmates. The child grew up believing that scars were bad, and that it was terrible if others would see their scars.

The massively disfigured person, on the other hand, is forced to come to terms with the altered appearance in reasonable time because of the constant stares of the public. The facially disfigured person must go through the stages of grief or the loss of self, just as though the person had died.

On the other hand, the person who can hide their burns is never forced to accept the change in body image and inwardly thinks of herself as no longer "Daddy's perfect little girl!"

Here are excerpts of a typical letter:

> I have just read an article you wrote in the Spring 1989 newsletter, The Icarus File. It was titled "The Hidden Burn." I am part of that group. I have really suffered emotionally and mentally since I was 11-12 years old. I was laughed at as a child by a fellow student. I basically went into a 16 year "hide." I didn't let anyone come near me (close). No one was able to really get to know me after that. My parents were not aware of my problem. I would still use my hand normally around them, but the minute I was around an outsider I would hide it. In college I dated a guy for one and half years. He never knew that I was burned. I guess you could say I became a pro at hiding my burns. I have recently started counseling and it has helped. My scars are on my stomach, leg, and hand. It has really put a damper on my dating life. I am 27 years old.
>
> Thanks

We also wondered why the unique problems of this group had not been recognized and addressed by the professional healthcare system except, perhaps, by a select group of psychotherapists who could have encountered some of them as patients. Realizing that the extent of the problem is not even recognized by the patient until a decade or more after suffering the initial trauma, there was little chance that the medical professional would become aware of it. They were pleased with the result of discharging from care, a little girl, fully functional, and with her scars healed.

The only way the professional caregiver could become aware of these patients would be by an extremely long prospective study, or by inviting long-term survivors to return to their respective burn centers. Our purpose in establishing National Burn Survivors Sunday as a reunion day for burn survivors and medical staff (including departed staff members), was to serve the purpose of bringing to the attention of care givers their successes and failures in treatment and rehabilitation. This would benefit both patient and professional.

Although we felt initially that the hidden burn problem affected only females, a case of a male survivor surfaced that matched all the characteristics. More of them have followed since. We then realized that the reason our data base was skewed so heavily female was because the initial exposure was in supermarket tabloids and morning and afternoon television talk shows. These are mainly seen by women! Men as well as women suffer this syndrome.

Nevertheless, women suffer more from the relatively minor scarring than men do because beauty is considered more important in a woman. Scars may be thought of as macho in a man (viz., tattooing).

One approach we use to help this suffering population is by first encouraging them to network with each other through exchange of addresses and telephone numbers. This enables them to contact others who share the same problem (mutual peer support) and they then realize they are not alone.

The next step is to teach them that scars were not anything to be ashamed of, that they had not done anything wrong; the harm was done to them!

We encourage them to expose their scars gradually. This is extremely difficult for many to do and accept. But once accomplished, the results are very positive. By not covering your scars, you are conveying to others that you feel comfortable with your appearance. They, in turn, will feel comfortable because you are obviously comfortable!

We advise parents of newly burned children about the long term negative effects of encouraging their children to hide their scars. They do so in the belief that they are protecting their child. We hope that professional caregivers will also emphasize this to families of burned children.

Burn survivors should be made aware of the new techniques available in surgery and paramedical cosmetology to help in removing or minimizing scars.

Those who have availed themselves of these new measures, especially tissue expansion surgery for scar removal, have had outstanding psychological improvement, totally turning their lives around for the better.

The Hidden Burn is a newly recognized population of burn survivor that should be identified and aided.

Burned children, especially female pediatric patients, should be encouraged to expose their scars in social situations to prevent this unfortunate and unnecessary condition from developing.

New surgical treatment to eliminate small scars, no matter their age, is now available.

When surgery is not an option, paramedical cosmetology may be used to minimize the appearance of the scars and accent the patient's attributes.

Alan Breslau

Chapter 34

Burns and Sexuality

As social creatures, people have always been relational beings. As human beings, originating from relations and sexual links between two persons (a man and a woman) we can only exist and develop in relation to others.

According to Conrad Van Emde Boas,[1] a famous Dutch sexologist, the human person and sexuality can be considered from four different but not separate dimensions:

1. capability of experiencing lust,
2. the establishment of relationships,
3. procreation, and
4. the social commitment within the human society (the institutional aspect).

The complete development of these four aspects of human nature supposes a long and never-ending learning process and personal development. This developmental process includes presented and seized opportunities to succeed on the one hand and risks of failure on the other hand. This is a personal history, with important emotional/psychologic experiences and contacts with the social world as well as biologic/physical aspects—*mens sana in corpora sano*—a healthy mind in a healthy body.

©January/February 1992 *Journal of Burn Care & Rehabilitation*. Reprinted with permission.

433

The body is an essential part of this complete sexuality. Through creative body language, emotions and desires may be expressed between partners with more subtlety and honesty. The sensory pleasure and the sexual tactility open a royal road to contact: from *"I can feel"* to *"now I can feel you."* In this way, the body communication and contact is the language of both the tactile and the tactful, of progressively learning how to feel and to sense one's own corporality as well as that of the other. The other is also experienced as a body—touched, but not found indifferent or touchy.[1]

This kind of tactile language is unknown in the present-day variation of lust (sensuality) inherent in "consumption" sex. Our society dates back to times with a strong repression of sexual lust. Sexual lust, which was seen as voluptuousness, was oppressed. Nowadays sexuality is not as oppressed, but rather imposed. In our consumption-oriented society, sexuality has become a commodity. As a matter of fact, for many persons, sexuality is the cheapest available stimulant.

It is therefore everyone's duty to open up in a tactful and pleasant way the different registers of the body and to steer these experiences as a master. To achieve this, sexual culture is necessary; this is not a liberation from but a liberation *to* sensual sexual contact: sexuality as "body communication," that is, language without words, and this dimension should not be reduced to a purely genital context.

Our recent Western past has pushed aside our skin and stressed the importance of the ear and eye—the senses that work at a distance. We must learn again how to feel our forgotten skin, which is our extended opportunity for contact.

Skin as a Means of Sexual Contact

The skin is the largest organ of our body. Of all of its functions, the skin's emotional function has been stressed over the last few years. In this field, the child psychologists, especially the child analysts, have done most of the essential research. Indeed, skin contact between the newborn baby and the mother seems to have an important emotional value for the child.

Lambrechts[2] considers the newborn baby as completely skin. This means, on one hand, that all other senses develop from the skin. In other words, the eyes, nose, and tongue feel in the beginning more than they see, hear, smell, or taste. This also means that the sense of touch is the basis of all sensory life. By feeling and caressing and by being touched and caressed, the child gradually acquires stability and coherence.

The basis of the relational life of every human being is also created through the sense of touch. We must remark here, however, that
our society and its strict medical hygiene do not make it easy for the
child in the search for (tactile) sensuality; since the baby is kept
wrapped, a part of the tactile experience is hindered at an early stage
and the child risks underdevelopment and atrophy of his or her tactile capacity.

The eroticism of the skin was described for the first time by Freud
in his "Drei Abhandlungen zur Sexualtheorie" in 1905. According to
him, the skin is the organ around which several stages—discovered
by him—in the development of a human being take place (the oral,
anal, and genital stages). In addition, there are strong individual differences among people where the eroticism of the skin is concerned.
We do not yet know whether these differences are hereditary or
whether they go back to the first skin contacts of the mother and father with the child. We do know, however, that a mother offers skin
contact to her child in a fixed pattern, identical in both quality and
quantity to the contact she received from her own mother. Musaph[3]
writes that English research from Anna Freud's school has shown on
film that the pattern of skin contact of a mother and her baby is similar to her contact with her partner, as well as to her skin contact with
her own body.

The significance of touching in interpersonal relations cannot easily
be overestimated. A handshake and a strike in the face clearly indicate different attitudes that one has toward the object of the touch.
The feelings between mother and child, between brother and sister,
or between two lovers are clearly illustrated by the ways in which they
hold and caress one another. In adult sexual contact, different forms
of touching and caressing are a part of foreplay, and this corporal contact is not exclusively limited to the genital zones. Freud made a distinction between sexuality and genitality. In cases of many couples
who ask for help with sexual dysfunction, the advice to ameliorate
and increase skin contact is an important means of breaking through
vicious circles of fear of failure and the need to perform.

Through skin contact, a range of various feelings, from appreciation, affection, and sympathy to envy and anger, may be expressed.
The way in which these feelings are expressed through skin contact
is strongly dependent on cultural pattern. In tropical and subtropi-
cal countries skin contact is more often offered than it is in our colder,
clothes-wrapped culture. Moreover, body and skin contact are heavily
impoverished by our idol "privacy." This is felt especially by older
persons who lack contact in their social isolation. For this reason, they

usually hold the hand of a visitor longer than a younger person would, and each form of body care—massage, pedicure, or whatever—is quite an experience for them.[3]

The communicative function of the skin is again stressed when we investigate the influence of the skin on first judgments of others. In our social contacts, we tend to accord positive characteristics to those with nice, smooth skin. A woman with nice skin is not only viewed as erotically desirable but is also unconsciously accorded better character traits. A girl with unattractive skin (for example, a skin covered with acne) clearly feels a handicap in her social contacts; not many people like to go out with her.

This is called the *halo phenomenon*. The corporal situation of the skin is extended to the characterologic situation. In addition, persons with nice skin are considered sexually attractive and charming. Our consumption-oriented society exploits this with thousands of bottles of skin creams, milks, and so on. The imputation of sexual attraction to nice, smooth skin is an example of the halo phenomenon.

The Burnt Skin: Risks and Opportunities for a Satisfying Sexual Relationship

Is life still possible after burn injury? Sexual life is indeed closely linked with the quality and even the possibility of life. The sexual, or libido, element in a human being strives for zest in living and development; in cases of danger to life, however, this libido eliminates itself so that all energy can be devoted to the struggle for life.

Living with a perilous burn, which entails much pain, long-term hospital treatment, and coping with the many remaining scars, requires a considerable amount of physical and psychologic energy. It is a sound and understandable principle that lustful genital contact with a partner, considering responsible parenthood, is suspended during a period of uncertain survival. Once survival has been guaranteed, however, life resumes and the person starts looking again for social contacts, sexual expression, and commitment. However, this is only possible to the extent to which sexuality is or is not hindered by physical limitations or emotional barriers.

It is well known that people with skin problems, especially when a normally uncovered part of the body is concerned, have great difficulty in contacting other people. This handicap is present in the intimate contact between two partners and between parents and children, as well as in first contacts with strangers. Therefore, a lasting skin defect demands the extreme assimilation capabilities of a person. This assimilation behavior is influenced not only by the degree of the skin defect itself but also, and especially, by the individual personality structure of the person. The way in which the handicap is experienced and assimilated, the quality of the relationships with partner, peers, members of the family, and colleagues, and the way in which relatives and friends react to the handicap (as viewed from their own personality structures) are all highly individual. Because of this, all counseling must be tailored; it cannot be ready-made but must be adapted to a unique person with specific social surroundings.

Herman Musaph[3] describes three typical assimilation patterns on the level of the psychosexual life of patients with psoriasis. According to this author, the observations of the patients with psoriasis can be extended to patients with other chronic skin defects. The psychosocial relations of patients with skin conditions do not depend so much on the medical (e.g., dermatologic surgical) diagnoses, on the social and psychosexual consequences of their skin problems.

Indeed, although skin contact with these patients can take place without medical problems, experience shows that all too often skin defects give the patient a feeling of being marked and impure, of being a freak. Often, irrational resistance also originates in the partner; the affected skin is considered "dirty."

The Exhibitionistic Rejection Form. The feelings of shame over the affected skin may be assimilated by the patient's determination to seem not at all bothered by the rejecting, sometimes even hostile, attitude of other people. The patient feels the desire to demonstrate that he or she is not affected by other people's reactions. Sometimes, even, as many people as possible are manipulated in a subtle way, to look at the skin and to care for it.

In other words, the patient wants to convince others, and thus himself or herself that the skin defect is unimportant and that he or she does not really suffer from anything. Another underlying motive for this behavior may be to test the other, asking the question, "Do you accept me the way that I am?"

The Dependent-Rejection Form. In this pattern, a patient tries to get as much profit as possible from the skin problems. The patient pretends to be severely handicapped, in need of help, and entitled to well-organized help. Many of other persons are thus manipulated in a clever way. Once mobilized, such will always find other meddlesome persons—"helpers"—who like to interfere and who will start a relationship with the patient because of a kind of "boy scout" mentality.

The Exaggeratedly Shamefaced Attitude. With this attitude, a patient lives in well-organized social isolation. In this way, the patient can avoid the confronting rejecting glances and remarks from others. The patient goes into hiding alone, and all erotic and sexual approaches are eschewed.

In the scientific literature about burns, virtually nothing has been said about burns and sexuality. We can only refer to an extremely limited number of publications. According to Hamburg,[4] sexual problems are not frequent in people with burns but are usually serious when they do occur. Burns to the genitals and to the perineum are not unusual, and their treatment is medically fairly simple in most cases. However, even minor burns in these areas are seen by many patients as worse than much more serious burns in other areas. Women are often concerned about fertility, especially when menstruation is interrupted, as is often the case.

According to Bernstein,[5] individuals react with personal adaption skills and coping styles. But physical and sexual attraction are close, and showing the scars is for people with burns often too demanding. This excludes them from the sexual market. Therefore, Bernstein pleads for techniques (in plastic surgery and in physiotherapy) to help bring the patient as close to reality as possible.

Goodstein[6] says that another reason that burns of the face and the genitals cause greater emotional problems is the symbolic significance of these areas. Goodstein mentions that before discharge the patient with burns on these areas often tests his or her capability of being loved by engaging in such behaviors as innocent but annoying flirtation with the staff. Goodstein also pleads for honest, simple, and hopeful answers to the patients questions about issues of sexuality, such as resumption of menstruation, capability of erection, fertility, and other areas of concern.

According to Bowden,[7] a retrospective survey in 1977 of about 350 persons who were treated in a burn center between 1956 and 1976 shows that the self-esteem of the patient with burns does not depend on the degree of the burn, nor does it depend on the part of the body affected. Rather, the chief determinants of self-esteem are the *age* of the patient when the burn occurred and the time elapsed since the burn. Patients who were between birth and eleven years of age at the time of injury and who were adolescents at the time of the survey had the lowest self-esteem, in contrast to patients whose burns occurred when they were between 10 and 49 years of age. The consequences for self-esteem (and consequently for sexuality?) only became apparent after six years had elapsed since the burn. The women with burns showed lower self-esteem than did the men; this difference was most striking between eleven and thirteen years after the burn.

Conclusion: Some Practical Considerations from the Sexologic Point of View

The near absence of scientific research that relates to the sexuality of persons with burns indicates the still-existing taboo regarding sexuality in the medical world. The research by Bowden on the self-esteem of persons with burns is important because it refers to the possibility and even probability of psychosocial and sexual problems surfacing in later life. This pattern is also clear from our own clinical experiences. We see that burns with remaining scars in a young child create the most problems when the child becomes an adolescent. We also notice that, even after years of recovery and learning to live with their damaged skin, many adults show other relational difficulties later. In the treatment of patients with burns, a first phase, survival and recovery, must be followed by a second phase, discharge from the safe hospital surroundings and return to family, neighborhood, school, job, and so on.

How does the patient's return to the sexual society happen? Is the mutilated skin anxiously covered and neglected; does the patient retreat to coitus under the blankets in the dark, as is still the case with many "healthy" couples? Or have both partners acquired a more open relationship with fewer taboos and more caressing and skin sensitivity because of frequent confrontation with body-cherishing contact, such as massaging of the naked skin with soothing oils? Have they acquired sexual contact more aimed at erotic feelings than at coital performance, or vice versa? Has sexuality for the greater part perhaps disappeared from their interests? Or have they developed a relationship based on an obsessional preoccupation about the burns and with a caring and patient-centered attitude of the partner?

Doctors are not necessarily experts on sex, and patients will not begin to discuss their sexual lives and problems with medical staff unless they are invited to do so. A doctor, a physiotherapist, or a nurse who shows an honest interest and who asks questions about sexuality in a gentle manner will be able to learn to what extent the patient and the partner are able to live together again in "lustful" contact. Reassurances (sexual life is possible again once all wounds have been healed; menstruation may be interrupted for a certain time but will start again spontaneously when the body has healed completely and the endocrine system is functioning properly again, and so on) combined with advice (such as a suggestion that the patient look for a coital position that does not involve leaning on the burned areas) are important. The healer should also discuss the resumption of contraceptive behavior, since asking about contraception implies the acceptance of sexual contact. Such an attitude also stimulates both partners to express their emotions—fear of being rejected, feelings of hesitation, fear of hurting—and in this way helps promote mutual communication.

An important psychosexual step in treating the patient with burns is the task of the partner (or the parent, in the case of a child with burns) of regularly rubbing the patient with almond oil. This skin contact has a double function; apart from aiding the recovery of and improving the skin texture, it also aids the recovery of and improves the sensitivity of the skin. Remembering that "the function makes the organ," a positive sensitivity of the skin is cultivated by touching, caressing, and massage. Moreover, this skin sensitivity is strongly influenced by emotional and relational factors because the patient is being caressed and massaged by another human being; the resulting satisfying (sensual) effect will create or enhance a relationship with the person who provides the stimulation. In this way, the patient will come to feel accepted again by the other, despite the mutilated skin, and will again experience the feeling of being united with another. The patient can, and is allowed to, feel good in his or her skin again. In this sense, the procedure in the burn center in Leuven is important from a psychosexual point of view. Even before the patient's discharge from the hospital, the partner is asked to learn how to rub the patient with burns with almond oil. (Here we would like to ask the manufacturers to produce an equally effective oil with a nicer smell!) In this way the partners are confronted with the painful or mutilated skin within their intimate relationship and the problems are literally touched and taken into account. This is a good way to overcome the touch taboo and to approach the threshold of the sexual touch.

This procedure is also followed by parents of children with burns. Extensive and frequent contact between parents, both mother and father, and the child is important here. This contact strengthens the child's feeling of unity and soothes the pain, sorrow, and grief. Speechless body contact during physical comforting passes on the love from parents to child without words, so that the child feels accepted again, and at the same time it heals and strengthens the skin and its sensitivity. For the parents, it is a heavy task to be regularly confronted with the pain, the mutilation, the limited future prospects of their child, and sometimes irrational feelings of guilt. Therefore it is also important for parents to be able to express their emotions and feelings, and to assimilate them by doing so, so that they will not pass on any feelings to the child without being aware of it.

Apart from the medical care, the treatment of patients with burns should also provide the possibility of a therapeutic dialogue. If nurses, doctors, or physiotherapists feel incapable of doing this, whether because of lack of time or feelings of incompetence, positive referral of the patient to a specialized counselor (a sexologist or a child psychiatrist, as appropriate) is necessary. This type of action presupposes intense teamwork among the various disciplines. Self-help groups are also valuable in such situations for exchanging information and experience.

References

1. Nijs P. (tegen) *Stromingen in de seksuologie.* Leuven: ACCO, 1979.

2. Lambrechts G. De Zinnelijke wereld van het kind een terugblik op onszelf In: Nijs P, et al., eds. *Cahiers voor Seksuologie.* Antwerpen, Amsterdam: De Nederlandsche Boekhandel, 1979.

3. Musaph H. De huid als seksueel orgaan. In: Mariette CT, Moors-Mommers, et al., eds. *Handbock seksuele hulpverlening.* Deventer & Antwerpen, Amsterdam: Van Loghum Slaterus, 1983. Volume 3, p. ll.B.5 MUS 1-12.

4. Hamburg DA. Clinical importance of emotional problems in the case of patients with burns. *N Engl J Med* 1953;248: 355-9.

5. Bernstein NR. Psychosocial results of burns: the damaged selfimage. *Clin Plast Surg* 1982;9:337-46.

6. Goodstein RK. Burns: an overview of clinical consequences affecting patients, staff, and family. *Compr Psychiatry* 1985; 26:43-57.

7. Bowden ML, Feller I, Tholen D, Davidson TN, James MH. Self-esteem of severely burned patients. *Arch Phys Med Rehabil* 1980;61:449-52.

—by Frida Bogaerts, PhD, and Willy Boeckx, MD

Leuven, Belgium

Chapter 35

When Is the Burn Injury Healed?

Psychosocial Implications of Care

The psychosocial and economic effects of burn trauma are profound, not only for the patients, their families, and the burn unit staff members, but also for society as a whole. Understanding the perception of stresses experienced by patients, families, and staff is discussed, and related strategies to help in reducing the stress are presented. A comprehensive psychosocial support system can help the nurse in reducing the psychosocial morbidity of severe burn trauma.

He appeared calm as he began the story of how he was burned and the experiences he had while recovering. Mrs. J. sat beside him, listening intently to his story with glistening eyes. Mr. J sustained a 60 percent total body surface area burn injury during a helicopter crash. In addition to partial and full-thickness injuries, he had fractures of both femurs.

As he retold the horror of the accident and the sensations he felt while his clothes, skin, and hair were burning, his voice was strong. He had told this story often. But his voice began to quaver as he described the weeks and months of painful treatments and the uncertainty of the future. The anguish of being dependent on others for so long was visually evident in his facial expressions.

Mrs. J described the shock of hearing the news of the accident, seeing her husband for the first time, and the uncertainty of the future.

©May 1993 American Association of Critical Care Nurses, *Critical Issues in Critical Care Nursing* Vol. 4, No. 2. Reprinted with permission.

He was transferred more than 2,000 miles to a burn unit within hours of the injury. She somehow found the strength to make child care and travel arrangements. She was fearful because she had never traveled more than 100 miles from home, and she knew she would be alone. Glimpses of the weeks of worry and depression were evident in her expressions as the story unfolded. She described the significant turning point for her in the long wait. Returning from a visit, her hope was diminishing because it had been so long since Mr. J recognized her. That night the nurse called her at 11 p.m. to give her a message of love from her husband; the message included the use of his pet name for her.

Many nurses who had cared for this man and his wife were deeply moved by hearing Mr. and Mrs. J.'s version of that long hospital stay. As I listened to the stories of Mr. and Mrs. J, I reflected on the role of the nurse in helping patients and families through such a tragedy. What does the patient worry about during the various stages of recovery? Are there ways for nurses to minimize the psychologic stress experienced by patients, families, and themselves? What are the family needs as they perceive them versus the perceptions of the nurses? Are they met? Could they be met better with different interventions? How do nurses cope with the demands of treating burn patients? I believe a psychosocial support program in a burn unit involves considering the answers to all these questions.

Why the Need for Comprehensive Psychosocial Support?

Approximately 100,000 patients with burn injuries require hospital admittance each year. As advanced technology and new interventions decrease mortality, quality of life issues become of greater importance.[1] The psychosocial and economic effects of burn trauma are profound, not only for the patient and family, but also for society as a whole.[2]

Initial data obtained while developing a burn-specific health scale indicated that the psychosocial performance of patients with major burns lagged behind their performance in other areas of the recovery process.[3] About two-thirds of patients have some psychologic disability that requires therapy at hospital discharge and for as long as six months afterward. The sequelae are mild to moderate in most patients and relate to issues of depression, anxiety, and alcoholism. There is evidence that some problems, if not treated, can persist for an extended period.[3, 4] The variance in psychosocial adjustment usually does not relate solely to the extent or degree of burn injury. It is the effect of other factors, such as anatomic location of injury, employment status, loss of family role, strength of family support systems, age at time of injury, and previous history of psychiatric illness, which correlates with psychosocial adjustment.[2, 4-9]

The role of various types of social support on the adjustment process was identified as a priority at the National Institutes of Health Consensus Conference on Burn Injuries.[10] The literature supports providing structured psychosocial help to patients and families during hospital stay and after discharge to reduce the psychosocial impact of burn trauma.[9, 11-18]

Comprehensive psychosocial support in a burn unit also needs to include providing support to the staff caring for the patient. Because nurses are the most constant feature of the patient's environment, the stress is observed most consistently in this group of health care providers.[19] Understanding the stresses of providing nursing care for burn patients and self-recognition of the manifestations of that stress are crucial to remaining an effective and compassionate nurse who can provide the support needed by the patients and their families. This chapter is intended to increase nurse awareness to the psychosocial implications of caring for burn patients and their families. Through knowledge, the true art of nursing can be realized in providing care to this special patient population.

The Patient's Perspective

A burn injury is one of the most traumatic, dehumanizing injuries an individual can experience. The adaptive problems that normally occur while recovering from burn injury are well described[20] (Table 35.1). Finding effective psychologic interventions remains a priority.[10.]

Table 35.1. Common Psychologic Adjustment Problems to Severe Burns

Threat to survival
Physical and psychologic pain from injury and treatment
Fear of disfigurement
Long recovery process/conflict with dependency
Separation from loved ones
Alteration in family roles
Effect of injury on future plans

The physical response and care for a severe burn injury occur in three phases: resuscitative, acute, and rehabilitative. It is helpful to consider psychologic responses to burn injury as stages of adaptation.[11] Table 35.2 lists seven stages of adaptation related to the phases of care, although patients do not move linearly through these adaptation stages. The emotional responses often are like a pendulum, moving in and out of "stages" as the patient undergoes a variety of treatments and procedures. All extensively burned patients have some manifestations of most of these stages as they physically progress through the phases of care.

Resuscitative Phase

The patient may be alert and oriented initially, but hemodynamic instability, analgesics, and sedatives may subsequently induce confusion and disorientation. Inappropriate behavior or uncooperativeness with treatments may occur. The use of restraints may compound confusion. The nurse needs to reassure the patient and explain why restraints are being used.[21] Patients questioned later about this period often do not remember it or have confused memories. The first stage of adaptation, survival anxiety, may begin on admission.[11] The patient is tremulous, startles easily, and may have difficulty in concentrating. Anxiety is related to the fear of dying.[9, 11] Effective interventions

Table 35.2. Stages of Psychosocial Adaptation in Burn Recovery

Stage of Adaptation	*Phase of Care*
Survival anxiety	Resuscitative Early acute
Adaptation to severe pain	Acute
Search for meaning	Acute
Investment in recuperation	Acute
Acceptance of losses	Acute, rehabilitative
Investment in rehabilitation	Rehabilitative
Reintegration of identity	Rehabilitative

From Watkins PN, Cook EL, May SR, Ehleben CM. Psychological stages in adaptation following burn injury: a method for facilitating psychological recovery of burn victims. J Burn Care Rehabil 1988; 9:376–384.

include providing information about prognosis, repeating instructions often, and orienting the patient to reality (day, time, place) frequently. This period of physical and emotional instability is short when resuscitation is successful.

Acute Care Phase

The longest period of adjustment occurs in the acute phase, which lasts until the burn wound is closed by healing or grafting. Patients say that their most vivid recollections are of the nurses and the care they gave.[22] Because most units limit family visitation, the staff becomes the patient's "significant other," and the patient begins a "career as a burn patient.[9, 22] Most or all of the adaptive problems previously identified can be expected as the patient moves through the seven stages of adaptation.

Survival anxiety may continue. As the patient's physical condition stabilizes, anxiety related to potential disfigurement and changes in future identity and roles may lead to depression, withdrawal, and regression.[11] Prognostic information is most important to the patient at this stage. Questions like "What happens next?" or "What will happen to me?" often are the first sign of their worries. Allowing expression of these worries and providing accurate information is essential in providing support.

A major problem during the acute phase is *adaptation to severe pain*.[11] Patients have trouble dealing with the pain when it is inflicted by the staff that they depend upon for support. Pain management strategies include pharmacologic and nonpharmacologic interventions to alleviate pain or help patients control it. Patients are anxious about their ability to cope with pain, so allowing them some control in the treatment process is an essential component of an effective pain management program. Simple patient education that focuses on what to expect during wound care and how to relax has been effective in reducing perceived pain.[13] Control also is an important element of the effectiveness of patient-controlled analgesia. The chapter on pain management in this volume describes specific pain interventions and their application.

Many patients say the pain was the worst part of their hospital stay.[16] Nurses must become knowledgeable in the use of pharmacologic and nonpharmacologic pain management strategies. Although this is a concern of most nurses who care for burn patients, few have adequate knowledge in this area. Thus, burn patients often remain undertreated for their severe pain. Effective pain management must become a major focus of nurses in meeting the psychologic needs of the patient.[9,21-23]

As patients become more alert, they *search for the meaning* of what has happened.[11] Detailed and repetitious recounting of the events of the injury occurs. The recounting is useful in desensitizing patients to the horror of what has happened and decreasing nightmares.[9,11,22] Nurses need to listen to the patient, provide support, and avoid judging the patient's explanation for the injury.

With the beginning of grafting procedures and wound closure, patients become more *invested in recuperation*.[11] They look to the staff for "bench marks" of progress and begin to acknowledge their new status as a burned person. Frustration and depression may be expressed regarding the slowness of recovery. Often, progress is made only to be lost because of additional surgical procedures and immobilization. Because the staff members are consistently optimistic about the recovery process, the patient does not always trust all of the information given. Specific progress information given by the surgeon becomes the most valued.[22]

Boredom becomes a major problem even when patients begin to socialize with each other. The routine becomes monotonous. When staff members plan special events, such as a pizza party, which alter the routine, morale improves. Inspirational tapes or visits from burn survivors may provide additional motivation for patients to work hard at the recovery program."

As patients are encouraged to become more independent, there often is resistance. The pain associated with increased activities may be interpreted as indicative of lack of progress. In addition, the patients and staff may have differing perspectives of "being independent." Expressions of dislike or hatred for individual staff members are not unusual.[22] At this point, it is important to establish a daily program with the patient that sets readily achievable goals so that recognizable progress can be attained. Motivation is increased with the attainment of such incremental goals.

When independence increases, the recognition of losses becomes clearer. *Accepting losses* is an emotionally difficult stage for the patient.[11] As socialization occurs, patients compare their situation with that of the other patients. Patients are comforted by their perceptions that their injuries are not as bad as someone else. It is during this phase that the patient may first see their scars and begin to grieve for their losses. Their fear of appearing as a "monster" to others produces anxiety when the patient leaves the burn unit for the first time. In addition, financial concerns and worry about the future can produce anxiety and depression. Tearfulness, decreased appetite, sleep disturbances, bargaining for release from activities, and depression are common manifestations of this stage.

Nurses should allow verbalization of these fears and validate that they are "normal." Nurses should support the patient during the grieving process. Taking trips away from the unit to the cafeteria or outside the hospital with family helps the patient to deal with the reactions of others.[15] Patient support groups are particularly useful in promoting the verbalization of the emotional reactions to such trips and helping the patient understand that such fears are not unusual.[14]Social service personnel and chaplains can help patients deal with financial planning for discharge and spiritual dilemmas.

Rehabilitative Phase

In the rehabilitative phase, patients renew their interest in the outside world. Although critical care nurses may not interact with patients during this phase, knowledge of the patient's concerns can help the nurse to prepare the patient/family for this stage. "Letting go" of the protective burn unit environment is not an easy task for the patient and may result in some "acting out" behaviors as discharge approaches.

The last two stages of adaptation (*invested in rehabilitation and reintegration of identity*) occur just before discharge, during outpatient treatment, or several months to years after discharge.[11] The goal of these stages is regaining the preinjury level of function. Providing reassurance that the patient will be able to adapt is the most helpful strategy. Providing information about additional needs for reconstructive surgery and therapy assists the patient in establishing realistic goals. Some facilities use group therapy and education to prepare patients before discharge for reintegration into the community and family roles.[15] Providing resource material about self-help groups can be vital in helping the patient make independent decisions related to additional psychosocial support. Once a person gives up the victim persona and accepts that they are a burn survivor, they are emotionally healed.

The Family Perspective

Having a family member who is severely burned and in the hospital for a long time messes with your concept of hope. You are living day to day or even hour to hour.

Burn patient's family member.

The acute nature of burn trauma frequently leads to a crisis for the family of the patient. Normal coping mechanisms are overwhelmed, and a state of disequilibrium occurs. There is a threat to survival of the family unit.[9, 21.] High levels of stress usually occur during the acute phase of the patient's hospital stay and generally recede during the recovery phase.[24] Strategies for reducing anxiety and promoting healthy coping mechanisms helps the family provide the crucial support needed for recovery. If the patient is not likely to recover, crisis intervention therapy can help the family make the necessary decisions related to the dying process.

An accurate assessment is important to effectively meet the family's needs. Although the needs of the families of critically ill patients are known, there is little published regarding the needs of burn patients' family members.[25] Because burn patients remain acutely ill for extended periods, the needs of the families may change as recovery proceeds through the various phases of care and the patient progresses through the stages of adaptation. Table 35.3 displays the most important needs identified by family members at the US Army Institute of Surgical Research within the first 72 hours after admission of the patient.[26] The eight needs indicated by asterisks continue to be important throughout the continuum of care, until the time of discharge from the burn center. As Mrs. J. suggested, the need to be

Table 35.3. Most Important Needs as Perceived by Family Members of Critically Burned Patients within 72 Hours of Admission

To know the expected outcome*
To have questions answered honestly*
To know how the patient is being treated medically*
To know specific facts about the patient's progress*
To feel there is hope*
To be assured that the best care possible is being given the patient
To be called at home about changes in the patient's condition*
To feel that hospital personnel care about the patient*
To know exactly what is being done for the patient
To be told about transfer plans while they are being made*
To see the patient frequently

*Needs that continue to be important until time of discharge.

told about changes in the patient's condition when they occur is an important need. This was the only need consistently identified (throughout a six week period) as important by the family member and the nurse caring for the patient.[26]

Nurses may be unaware of the specific needs of individual family members. Consequently, a careful assessment of each family's needs as perceived by the family members is needed. This becomes the foundation for structuring relevant interventions to provide the psychosocial support required.

Just as patients go through stages of psychologic adaptation, so do the family members.[27] Initially, families seek assurances and honest information concerning the prognosis. There is an overwhelming need for hope and information. Specific information about the medical treatment and patient progress is most important in the beginning stages of the acute care phase. When family members first visit the patient, they are relieved to find that the patient is alive. Orienting the family to the burn unit is helpful in preparing them for the different environment and for the appearance of the patient. Because of the continuing fear of death and the appearance of the patient, family members often exhibit a great deal of anxiety. The confusion and disorientation of the patient are disturbing, and the family members require reassurance that delirium is a common occurrence during this phase.[1, 27]

As the patient's recovery progresses, the family members often come to view themselves as an advocate for the patient and a "cushion" from the staff.[22] The "pain problem" is a major source of stress. Family members feel helpless and frustrated. Expressing their angry feelings to the staff is difficult because of concern that it will jeopardize the patient's relationship with the staff.[27] It is important that the family perceive that the staff members care for the patient because the advocacy role becomes more stressful as the patient regresses psychologically.[26-28] Allowing the family members to express their feelings is crucial. Support groups can provide a safe environment for such expressions and allow for discussion of strategies for being an effective advocate for the patient.[17, 18]

During the acute phase, the family has many questions concerning the treatment regimens and prognosis. At this point information from the surgeon is important.[26] The use of a variety of educational strategies is helpful in meeting needs quickly. Video presentations about treatment protocols can be shown when it is appropriate to the care of a specific patient. Written information containing definitions of commonly used terms and descriptions of expected care can help in understanding explanations given by the staff.

As patients begin to need to express their feelings, relatives have difficulty in dealing with those feelings. They often discourage such discussions.[27] Additional stress occurs with role reversal in the family dynamics.[22, 28] This phenomenon contributes to the patient's dependence/independence conflicts as discharge approaches.

As discharge approaches, the family needs to learn how to provide care at home. Because of their limited involvement in direct care of the patient during the hospital stay, family members of adult patients often find this to be a very stressful period. Parents of children usually are more involved in direct care and thus better prepared at the time of discharge. To reduce the anxiety and stress caused by discharge, early involvement of the family in care is helpful.[9, 22, 27] More contact between the staff and family for discharge education occurs when visiting hours are extended. As family members learn to apply compression dressings to the legs, treat small open areas, evaluate the healed skin, and apply the pressure garments, they gain confidence in their ability to provide care at home. This type of education for one or two weeks before the estimated discharge date can be reinforced by providing written material concerning home care. Allowing the patient to take short day or overnight trips outside the hospital provides time for the family to adapt to the reactions of others to the patient's burn scars. Families also may need assistance with financial problems. Additional information concerning self-help support groups in the community can aid the family in seeking help after discharge.

The patient and family are a unit. Meeting the family needs is important to the psychologic recovery of the family unit. The saying "they also serve who only sit and wait" is descriptive of the role family members often must take during the acute phase of the patient's hospital stay. For the family, the stress of waiting can be as psychologically severe as the burn injury is for the patient. Nursing personnel must consider ways to support the patient/family unit to reduce the emotional stress of the burn injury and the hospital experience.

The Staff Perspective

There are three general areas that provide a framework for examining the stresses experienced by nurses in burn units[21]: the trajectories or expectations of recovery or death; the issue of control in the work environment; and the engagement of burn patients/families in a social-emotional bonding.

Trajectories

At the time of the patient's admission, the nurses quickly develop expectations regarding the patient's recovery or death. This serves as a way to organize their work. Because burn care requires the efforts of a variety of practitioners, conflicts may occur. Each group has different expectations and methods of organizing work. All members of the team soon learn that their personal fund of information is incomplete and that additional information must come from the other disciplines. Without the missing information, nurses become stressed when their expectations of the patient's progression are not met and they find that they do not know what to tell the patient and patient's family about what is happening. These interactions, which may occur any time throughout the day, are stressful and may lead to avoidance behavior.

Regular (at least weekly) multidisciplinary conferences are essential to the establishment of a consistent and accurate plan of care known to all members of the burn team. Daily medical rounds that provide data on the patient's medical status throughout the past 24 hours and project the day's plan of care can be useful to nurses. The discussions during the rounds may impart an appreciation of the concerns of the physicians for specific problems and enable nursing personnel to organize their work based on the projected care for the day. The benefits of this knowledge are twofold. Nurses can monitor and evaluate the patient more accurately for expected outcomes, and care can be organized to promote rest periods for the patient.

When a patient dies, the nurses respond based on the circumstances surrounding the death.[22] Was it unexpected? Was it a long, lingering death, with the outcome certain for several weeks? Was it an expected death that occurred quickly? Providing an opportunity for nurses to talk about the death and grieve, if necessary, is important. Otherwise the issue is not resolved, and chronic stress can develop. Nurses sometimes form a strong bond with patients and their families, and attending the funeral or sending sympathy cards can help bring closure in the grieving process.

Control in the Work Environment

There are three issues of control nurses face constantly in providing burn care.[22] The first revolves around the dependence/independence continuum of the patient's recovery. The goal of burn care is to return the patient to independent function. Tension occurs as nurses promote patient independence because of the dependent nature of burn care and the different meaning of independence to the nurse and patient. Patients often are not in control of their daily activities because of the location of their injuries or the immobilizing effects of treatments. They must be bathed, fed, walked, turned, and dressed. The frustration this dependence causes often leads to inappropriate or manipulative behavior by the patient. Nurses must set limits and structure the environment to "control" such behavior. Additional stresses may come from the family trying to function as a patient advocate. When the patient and family are included in the planning of care, they are given accountability and responsibility for some aspects of care and the goals to be achieved. This action promotes independence and a perception of being in "control" of the situation because they are involved actively, rather than passively.

Pain management often becomes an issue of control. Nurses must understand that the authority on the patient's pain is the patient. Only the patient can tell the nurse about the pain experienced. As nurses develop strategies that allow patients some control over their pain management, the stress of inflicting pain will be reduced.[23.]

The second area of control relates to patient compliance with the treatment plan.[22] Early in the hospital course, nurses socialize burn patients to their role as patients. They creatively try to "hook" the patient into the program.[22] Calling the patient by the name chosen by the patient, providing frequent explanations of the goals of care, and establishing progress bench marks can facilitate patient compliance. The nurse invests a great deal of energy in obtaining patient compliance. Thus, the nurse may experience a sense of failure or frustration when the patient regresses or gives up. One way of sensitizing staff to their reactions to the stresses involved is through videotaped interviews with patients and staff. The tapes of interviews about the stress experienced in the burn unit are useful in stimulating discussion at staff conferences.[29.]

Nurses also become involved in creating an optimistic and positive environment for themselves and the patients.[22] They celebrate birthdays, achievements, and holidays. Planning frequent social events is common. Promoting a professional environment centered on the patients' needs helps to reduce conflicts. When the patient and family know the staff care and are working toward mutually established goals, conflicts are reduced.

A third source of conflicts or stresses related to control is the multidisciplinary nature of burn care.[22] Individuals in each discipline attempt to organize care to make their work go smoothly. Conflicts arise every day because of the interdependence of the work: the physician comes into the unit at 11:00 a.m. and wants to see the burn wounds just after the nurse has spent two hours bathing the patient and reapplying creams or dressings; the nurse does not coordinate morning care with the physical therapists, thus limiting the patient's exercise time with the therapists; care is not completed before visiting hours, which causes a delay in the visit or a less-than-optimal visit because the patient is uncomfortable. Once the nurse knows the physician's plan of care as outlined in morning rounds, care can be coordinated by taking time each morning to discuss plans with individuals from all other disciplines involved in the care. The person who really suffers from uncoordinated care is the patient. The stress that this engenders in the nurses comes from a sense of failure toward the patient in easing the pain of care.

As staff members become oriented to burn care, they need to understand the differences in each team member's work and the types of stresses generated. Understanding and communication promote respect and value for the role each team member has in the caring process.

Engagement in Bonding with the Patient/family

In the burn unit, the nurses are a constant in the patient's life.[22] The nurses are the people who encourage, praise, and enable patients to follow the treatment plan toward independence. It is not unusual for strong emotional ties to develop between the patient/family and the nurses. As discharge approaches, the nurses face the stress of breaking those ties. If rapid healing occurs or a rehabilitation bed becomes available, the day of discharge arrives with little warning, and the patient leaves without closure occurring. Frustration, sadness, or a sense of loss are common reactions among nurses to this situation. It is uplifting when the patients and families write to the unit or return for a visit. Seeing the patients do well increases the morale and makes all of the work worthwhile.

Conclusion

We can't be more than we are, but what we are is so much more than we believe.

Anonymous.

The psychologic and physical effects of burn trauma are severe, but in all experiences, there is an opportunity for emotional growth. Many patients and family members are proud of their courage during the recovery process and are made stronger by this life-altering event. When provided consistent and planned emotional support during the hospital stay, patients and families may discover their "reservoirs of strength."[30] Comprehensive psychosocial support of burn patients and their families is essential in reducing the morbidity of emotional problems resulting from the trauma of burn injury and treatment. In understanding the stresses faced by the patient, family, and staff, nurses can use strategies to reduce anxiety, conflicts, and emotional distress during the phases of recovery. The challenges of providing psychosocial support in the burn unit are many; the rewards are great!

References

1. Ariz CP. Psychological considerations. In Artz CP, Moncrief JA, Pruitt BA Jr., eds. *Burns: A Team Approach*. Philadelphia: WB Saunders; 1979:461465.

2. Shenkman B, Stechmiller J. Patient and family perception of projected functioning after discharge from a burn unit. *Heart Lung* 1987; 16:490-496.

3. Blades B, Mellis N, Munsteer AM. A burn specific health scale. *J Trauma* 1982; 22:872-875.

4. Wallace LM, Lees J. A psychological follow-up study of adult patients discharged from a British burn unit. *Burns incl Therm Ini* 1988; 14:39-45.

5. Cobb N, Maxwell G, Silverstein P. Patient perception of quality of life after burn injury: Results of an eleven-year study. *J Burn Care Rehabil* 1990; 11:330-333.

6. Berry CC, Patterson TL, Wachtel TL, Frank HA. Behavioral factors in burn mortality and length of stay in hospital. *Burns incl Therm Inj* 1984; 10:409-414.

7. Browne G, Byrne C, Brown B, et al. Psychosocial adjustment of burn survivors. *Burns Incl Therm Inj* 1985; 12:28-35.

8. Tucker P. Psychosocial problems among adult burn victims. *Burns Incl Therm Inj* 1987; 13:7-14.

9. Goodstein RK. Burns: An overview of clinical consequences affecting patient, staff, and family. *Compr Psychiatry* 1985; 26:43-57.

10. Knudson-Cooper M. What are the research priorities in the behavioral areas for burn patients? *J Trauma* 1984; 24:SI97-S202.

11. Watkins PN, Cook EL, May SR, Ehleben CM. Psychological stages in adaptation following burn injury: A method for facilitating psychological recovery of burn victims. *J Burn Care Rehabil* 1988; 9:376-384.

12. Miller WC, Gardner N, Mlott SR. Psychosocial support in the treatment of severely burned patients. *J Trauma* 1976; 16:722-725.

13. Tobiasen JM, Hiebert JM. Burns and adjustment to injury: Do psychological coping strategies help? *J Trauma* 1985; 25:1151-1155.

14. Vanderplate C. A personal adaptation group for burn injured hospital patients. *Int J Psychiatry Med* 1982; 12:237-242.

15. Goggins M, Hall N, Nack K, Shuart B. Community reintegration program. *J Burn Care Rehabil* 1990; 11:343-346.

16. Kolman PBP. Managing psychopathology in burn patients. *J Burn Care Rehabil* 1984; S:239-243.

17. Bailey EW, Moore DA. Group meetings for families of burn victims. *Topics in Clinical Nursing* 1980; 2:67-75.

18. McHugh ML, Dimitroff K, Davis ND. Family support group in a burn unit. *Am J Nurs* 1979; 79:2148-2150.

19. Roberts ML, Pruitt BA Jr. Nursing care. In Artz CP, Moncrief JA, Pruitt BA Jr., eds. Burns:—A Team Approach. Philadelphia: WB Saunders; 1979:382389.

20. Andreason NJC, Noyers R Jr., Hartford CE. Factors influencing adjustment of burn patients during hospitalization. Psychosom Med 1972; 34:517-525.

21. Summers TM. Psychosocial support of the burned patient. *Crit Care Clin North Am* 1991; 3:237-244.

22. Mannon JM. *Caring for the Burned* Springfield, IL: Charles C. Thomas; 1985.

23. Molter NC. Pain in the burn patient. In Puntillo KA, ed. *Pain in the Critically Ill*. Gaithersburg, MD: Aspen Publishers; 1991:193-209.

24. Cella DF, Perry SW, Kulchycky S, Goodwin C. Stress and coping in relatives of burn patients: A longitudinal study. *Hosp Community Psychiatry* 1988; 39:159-166.

25. Hickey M. What are the needs of families of critically ill patients? A review of the literature since 1976. *Heart Lung* 1990; 19:401-415.

26. Molter NC. Research data. 1991: unpublished.

27. Brodland GA, Andreasen NJC. Adjustment problems of the family of the burn patient. *Social Casework* 1974; 55:13-18.

28. Reddish P, Blumenfield M. Psychological reactions in wives of patients with severe burns. *J Burn Care Rehabil* 1984; 5:388-390.

29. Pauker SL. A new use for videotape in liaison psychiatry: A case from the burn unit. *Gen Hosp Psychiatry* 1986; 8:11-17.

30. Tempereau M, producer. *Reservoirs of Strength*. Bravo Entertainment; 1989.

Nancy C. Molter, RN, MN, CCRN

United States Army Nurse Corps and the United States Army Institute of Surgical Research, Fort Sam Houston, Texas.

Chapter 36

Burn Camp:
Where Scars Don't Matter

Burn patients have a much higher survival rate than ever before. But that poses psychological problems for seriously burned kids: How do they return to normal life? How do they handle stares and taunts?

Children who survive severe burns face a long haul of physical and psychological healing. In West Virginia, there's a place to help them: Burn Camp.

In his summer camp's horse corral, Stevie, 8, refuses to get on a pony. "Come on!" campers keep shouting. "I didn't know how big a horse really is," Stevie says, looking pale and terrified. Finally, J.D., 15, a junior counselor, motions Stevie over. They talk quietly. "You've seen people riding horses on TV, haven't you?" J.D. reasons with Stevie. "Just pretend it's someone else getting on the pony."

Stevie gets on and rides. He is triumphant. "I didn't know riding a horse was that much fun!"

For Stevie and J.D. this is a small but significant moment. Both boys are survivors of severe burns. At Western Pennsylvania Hospital's Summer Camp for Burned Children, held at the Emma Kaufmann Camp at the upper end of the Blue Ridge Mountains near Morgantown, West Virginia, campers learn to readjust to life, to gain self-confidence, to realize that they can overcome their physical and emotional traumas. Stevie, who was burned on his arm and chest when he ran into his dad, who was carrying hot liquid—discovered that he could conquer his fears. J.D. was 10 when he tripped and overturned a deep fryer, severely burning his arm, shoulder and chest.

©August 10, 1997. *Parade Magazine*. Reprinted with Permission.

This was the eleventh year the Western Pennsylvania Hospital Foundation had invited children, aged 5 to 16, for the four-day camp in June. Children can attend for two years after their release or once they turn 5. This year, 24 campers from Pennsylvania, Ohio and West Virginia attended. The cost, approximately $450 per camper, is financed by a Pittsburgh-area can recycling program called Aluminum Cans for Burned Children and by donations and grants. There is no charge to the children's families. Many of the camp's all-volunteer counselors are nurses or firefighters.

Skin that has been burned loses much of its elasticity, and a crucial part of recovery is to keep campers moving so that skin grafts will take more easily and joints don't become frozen by the tightening skin. For many months after skin grafts, kids have to wear tight elastic pressure garments to flatten out scarring. But the garments are tough to get on, and they can get hot. Counselors motivate children to keep moving and to wear their garments.

When necessary, nurses change dressings on wounds. Severely burned skin has lost its sweat glands, and counselors must keep the kids from overheating. The children drink plenty of fluids.

Many of the children undergo periodic surgery to open scar tissue and make room for growth. Tammy, 6, was extensively burned. She lost part of her pinkie finger and hair follicles on top of her head', leaving her with large bald spots. Tammy won't be able to have complete hair transplants until she stops growing. At school, she was shunned. But here in camp, Tammy is affectionate, always hugging the other children and counselors.

Every day is filled with traditional camp activities: swimming, canoeing, kayaking, arts and crafts, hiking and making ice cream sundaes. And there are many special challenges. Some campers go tubing-sitting in an inner tube as they're pulled by speedboat around the 17-mile-long Cheat Lake. There are exercises in trust and working together to solve problems, such as how to get 12 children and adults crowded onto one car tire in the playground.

Campers find time to play practical jokes on counselors and have pillow fights. They get to act silly. But counselors are careful not to spoil the kids—and to maintain a healthy sense of humor. "No cuts! No bruises! Come back alive!" a counselor yells to children going off on a supervised bicycle trail ride. "The whole purpose is to make it a safe place but to keep it lively," says Linda Leonard, a burn-unit nurse who was one of the camp's founders.

The Phoenix Society for Burn Survivors says approximately 1.25 million Americans are severely burned each year—about half of them children. More than 5000 Americans die each year from burns or smoke inhalation. Children under 5 and older persons are most frequently burned.

"You need to see what these children have gone through before they get to camp," Arlene Snyder, president of the Western Pennsylvania Hospital Foundation, said to me as we toured the state-of-the-art burn unit at the hospital the day before I left for summer camp. As we entered the treatment suite, a 2-year-old boy with a burned face was being led back to his hospital bed. To me, he looked unbearably sad.

It's tough for some children to let other people see their burns. Frankie, 6, keeps circling the swimming pool but won't take off his shirt. "Come on, Frankie!" a lifeguard urges. When Frankie was 3, he played with matches in his bedroom. Firefighters found him curled up in a closet, with burns over 70 percent of his body He and his baby brother, Alonzo, were flown by helicopter to Western Pennsylvania Hospital in Pittsburgh. Frankie made it; Alonzo didn't. "Frankie never talks about his own burns," one nurse says. The nurses worry about his feelings of guilt. After much gentle persuasion, Frankie jumps in and struts around the pool. "At least I'm in now!" he shrieks, delighted.

Tall, gentle Raya, 12, suffered third-degree burns over most of her body and lost several toes in a fire that destroyed her home. Two of her cousins died, and her sister suffered from smoke inhalation. Three months after her release from Western Pennsylvania Hospital, Raya began to lose her hearing—a side effect of the antibiotics she had received. Last year at camp, Raya was shy. This year, after attending a school for the deaf and receiving a cochlear implant, she has blossomed.

Burn patients have a much higher survival rate than ever before. But that poses greater psychological problems for burned children: How do they return to a normal life? How do they handle the inevitable stares and taunts?

"We get them to realize that it's not just their scars that make them unique," says Diane Demarest, the camp's child-life specialist. "Challenging camp activities help them build confidence that they carry into the world."

For years, people have stared at Veronica, 9, who was burned from head to foot as a baby. "Did we do her a favor, saving Veronica's life?" a nurse once asked. "Veronica has a real strong will that challenges everybody," says one counselor. "But, hey, that's why she's here."

"The ones who survive are strong," adds another counselor. "It's worth getting through the hard parts because there is quality of life."

The counselors bring a special passion to their work. Maggie Hyder had been the nurse for several of the kids until recently becoming a

flight nurse for an emergency helicopter service. "Burns are so devastating," Hyder says. "It just hurts so bad. But here the children don't
have to care about being scarred."

"Camp is good for me too," says Linda Leonard. "I see that what I
do on the burn unit is worthwhile. This is where everything makes
sense. Seeing these kids be kids—that's what helps me cope with what
I do for the next burned kid who comes to the unit."

"You hope camp made a difference for them. Then you see a big
smile on a kid who's been so unhappy. And you know that it did."

For information on the camp, write to: Western Pennsylvania Hospital Foundation, Dept. P, 4818 Liberty Ave., Pittsburgh, Pa. 15224. For
a list of other camps for burned children around the world, write to:

Phoenix Society for Burn Survivors, Inc.
National Headquarters
33 Main Street, Suite 403
Nashua, New Hampshire   03060
(603) 889-3000; (603) 889-4688 Fax
888-BURN (2876) (toll free for burn survivors)
email: information@burns-phoenix-society.org
web page: www.burns-phoenix-society.org

—by Lou Ann Walker

Chapter 37

Study of Hope in Patients with Critical Burn Injuries

Abstract

The purpose of this study was to determine which factors patients with critical burn injuries would identify as affecting their feelings of hope; specific attention was given to the influence of nursing actions on these feelings. The non-probability purposive sample consisted of nine white male patients who had been admitted to a large burn center in the Southwest. Content analysis technique was used to determine the nursing behaviors that influenced the patients' levels of hope. Hope in this study is viewed as a dynamic process with past, present, and future dimensions. The majority of factors that subjects identified as affecting their levels of hope evolved from the present dimension. This study indicates that factors that affected each subject's level of hope were contingent upon where the patient was in the psychological recovery process that occurs after burn injury. Accordingly, the efficacy of specific nursing actions is contingent upon consideration of these same factors. (J BURN CARE REHBIL 1993;14:207-14)

Hope is that framework of thought processes, affect, and spirituality through which people view the world when they have a specific goal and feel some sense of probability in regard to attaining it.[1] Empirical evidence suggests that the concept of hope plays a major role in the recovery and sustenance of critically ill patients. Engel[2]

463

observed that the onset of illness and, in some cases, death is preceded by a psychologic state that he calls "the giving in-giving up complex." This psychologic state is characterized by the patient's feeling of hopelessness. Hopelessness has been tied to sudden death phenomena in humans,[3] whereas hope has been linked to healing rituals and invocation of the placebo response.[4]

As nursing knowledge of the complexity of disease increases, so does appreciation for the role that psychosocial factors play in the disease process. Hope is one concept that has been witnessed empirically in the critical care area, yet mastery of its deliberate use has not been demonstrated. Indeed, if by technical standards, there is no hope of curing a patient, often the concept is ignored completely and such patients receive the least amount of support.[5]

Critical care nurses are in a unique position to convey hope to those patients who are most critically ill. In order to convey hope to patients and to identify appropriate nursing skills, adequate knowledge of the hope process must be acquired.[6]

One type of critically ill patient who needs supportive hope is the patient with burns. A major burn is one of the most devastating insults that a person may experience. Patients who have sustained major burn injuries confront actual threats to survival, fear of disfigurement, prolonged physical pain, and an extended convalescence.[7] Both psychologic and physiologic needs of the critically ill patient are amplified in the patient with burns. It is for this reason that this patient population was determined to be most representative of critically ill patients.

The purpose of this study was to examine factors that affect hope in the patient with critical burn injuries in order to identify specific nursing actions that influence the presence of hope in those patients. Specifically, what factors do patients with critical burn injuries identify as affecting their feelings of hope and what specific nursing actions do these patients report as affecting their feelings of hope?

Conceptual Framework for the Study

Concepts. The conceptual framework that emerged in this study was the result of the investigators' interpretation of the hope process as supported by the literature and articulated in the nurse-patient relationship. Three concepts were cogent to the framework of this study on the basis of the view that the patient has a perceived need for change. (1) The nursing process is the prescriptive plan for the nurse's role in the facilitation of hope, (2) the hope process is the shared product of the nurse-patient interaction, and (3) the nurse is facilitator of this process.

Dimensions. Within the conceptual framework, hope was viewed as a dynamic process, the impetus for which is a perceived need for change. Hope consists of a past, a present, and a future dimension, as identified by Stotland.[1]

The past dimension of hope is the summation of the individual's life experience. This dimension provides the explanation for the patient's present interpretation of the situation. Coping mechanisms that have previously worked may also be drawn from this dimension. Much of the covert action that is associated with hope may be the product of experiences from the past dimension.

The present dimension of hope is the part of hope that is based on interpretation of present circumstances. It is influenced by what the patient finds when the reality of the present situation is surveyed, and it may influence covert or overt action. Covert action may be evidenced in this dimension of hope by the acceptance of alternative goals, such as hoping for a better quality of remaining life or taking one day at a time.

The future dimension of hope consists of the patient looking ahead for possibilities. This part of hope can be brought to fruition only through some change that will occur in the future.

The three dimensions of hope are not fixed in proportion or importance but rather interact as parts of a whole and are influenced by the way in which the patient perceives life, present circumstances, and future possibilities. One dimension may become more important than another, but the patient's hope system is the product of the interaction of all dimensions. The fluid and dynamic nature of the hope process is shown in Figure 37.1. Any one dimension may predominate

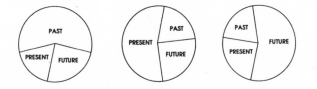

Figure 37.1. The three dimensions of hope: past, review life and search for meaning in life; present, determine meaning of illness and take "one day at a time;"future, look ahead, as in "hope for recovery."

at a given time, depending on which intervening variables are influencing the patient's level of hope.

In the investigators' conceptualization of the hope process, the nurse is viewed as a facilitator of hope in patients. Once the need for nursing intervention has been identified by means of an assessment of the patient, the nurse should collect enough data about the patient's personality, past experiences, social support system, present perceptions, and future expectations to know which of these intervening variables might be supported in order to facilitate hope. By assessing the three dimensions of the patient's hope system, the nurse may build a plan of care that is appropriate for the specific patient. This process is depicted in Figure 37.2.

Inherent in the conceptualization of the framework of this study is the supposition that the nurse may play a crucial role in facilitating hope in the patient by accurately assessing the patient's hope system and communicating hope for the patient in a manner that is appropriate to the patient's situation. Although the hope process is shared by both the nurse and patient, it is the nurse who facilitates this process by initially communicating hope to the patient. The nurse is in a unique position to support the process of hope.

Psychology of Hope. The uniqueness of burn injury must be considered as it relates to the impact it has on the psychological integrity of the individual. Psychological recovery occurs in three phases

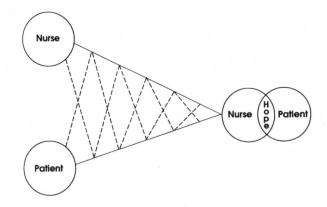

Figure 37.2. Nurse's role in facilitation of hope.

in patients with burns.[8] Patients with burns proceed through these psychological phases at their own rate, dependent upon factors that are unique to each patient's condition such as age, degree of burn injury, affective and cognitive development before the injury and available social support.

All patients with burn injuries are faced with the task of adapting to the threat to survival, fear of disfigurement, prolonged physical pain, and a long and tedious convalescence.[9] As these major difficulties are confronted, problems that are secondary to such adaptation may occur. These adaptations are manifested in the patient's behavior and appear to occur in three phases of psychological adjustment.

The first phase is referred to as the initial, early, or acute burn phase and may be characterized by denial of the injury, repression of feelings, and at times, manifestations of periods of delirium, which can be either physiological or psychological in origin. This phase may last for several weeks and is distinguished by the egocentricity of the patient as the fight for survival continues.[10]

The second phase is referred to as the intermediate or reactive phase and consists of the patient's attempts to make sense of the environment and of what has happened. Robertson, Cross, and Terry[10] identify the three major behavioral cues that occur during this phase as pain, depression, and regression. This phase is construed as beginning when the patient becomes stable, and it may last for several months.

The third and final phase is referred to in the literature as the rehabilitative phase, and it is a period of transition from the hospital to the real world. Patients begin to focus on physical disabilities and appearance. Anxiety regarding reestablishment of life roles is typical during this period.

Although the purpose of this study was to examine factors that the subjects identified as affecting their feelings of hope, these findings must be interpreted in the context of the psychological framework of the patient with burns.

Methods

Sample. The convenience sample that was selected for this study consisted of nine male Caucasian patients who had been admitted to a large southwestern regional burn center after injury. Six patients were involved in gasoline explosions, two were involved in motor vehicle accidents, and one was injured in a missile explosion. Burn size varied from 23% to 70% of body surface area. Patients ranged in age from 18 to 58 years, with a mean age of 31.3 years. Formal educational level varied; one patient had completed 10 years of school and two patients had master's degrees. All spoke English as their primary language. Five of the patients were married and four had never been married. All but one patient identified a specific religious preference; this patient preferring not to answer that question because it was an area of concern between his spouse and himself. Later he identified his wife as a Christian Scientist.

This qualitative study was cleared through the institutional review process, and statements of informed consent were obtained from all participants.

Setting. After the patients consented to participate, demographic data were obtained and audiotaped interviews were conducted by the primary investigator. Interviews of the patients were semi-structured, and open-ended questions were used to provide flexibility and allow for unanticipated responses. In the initial moments of the interview, each patient was asked to describe how the injury had occurred and how much time he had spent in the intensive care unit. Once the patient appeared to be comfortable with the tape recorder, the investigator asked an open-ended question regarding a hope experience. The investigator's initial comment was "think back about something that someone did for you or to you or something that happened to you or around you since you've been in the hospital that made you feel more hopeful or less hopeful. I want to know about someone or something that influenced your level of hope." The interviewer guided the remainder of the interview by using semi-structured questions.

Data Analysis. Data that were collected in this study were analyzed by content analysis. Content analysis is a method that allows for the investigation of problems when verbal or written communication is the source of data.[11] In this study, the coding definitions were derived from the study subjects' conceptualizations of hope and were consistent with current literature and existing theory.

The data were coded by the primary investigator who, immediately after conclusion of an interview, took each datum (a verbatim response or comment from a subject) and placed it in the emerging coding category. It was through this coding process that specific themes evolved. Although categories of past, present, and future dimensions of hope were well defined, subcategories evolved within the present dimension of hope. There was evidence that hope was both negatively and positively influenced in all three dimensions. Data cited reflect both positive and negative influences on hope. The study findings are presented in three major coding categories: past, present, and future dimensions of hope.

Validity of Coding Categories. Content validity was established according to the informed judgment of the investigators. If the data fit into the coding categories easily and realistically and the results were consistent with existing theory, content validity was supported.

Reliability of Coding Categories. Reliability in the use of content analysis reflects the extent of agreement between the coder and an independent judge.[11] The reliability of the coding categories that were used in this study was measured by means of intercoder agreement. Another nurse researcher who was not involved in the investigation randomly selected three data sets with the use of a table of random numbers. After a brief training session with the investigators, the independent nurse researcher coded data from the randomly selected tapes. The independently coded data were compared with the same data as coded by the investigators. Reliability was quantified by percentage of agreement. The overall percentage of intercoder agreement was a mean of 94.8% for the three categories of hope—past, present, and future dimensions.

Results

Past Dimension of Hope. The past dimension of hope consisted of content that reflected a sense of continuity with the past. It was as if something that a patient had learned in the past was responsible for his reaction in the present. This took the form of successful coping mechanisms, ideology, religious faith, or basic trust. It was from this dimension of hope that several of the patients extrapolated in such a way as to lend meaning to their present injury. Examples of comments that are drawn from this dimension of hope are: "Good humor will take you a long way," and "I pray to God every night. I know he will help me." These comments are evidence of thought processes that were formulated in the past but drawn on in response to the stimulus of the burn injury. Although all patients stated that they had attempted to find meaning in their injuries, not all had been able to do so. Those patients who could translate the injury into a meaningful experience appeared to be more comfortable with their situation, as reflected in comments such as "There are times when the question becomes, 'How come?' and the answer is, 'God did it.'" Although the presence of the patients' prior belief systems or thought process was obvious, it was not apparent whether significant others or environmental factors had invoked such thinking. The fact that such cognitive schemas presented themselves, however, is consistent with Stotland's theoretic framework of hope, which suggests that such cognitive structures account for assessment in the patient's hope process.[1]

An unanticipated finding was the infrequent citing of religion as a source of hope by many of the patients. Although one patient spoke of God's influence throughout the interview and another patient mentioned that God had been a sustaining force, the remaining eight patients did not credit religious values or beliefs as affecting their level of hope. This was particularly surprising in light of the fact that they had been asked for religious preference initially during the collection of demographic data and 9 of the 10 had indicated a preference. Religious faith has been positively correlated to levels of hope in earlier studies.[12-14]

It was not evident that schemas from the past were deliberately invoked or facilitated by caregivers. It was obvious, however, that this was a contributory factor to the patients' feelings of hope. Schemas from the past appear to be part of the hope process that needs assessment by caregivers. Those schemas that have positive influences on a patient's hope process could be supported and those that have negative influences could be appropriately addressed.

Present Dimension of Hope. Originally, the present dimension of hope was believed to include those matters that appear to be the product of current experiences. Factors that were identified by patients as relating to the present dimension of hope were related to areas of perceived support and powerlessness. As data collection progressed, the following eight subcategories emerged: (1) nurturance of the patient, (2) validation of worth, (3) feelings of powerlessness, (4) trust in significant others, (5) support of other patients with burns, (6) reality surveillance, (7) treatment affiliation, and (8) sick role responsibilities. These categories overlap and interact with one another. A comment made by a patient such as, "I didn't know if the nurse was that busy or if I was that low a priority," might reflect a need for nurturance and validation of worth and feelings of powerlessness. It is interesting that all patients identified the caregivers rather than a significant family member as having the most influence on their levels of hope. The following discussion details development of the subcategories that evolved in the present dimension.

Nurturance of the Patient. All of the patients identified nurturance as a major influence on their levels of hope. Most of the comments reflected the amount of caring that was transmitted by the caregiver to the patients. In four cases, the patients said that nurturing was provided by spouses, siblings, or parents, but all focused on this aspect of the caregiver. Patients in the study made frequent references to the need for nurturance and caring from caregivers. Because the majority of these patients had been hospitalized for a long time and saw their significant family members or friends for only a few hours a day, perhaps the caregiver assumed the "attachment" role about which Weiss[15] writes. In this way, caregivers become significant others for the period of hospitalization during which patients are so critically ill. If the patients perceive that these needs are being met through social and emotional interactions, then they feel sustained and hopeful. If they believe that these needs are not being met, they may feel, as one patient stated, "emotionally isolated." Six of the patients reported that caregivers were unable to talk with them as much as they would have preferred, and they attributed this to the fact that the caregivers were too busy.

Validation of Worth. The subcategory of validation of worth evolved as comments surfaced regarding continued worth as a competent human being. Weiss[15] defines validation of worth as a sense that one is competent in one's role, is appreciated and admired, and is respected as a person of value. Perceptions were sometimes based on comments that were made to the patient by caregivers. These comments were based on direct evidence of continued worth as the patients perceived it. All of the patients drew on this experience as a sphere that affected their levels of hope. Examples included such comments as "I thought I was just a vegetable," or "I used to hate it when all the doctors would come around and look at me. It made me feel like a freak."

All patients made remarks that alluded to validation of worth. Most significant in this subcategory was whether or not patients perceived that they were important to the caregivers and were contributing members of the burn unit. If the patients perceived that caregivers listened to them, feelings of satisfaction and worth increased. If they were able to help other victims by providing emotional support or physical assistance, self-esteem increased. Both of these experiences were related by patients as affecting their levels of hope.

Feelings of Powerlessness. Powerlessness was a predominate theme in all of the interviews. Much of this theme had to do with the

471

frustration and the feeling of uselessness that are associated with the limitations imposed by the burn injury itself. Roberts and Pruitt[16] state that burn injury robs the patient of autonomy over his or her body for an extended period of time. Patients were not only demoralized over not being able to do for themselves but also stated that not being able to have input into their care resulted in a decreased level of hope. Indeed, one patient stated that his greatest achievement was convincing a nurse that there was more than one way to skin a cat." Although it is obvious that the input patients with burns can be allowed to have in regard to treatment is limited, input in general can be significant and frequent. Robertson et al.[10] recommend making the patient an active participant in his or her own care, which thereby increases a sense of control and decreases the amount of anxiety related to painful treatment that is performed by others. Although most people may see a feeling of powerlessness as a concept with which they can easily deal, someone who has lost identity, significant relationships, roles in life, and autonomy sees a feeling of powerlessness as a formidable obstacle.

Trust in Significant Others. Comments in this subcategory were related to the patient's faith or trust in comments that were made by significant others about the patient's progress. Although it appeared that the amount of trust in a relationship sometimes depended on past experiences with the significant other, it was expressed as a present influence on the level of hope. All patients identified this subcategory as affecting their levels of hope. Much of the content of these comments concerned trust in the staff members as competent caregivers. One patient judged such competency by the organization of the caregiver. Several judged competency on the basis of whether caregivers followed through on what they said they would do. Although this finding may be evidence of invocation of schemas regarding faith in competent caregivers, it may also be that it was the result of the fact that caregivers were physically present more often and were thus able to provide encouraging feedback more frequently. Hamburg et al. [17] suggest that the patient should be reassured repeatedly by someone with whom the patient has formed a trusting relationship.

Support of Other Patients with Burns. Six patients cited this subcategory of the present dimension of hope as influencing levels of hopefulness. All of the patients who cited this subcategory as affecting hope were out of the intensive care unit and on the ward. Physical closeness was greater on the ward, and patients tended to be more mobile than they were in the intensive care unit. This increased mobility and close approximation to one another appeared to increase the facilitation of hope. Patients in the study stated that seeing patients who were worse off than they were increased their level of hope sometimes and at other times decreased it. It appeared that if a patient had contact with another patient who was more severely injured but was coping well, it exerted a positive influence. If the other patient was not perceived as coping well, even if he or she was physiologically stable, then such contact was interpreted as a negative influence. Indeed, one patient avoided another who always had the "blues." Although some burn units deliberately use contact with other patients with burns as a therapeutic tool,[8] the findings of this study indicate that such a strategy may be used successfully only on a selective basis.

Reality Surveillance. Reality surveillance was another theme that surfaced in the interviews. Wright and Shontz[18] define reality surveillance as a continual reorientation to reality. Initially, this action resulted in a decreased level of hope in the patients in the study when they realized their limitations. An example was when one of the patients finally realized that he had lost an arm. As improvement could be seen, reality surveillance became a positive influence on the patient's hope process. When patients were unable to interpret signs of healing, the caregivers became the interpreters of progress. Reality surveillance that was effected by the caregiver and conveyed to the patient resulted in an increased level of hope. In this way, reality surveillance may be used in a therapeutic manner by caregivers.

Treatment Affiliation. All patients made frequent reference to treatment-related factors that affected their feeling of hope. Because pain was associated with treatment, it influenced the presence of hope in a negative way most frequently. Additionally, when patients spoke of treatment, they cited the difficulties and discomfort associated with it. Examples of patients' perceptions in this subcategory are: "Nothing helps the pain" and "Trying to use the bedpan can be very rough; rough treatment is uncalled for."

Sick Role Responsibility. Comments arising from the subcategory of sick role responsibility were made by six of the patients and related to their perceptions of their responsibilities as patients. If patients perceived they were responsible for rough treatment, they voiced fear and confusion: "When someone would be rough with me,

I wondered, What did I do wrong?'" Responsibility for taking an active part in rehabilitation also arose from this category.

Future Dimension of Hope. The element of positive expectation of goal attainment, as delineated in Stotland's theory,[1] was apparent in the hope processes of patients in this study. All patients referred to future goals in conversation. Most of the future goals that were mentioned were global in nature such as "becoming a person again" or "being me again and getting on with my life." Specific plans that were related by study patients demonstrated that realistic goals had been formulated. The part that caregivers played in formulation of these goals was evident in such statements as "They've [caregivers] told me that I won't be able to run for a while" and "I'm going to have to work at walking for a long time." In this case, the patient had received information from both his own reality surveillance and that of caregivers.

Future hopes appeared to reflect events on or around discharge from the hospital. Patients in the study did not speak of hope for the distant future, which may have reflected the fact that most of them were in the intermediate stage of postburn recovery. The one patient who might have been considered to be nearing the rehabilitative stage talked of "acceptance into his peer group" and of concerns about still being attractive enough to "meet girls." This particular patient was within 2 weeks of discharge and was not typical of the majority of patients in the study population.

Support of future goals in the study population appeared to be implied through the active rehabilitative efforts in the present. Encouragement of short-term goals then may be the foundation for the formulation of long-term goals. Perhaps it is only through the day-to-day encouragement of specific goals and through the conveyance of realistic information that alternative goals may be appropriately formulated. If such is the case, then the ability of patients to deal with goal formulation is contingent upon their existing emotional and cognitive states.

Accordingly, accurate assessment is vital to determine where the patient is in terms of postburn recovery.

Discussion

Findings of this study support existing theory only in part. Stotland's theory is based upon the proposition that "an organisms's motivation to achieve a goal is a positive function of its perceived probability of attaining the goal and of the perceived importance of the goal."[1] This proposition was supported by the findings in this study in that the future goals formulated by the patients evolved from the personal limitations that resulted from the burn injury and the values that patients had before the accident. Thus when one patient who had been physically active before both of his legs were burned stated that his hope for the future was "to learn to walk again," this reflected both a realistic and a personally valuable goal.

Stotland[1] describes the cognitive aspect of hope as a schema, which he defines as cognitive structure that consists of association between concepts. Evidence of the invocation of schemas in study subjects included trust in caregivers, previous association with burn injury, and verbalized attitudes about succeeding in the face of adversity. Such schemas did not contribute to the major part of the hope process as reported by study patients; rather, current events were reported as having the greatest impact on patient's hope processes. It is here that findings from our study diverge from Stotland's framework.

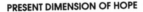

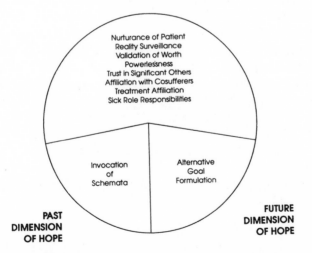

Figure 37.3. Hope in critically ill patients. Factors from the present dimension of hope are listed in order of perceived importance; nurturance of the patient is identified as most important.

Table 37.1. Suggested nursing actions for support of hope. *Importance of the nursing action to the patient is denoted by the presence of one X under the appropriate stage. Two Xs indicate greater importance for that particular stage. Importance was established according to frequency of responses in established subcategories.

Nursing action	Stage of recovery*		
	Acute	Reactive	Rehabilitative
Assess patient's level of hope	xx	xx	xx
Assess patient's coping history	xx	x	x
Listen to patients in an unhurried manner	x	xx	x
Be as gentle as possible with physical care	x	xx	x
Minimize pain as much as possible through medication, psychologic support	xx	xx	xx
Increase number of social interactions with patient	xx	xx	x
Allow patient choices in care	x	xx	xx
Keep promises made to patient	xx	xx	xx
Explain all procedures, share information with patient	xx	xx	xx
Do not threaten patient with procedures	xx	xx	x
Offer constant verbal encouragement of short-term goals	x	xx	xx
Assign a primary caregiver to patient	xx	xx	x
Deliver care in organized, competent manner	xx	xx	x
Give constant verbal feedback regarding healing	xx	xx	x
Assist with alternative goal formulation	—	x	xx
Encourage independent functioning	x	xx	xx
Monitor ancillary help's treatment of patient	xx	xx	xx
Assess outcome of hope-related nursing interventions	xx	xx	xx

Stotland[1] proposed that much of a person's hope structure evolves from an interpretive process through which new events are filtered. Depending on a patient's past experiences, an event is perceived in a particular way. Although the influence of past schemas was evident in this study, the majority of factors that patients in the study identified as affecting their levels of hope related to the experience of the present.

Interacting subcategories were present in the hope structure of the study population, which have been addressed only individually in the existing literature on hope. It may be that subcategories such as feelings of powerlessness, nurturance, and trust could be considered schematic variables that affect the level of hope. Viewed in this way, the hope structure that is presented here may resemble Stotland's theoretic framework. We suggest that the hope structure that was presented by the patients in this study is a "window" through which the patient who is recovering from burn injury views his or her world (Figure 37.3). What patients see when they look out that window depends on where they are in the recovery process. In this study of the hope process, it became evident that this framework of affect and spiritual thought processes operated within the context of the stages of psychological recovery as reported in the works of Miezala[8] and Robertson, Cross, and Terry.[10]

Recommendations and Conclusions

Findings from this study indicate that the factors that affected the patient's level of hope were contingent upon where the patient was in the psychological recovery process. Accordingly, the efficacy of specific nursing actions is contingent upon consideration of this same factor. Table 37.1 lists specific nursing actions that seem appropriate for the support of hope in the patient with burns. The specific nursing actions that are based on the findings of this study are presented in the context of the psychological recovery through which the patient with burns progresses.

Other recommendations regarding the support of hope are: (1) caregivers must assess their own feelings about the amount of hope that they believe is appropriate for any given patient. They too may need to formulate alternative goals for a particular patient. (2) A thorough nursing assessment that is relevant to the patient's hope structure should be made. (3) Outcome criteria for the evaluation of the therapeutic support of hope should be developed on an individual basis; the patient's history should be considered. The assessment of hope as a variable that affects patient outcomes is an area that requires further investigation. Only through formulation of such a data base may nurses intelligently and therapeutically facilitate the hope process in patients.

—by Frances D. Anderson, RN, PhD, CCRN, LTC, Army Nurse Corps, Joseph P. Maloney, RN, PhD, COL, Army Nurse Corps, and Alice R. Redland, RN, PhD San Francisco, California

References

1. Scotland E. The psychology of hope. San Francisco: Jossey-Bass, 1969.

2. Engel GL. A life setting conducive to illness: the giving in giving up complex. Bull Menninger Clin 1968;32:355-65.

3. Richter CP. On the phenomenon of sudden death in animals and man. Psychosom Med 1957-19:192-8.

4. Frank J. The role of hope in psychotherapy. Int J Psychiatry Med 1968;5:383-95.

5. Schneider JS. Hopelessness and helplessness. J Psychiatr Nurs Mental Health Serv 1980;18:12-21.

6. Brown P. The concept of hope: implications for care of the critically ill. Crit Care Nurse 1989;9:97-105.

7. Artz CP. Psychological considerations. In: Artz CP, Moncrief JA, Pruitt BA, eds. Burns: a team approach. Philadelphia: WB Saunders, 1979:461-5.

8. Miczala P. Postburn psychological adaptation: an overview. Crit Care Q 1978; 1: 93-111.

9. Weinberg N, Miller NJ. Burn care: a social work perspective. Health and Social World 1983;7:97-106.

10. Robertson KE, Cross Pj, Terry JC. The crucial first days. Am j Nurs 1985;85:30-47.

11. Holsti OR. Content analysis. In: Lindzey G, Aronson E, eds. The handbook of social psychology. Reading, Massachusetts: Addison-Wesley Publishing Co, 1968;596-692.

12. Dufault KJ. Hope of elderly persons with cancer. Cleveland, Ohio; Case Western Reserve University; 1981. Dissertation.

13. Stoner MJH. Hope and cancer patients. Boulder, Colorado; University of Colorado; 1982. Dissertation.

14. O'Conner AP, Wicker CA, Germino BB. Understanding the cancer patient's search for meaning. Cancer Nurs 1990; 13:167-75.

15. Weiss RS. The provision of social relationships. In: Rubin Z, ed. Doing unto others. Englewood Cliffs, New Jersey: Prentice-Hall, 1974;141-67.

16. Roberts MI, Pruitt BA. Nursing care and psychological considerations. In: Artz CP, Moncrief JA, Pruitt BA, eds. Burns: a team approach. Philadelphia: WB Saunders, 1979:380-4.

17. Hamburg DA, Artz CP, Reiss E, Amspacher V7H, Chambers RE. Clinical importance of emotional problems in the care of patients with burns. N Engl J Med 1953;248:355-9.

18. Wright BA, Shontz FC. Process and tasks in hoping. Rehabil Lit 1968;29:322-31.

Part Five

Safety and Prevention

Chapter 38

Fire and Burn Prevention Checklist

Most burn injuries happen in the home. This checklist will help you evaluate your home environment and develop good burn safety habits.

Kitchen

Do you

- Avoid wearing loose-fitting long sleeves when cooking?
- Know what to do if your clothing should catch fire?—Drop, Roll & Cool
- Have good lighting in kitchen and work areas?
- Always keep pot handles turned inward?
- Keep a large lid within reach when frying, to extinguish grease fires?
- Use large potholders or oven mitts?
- Avoid leaving food to cook unattended?

Electrical Appliances

Do you

- Dry your hands before using electrical appliances?

- Use electrical appliances on dry surfaces away from water?
- Unplug appliances when not in use?
- Check lamp and appliance cords for fraying and/or brittle insulation? Replace worn cords.
- Avoid overloading outlets?
- Use extension cords only for temporary connections?

Smoking Materials

Do you

- Use caution with smoking materials?
- Avoid smoking when in bed, tired, ill, or when consuming alcohol, or medication that makes you drowsy?
- Use large, safe ashtrays with islands?
- Have safe ashtrays in all smoking areas?
- Have smoke detectors in rooms frequently used by smokers?
- Empty ashtrays into a metal container?
- Check areas where people smoke for live cigarettes or ashes?

Housekeeping

Do you

- Keep fire escape routes free of clutter?
- Store matches and lighters out of the reach of children?
- Store combustibles /flammable materials such as paint thinner and solvents in original, tightly-closed containers, away from ignition sources?
- Unplug all electrical tools when not in use?

Emergency Procedures

Do you have

- Emergency phone numbers and other pertinent information posted close to your telephone?
- An emergency escape plan for your home—and practice it frequently? If you live with others, does it include an outdoor meeting place?
- Alternate routes for your escape, if the main routes are blocked?

When you report a fire

- Give your name and telephone number.

- Identify the problem—fire, number of people trapped, etc.
- Provide address and location—including house number, street name and municipality.

Smoke Detectors

Have you installed smoke detectors

- On each level of your home?
- On the ceiling just outside your bedroom door?
- In rooms frequently used by smokers?

Do you

- Test battery-operated smoke detectors every month?
- Change smoke detector batteries each year?

Protect your loved ones from burns. Share this information with your family and friends.

Chapter 39

Common Products that Cause Uncommonly Severe Burn Injuries

The problem often goes unrecognized, but thousands of people are burned every year by products they use every day.

During 1993, about 238,000 people were treated in hospital emergency rooms for thermal, electrical, and scald burns.

Members of the fire protection community know from experience that. Smoke inhalation, not burns, is the primary cause of deaths in structural fires. In fact, the percentage of fire-related deaths attributed primarily to smoke inhalation has been well documented as have the major causes of these fires.

But there is a related, if somewhat different, problem we tend to overlook: nonfatal burn injuries. One reason this type of injury often takes a back seat to smoke inhalation injuries is that most burns don't actually occur in incidents attended by the fire service.

Indeed, many burns, such as those resulting from scalds and touching hot surfaces, aren't even flame-related. Nevertheless, they represent a "related" hazard that's of significant concern to both the NFPA and public health officials.

The fire protection community generally acknowledges that severe burns are among the most excruciating of all injuries, often requiring long periods of rehabilitation, multiple skin grafts, painful physical therapy, and residual disfigurement that leaves victims with life-long psychological and physical trauma.

Every now and then, such injuries capture the attention of the media. Michael Jackson got a lot of coverage when he was burned while filming a commercial, as did Richard Pryor when he was severely burned while freebasing cocaine. But the attention never lingers for long, even within the fire protection community, and many thousands of individual tragedies arc undocumented altogether.

A recent article in the *Journal of Burn Care & Rehabilitation* notes that there are slightly more than a million burn injuries a year, based on the U.S. government's National Health Interview survey, which asks people in their homes to self-report health problems of all types.[1] Nearly a quarter-million of those burn injuries are serious enough to lead to an emergency-room visit, and nearly one-tenth of those are serious enough to lead to hospitalization. In recent years, hospitalization has more and more often meant admission to a specialized burn-care center, where the typical stay is nearly twice as long as it is in a typical hospital and the costs per day are much higher, Small wonder that several different studies have shown the cost of burn injuries running into billions of dollars per year.

This chapter will provide a brief overview of a particular part of the burn injury problem—the part that passes through hospital emergency rooms and involves identifiable products. For more than two decades, the U.S. Consumer Product Safety Commission's (CPSC's) National Electronic Injury Surveillance System (NEISS) has tracked hospital emergency room injuries, focusing, in particular, on product involvement, the Commission's legally mandated area of responsibility.

During 1993, about 238,000 people were treated in hospital emergency rooms for thermal, electrical, and scald burns (see Table 39.1). Of these, 151,000 were the victims of thermal burns, 6,100 of electrical burns, and 77,700 of scald burns. Although scald burns were far

Table 39.1. Total Burn Injuries for 1993

Kind of of Burn	Number of Emergency Room Injuries	Number of Victims Hospitalized	Percent Hospitalized
Thermal	151,000	11,100	7.3
Scald	77,700	9,700	12.5
Electrical	6,100	600	10.5
Not specified	2,900	200	6.1

less frequent than thermal burns, they required substantially more care, with a hospitalization rate 70 percent higher than that of thermal burns. Forty-nine percent of the thermal victims were under 15 years old (see Table 39.2). Only 4 percent of thermal burn patients and 7 percent of scald burn patients were 65 years or older.

The hospitalization rate was extraordinarily high for young scald victims and for older thermal burn victims.

Table 39.2. Percentage of Victims Hospitalized by Age in 1993

	Total	Under 5 Years	5 to 14 Years	15 to 64 Years	Over 65 Years
Thermal burns	7.3	4.7	9.0	7.7	21.3
Scald burns	12.5	26.4	10.9	4.8	14.7

Products Associated with Thermal Burns

In 1993, more thermal burns—16,300—were the result of hair curlers and curling irons than any other product among all ages (see Table 39.3). Children under 15 suffered most—10,400—of these injuries.[2] Fortunately, most of the burns appear to have been relatively minor:

Only 100 of the victims required hospitalization.

Room heaters, primarily kerosene heaters and wood or coal stoves, were the second leading cause of burns. Overall, room heaters injured 15,900 people in 1993. Kerosene heaters were responsible for 5,600 injuries and wood or coal stoves for 4,100.

The third leading cause of burns in 1993 was cooking ranges, which injured 14,900 people. Although the kind of range involved wasn't usually identified, the data indicate that electric ranges were most often responsible for children's burns and gas ranges for adults' injuries. Ovens were associated with an additional 7,200 thermal burn injuries. If ranges and ovens were combined into a single category, they would constitute the leading cause of thermal burn injuries.

Table 39.3a. Products Most Frequently Associated with Thermal and Electrical Burn Injuries Treated in Hospital Emergency Rooms in 1993 in Rank Order. (Continued on next page.)

Product	Total ER Visits	Number Hospitalized	Percent Under Age 15	Percent Over Age65
Total thermal burns	151,000	11,100	49.39	3.9
Total electrical burns	6,100	100		
Hair curlers, curling Irons	16,300	100	61.7	0.3
Heaters	15,900	600	75.4	4.2
–Kerosene	5,600	300	84.2	0.0
–Wood, coal stoves	4,100	100	82.4	1.5
–Gas, LP-gas	1,600	100	40.44	12.0
–Electric	600	0	97.2	0.0
–Other or not specified	4,200	100	67.8	9.7
Ranges	14,900	800	50.5	5.8
–Gas	1,600	200	17.9	6.1
–Electric	1,200	0	90.0	0.0
–Other or not specified	12,200	500	51.0	6.3
Irons	13,700	900	83.1	1.9
Gasoline	8,800	2,500	20.5	8.1
Cookware, nonelectric[1]	8,400	300	22.3	4.5
Ovens	7,200	200	44.9	0.5
–Gas	1,300	100	7.9	0.0
–Electric	300	0	90.9	0.0
–Other or not specified	5,600	100	53.0	0.0
Fireworks	7,200	600	57.7	2.3
Grills	6,700	300	44.7	0.3
–Gas, LP-gas	2,000	100	33.2	0.8
–Charcoal	1,600	100	39.3	0.0
–Other or not specified	3,000	100	55.0	0.0
Cigarettes	6,600	800	54.7	5.3
Clothing	5,000	1,000	32.3	8.1
–Daywear	3,200	600	35.1	4.9
–Nightwear	700	100	35.7	22.7
–Other or not specified	1,100	300	17.9	8.1

Table 39.3b. Products Most Frequently Associated with Thermal and Electrical Burn Injuries Treated in Hospital Emergency Rooms in 1993 in Rank Order. (Continued from previous page.)

Product	Total ER Visits	Number Hospitalized	Percent Under Age 15	Percent Over Age65
Cigarette lighters	4,300	400	45.3	1.2
Electric outlets, receptacles*	2,800	300	73.2	0.0
Candles, fuel-burning lights	2,600	200	21.5	16.7
Matches	2,300	400	36.1	5.2
Furnaces	2,400	200	26.1	0.0
Lawn mowers	2,200	<50	64.2	0.0
Welding, soldering equipment	2,60	0	12.5	4.7
Radiators	1,900	400	78.1	4.6
Floors	1,600	100	77.7	8.1
Charcoal	1,600	100	68.4	0.0
Household containers, packages[2]	1,300	200	34.5	4.8
Beds	1,200	100	84.2	1.4
Cutting torches	1,200	0	0.0	0.0
Electric heating pad	1,200	<50	9.4	26.7
Electric wire, wiring systems*	1,100	100		
Aerosol containers	1,100	300	52.7	0.0
Water heaters	1,000	0	28.0	0.0
Tableware, flatware	1,000	100	37.6	0.0
Light bulbs	1,000	0	77.3	1.8
Microwave ovens	900	0	16.1	13.5

1.   Includes bowls, canisters, and metal and nonmetal cookware.
1.   Includes metal, plastic, and wood containers.
* Denotes products with primarily electrical burn injuries. Electrical burns have been combined with thermal burns here because they form a relatively small subset.

Note: All estimates have been rounded to the nearest 100, and products with low frequencies have been excluded. Therefore, product detail doesn't add to the total. The estimates shown aren't necessarily mutually exclusive. A single accident might involve two products—for example, a cooking stove and cookware—and would be included in estimates for both products. Source: NEISS

Table 39.4. Products Most Frequently Associated with Scald Burns Treated in Hospital Emergency Rooms in 1993

Product	Total ER Visits	Number Hospitalized	Percent Under Age 15	Percent Over Age65
All scald burns	77,700	9,700	40.5	6.7
Hot water	22,300	1,800	25.5	7.2
Cookware (non-electric)[1]	14,100	1,900	37.0	7.2
Tableware (non-electric)[2]	10,500	1,300	81.5	4.2
Tap water	5,100	1,400	73.5	11.4
—Bathtubs and showers	3,200	1,100	59.5	17.8
—Sinks	1,300	200	94.1	2.6
—Faucets and spigots[3]	800	200	89.7	0.0
Ranges	3,900	700	52.8	4.9
Coffee Makers, All Kinds	3,300	300	40.2	12.5
Tables	2,800	600	93.8	0.0
Microwave Ovens	2,500	100	55.7	3.5
Pressure Cookers	2,300	200	1.6	1.5
Ovens	1,200	<50	18.0	31.1
Floors	1,200	400	40.3	11.3
Candles, etc.	900	100	38.8	4.6
Clothing	800	300	56.3	2.0
Slow Cookers	800	100	40.3	0.0
Adhesives	700	0	35.0	0.0
Counters, countertops	700	200	95.1	0.0
Antifreeze	700	0	0.0	0.0
Bottles and Jars	700	100	11.6	0.0
Irons	600	100	60.6	2.7
Drinking glasses	500	<50	72.7	9.1
Vaporizer, humidifier	500	<50	68.3	0.0
Radiators	500	100	10.8	7.3
Baby bottles	400	100	40.8	0.0

1.   *Includes mixing bowls, canisters, and metal and nonmetal cookware.*
2.   *Excludes drinking glasses*
3.   *Type of appliance not identified.*

Irons and gasoline injuries rounded out the top five products as-sociated with thermal burns, being responsible for 13,700 and 8,800 injuries, respectively. Injuries associated with gasoline were the most serious, resulting in 2,500 injuries that required hospitalization. This is more than twice as many injuries requiring hospitalization than any other product caused.

Fireworks were also a major source of burns, resulting in 7,200 such injuries in 1993. And this figure doesn't include the 5,400 other fireworks injuries that weren't thermal or chemical burns.

Clothing ignition injuries were relatively infrequent—there were 5,000 in 1993—but they were serious. In fact, clothing was the second most common product associated with injuries that re-quired hospitalization, of which there were 1,000. Although the proportion of clothing injuries involving children was similar for both daywear and nightwear, the overall frequency of burns involv-ing daywear was higher. Nightwear injuries were particularly likely to involve the elderly, compared with other consumer prod-ucts.

Other products involved in fires that injured a high proportion of elderly victims included electric heating pads, as well as candles and other fuel-burning lights. Children, on the other hand were especially prone to injuries involving heaters and irons. For each product, more than three-fourths of the victims were under 15 years old.

Products Associated with Scald Injuries

Table 39.4 shows, in rank order, the estimated number of scald burns associated with various consumer products that were treated in emergency rooms. The product at the top of the list, hot water, isn't very useful for identifying possible remedial action, since it's not clear whether this refers to *heated* water or to hot tap water. The comments associated with hot water injuries suggest that most involved heated water, but without a special study, it's impossible to know for sure. However, hot water injuries have been included in the table because they are identified with so many scald injuries. If a substantial pro-portion of these injuries involve hot tap water instead of heated wa-ter, the size of the problem associated with tap water scalds would assume greater importance.

The products most frequently associated with scald injuries were cookware, which resulted in 14,100 injuries, and tableware, which resulted in 10,500. Tap water, primarily in bathtubs and showers, was the third major contributor, resulting in 5,100 injuries. Almost three-quarters of the victims were children under age 15, and the hospitalization rate was extraordinarily high, about 28 percent.

Ranges and coffeemakers rounded out the top five products associated with scald injuries. They caused 3,900 and 3,300 injuries, respectively. Microwave ovens also accounted for a fairly large number of injuries—2,500—although the hospitalization rate for these injuries was relatively low.

The distribution of product-related scald burns among children wasn't remarkably different from the distribution among other age groups, except that there were more injuries from tableware than from cookware. Cookware injuries were somewhat more serious, however, requiring more in-patient care.

To Summarize . . .

In summary, then, the major sources of thermal, electrical, and scald burn injuries are ranges and ovens, hot water scalds, hair curlers and curling irons, cookware and tableware, gasoline, heaters, and irons.

Taken together, ranges and ovens claim more thermal burn injuries than any other product group, while the most important cause of scald burns is hot water—even though hot water isn't a "product." We don't know how many hot water scald burns can be attributed to hot tap water, as opposed to heated water, but the tap water scald problem may be larger than we originally supposed.

Cookware and tableware are also associated with a large number of scald burns. In fact, tableware is the largest source of product-related scald burn injuries among children.

A majority of the victims of burns inflicted by hair curlers and curling irons are children, too, as are a large number of those burned by irons.

While gasoline isn't responsible for the largest number of burn injuries overall, it is responsible for the largest number of burns that are serious enough to require hospitalization.

What We Can Do

Although this chapter focuses on the role of specific products in burn injuries, it isn't intended to set a specific agenda for the CPSC, NFPA, or any other organization. Those decisions will rest not only on the absolute size of the problem, but also on the number of products in use, the impact the problem has on particularly vulnerable parts of the population, and the nature and feasibility of any proposed corrective action.

Cold statistics do not easily translate into the suffering that many of these injuries entail. A visit to a burn care center and encounters with a few of the patients and the dedicated specialists who treat them would undoubtedly tell a more eloquent story. But perhaps these numbers will raise our awareness of the size and characteristics of America's burn problem and, in so doing, make us more aware of its importance.

For additional information on past or current efforts to reduce the toll that burn injuries exact, contact the CPSC or NFPA. Become a part of the solution.

1. Brigham and McLoughlin, *Journal of Burn Care and Rehabilitation,* Jan/Feb. 1996.

2. Hair curlers and curling irons constitute a single product group in NEISS coding; the proportion attributable to each is, by itself, unknown.

—Beatrice Harwood

Beatrice Harwood retired from the U.S. Consumer Product Safety Commission as supervisor statistician in 1998.

Chapter 40

Flammable Fabrics

The U.S. Consumer Product Safety Commission estimates that each year there are thousands of deaths and injuries from burns associated with flammable fabrics. Here are some accident patterns:

Six-year-old Tommy found some matches on a coffee table in his home. He lit one of the matches and dropped it on his shirt, which ignited. Tommy received severe burns over 40 percent of his body and had to be hospitalized for six months.

Grandpa McIntire was using gasoline in his basement to clean some paint brushes. He was smoking while he worked, and some sparks and ashes fell on one of the brushes and ignited the flammable vapors. Some of the gasoline had spilled on his pants and the flames quickly spread to his clothing. He was burned severely and hospitalized for months.

Several pots were heating on the gas range. Susan reached over a lit burner to stir something in a pot on a back burner. Her

Consumer Product Safety Commission, Fact Sheet No.17: Flammable Fabrics, Washington, D.C. 20207 Revised May 1975. This document is in the public domain. It may be reproduced without change in part or in whole by an individual or organization without permission. If it is reproduced, however, the Commission would appreciate knowing how it is used. Write to the U.S. Consumer Product Safety Commission, Bureau of Information and Education, Washington, D.C. 20207. Although somewhat old, the information in this chapter is still applicable and is currently circulated as a CPSC Fact Sheet.

long-sleeve robe ignited and the flames began to travel up her arm. Fortunately, she dropped to the floor immediately and rolled to smother the flames. She suffered burns on her arm and part of her face.

One night, 38-year-old Roberta Smith got into bed, lit a cigarette, and opened a favorite magazine. She fell asleep and dropped the lit cigarette on the bed. The cigarette burned through the sheets and began to smolder on the mattress. Several minutes later, Roberta awakened because she was having trouble breathing. She dropped to the floor and crawled out of the room. She suffered from severe smoke inhalation.

These illustrations represent some of the accident patterns associated with flammable fabrics:

1. Playing with, or using, matches and lighters. Children and adults can misuse matches and lighters although children are the more frequent victims.

2. Using flammable liquids. Smoking or using any other ignition source while using flammable liquids is very dangerous. Most people don't realize that vapors from flammable liquids can travel all the way across a room and be ignited by a distant pilot light.

3. Using kitchen ranges. Both gas and electric ranges can ignite clothing, especially garments that are loose-fitting with floppy sleeves.

4. Smoking in bed. Smoking is the most common cause of fires associated with bedding, mattresses, and upholstered furniture.

There are many other frequent ignition sources: space heaters, bonfires, fireplaces, and coal and wood burning stoves. The involvement of clothing usually increases the severity of body burn.

Recently, there have been some "success stories" in which flame retardant sleepwear has saved a child from what would have been severe burns if the child had been wearing flammable sleepwear.

These cases demonstrate the effectiveness of the new flame retardant fabrics. But "flame retardant" does not mean "flame proof," and precautions still need to be taken to avoid fires.

Fire is especially dangerous to the very young, the very old, and the handicapped because they do not know how or do not have the physical abilities to respond appropriately. However, the hazards of flammable fabrics affect us all since the majority of fabrics used in today's clothing will burn quite easily.

The Federal government has taken several steps to make fabrics less flammable. Standards have been set for the flammability of carpets and rugs, mattresses, and children's sleepwear in sizes 0 to 6X. A recent decision by the U.S. Consumer Product Safety Commission established a flammability standard for children's sleepwear in sizes 7 to 14, and this standard took effect in May, 1975.

The Commission has the following suggestions for the purchase, use, and proper laundering of flame retardant fabrics and some first aid tips if you do get burned.

Purchase

Buy flame retardant clothing for your children. Safer sleepwear should be available up through size 14, and some stores will be selling other articles of children's clothing made with flame retardant fabric.

If you sew, buy flame retardant fabrics to use in the garments you make.

Consider the following factors in purchasing all garments.

- Construction
  - Tightly woven, heavy fabrics (such as denim used in jeans) will ignite and burn more slowly than sheer, lightweight and loosely woven fabrics (such as cotton broadcloth used in shirts).
  - Napped fabric (such as cotton flannel) with air spaces between the loose fibers will ignite much faster than a smooth surfaced material (such as denim).
  - A fluffy high pile fabric (such as some sweaters) will ignite and burn faster than a close knit, low pile fabric (such as most pants).

- Design
  - Close-fitting garments are less likely to ignite than loose-fitting garments (such as robes, housecoats, blouses, shifts, and nightgowns with bell-type sleeves, ruffles, and trims).

Use—Be aware of the hazards of ignition sources and of flammable liquids:

- Kitchen ranges

  — Keep young children from climbing on top of stoves and igniting their clothing from a lit burner.

  — Don't try to keep warm by leaning against a stove because your clothing may ignite. Even an electric stove which has been turned off can ignite clothing if the stove is hot enough

  — Don't wear loose-fitting sleeves when you reach across lit burners either to operate control knobs or to reach for pans because your sleeves can ignite.

  — Use a potholder instead of a towel to remove a pan from a lit burner because a towel can touch the burner, ignite, and then ignite your clothing.

- Cigarettes

  — Don't smoke in bed because you might fall asleep and the lit cigarette could start a fire.

  — Be *aware* that elderly and handicapped people are likely to drop lit cigarettes or ashes on their clothing and, because of their disabilities, they may be unable to react to help themselves.

- Matches and Lighters

  — Be aware that elderly and handicapped people often drop matches on themselves when lighting cigarettes, cigars, or pipes, resulting in ignition of their clothing.

  — Be aware that many people, especially the elderly and handicapped, spill lighter fluid on their clothing when refilling a lighter, and the fluid may ignite when the lighter is lit, resulting in clothing ignition. Elderly and handicapped people should not use matches and lighters when they are alone.

  — Keep matches and lighters locked up away from children because children often ignite their clothing while playing with matches and lighters. Children usually find matches where their parents have left them:

- Flammable Liquids
  - Remember that the heavier-than-air *vapors* from flammable liquids can travel invisibly across a room and be ignited by a distant flame or heat source, such as matches, lighters, cigarettes, or pilot lights from water heaters and stoves.
  - Store flammable liquids in tightly-capped safety containers and keep them away from your living quarters—in an outdoor shed and out of children's reach.

Laundering Procedures for Flame Retardant Fabrics

Flame retardant fabrics should have permanent care labels. In order to maintain the flame retardant qualities, always follow the care instructions. Most recommend the following:

- Use phosphate-based detergents, not soaps or non-phosphate detergents. (If you live in an area where phosphates are banned, use a heavy-duty liquid laundry detergent.)
- Use warm water, not hot water.
- Do not use chlorine bleach.

(For more information, see Fact Sheet No.24; Laundering Procedures for Flame Retardant Fabrics.)

First Aid for a Burn

- Cool the burn with cool water; this reduces pain and stops further damage to the skin.
- Cover a large burn with a clean, dry sheet or other freshly ironed linen.
- Do not try to clean the burn.
- *Do not* put grease, butter, or ointments on a burn. Grease or butter can make a bad burn worse.
- Do not pull clothing over the burn.
- Do not try to remove pieces of cloth that stick to the burned area.
- Do not break blisters.
- Call a doctor immediately—even small burns can become serious if they are not properly treated.

Talk to your children about the dangers of fire and tell them what to do if their clothing does catch fire:

- Never run!
- Do not remain standing.
- Drop to the floor immediately and roll to smother the flames.

Plan emergency escape procedures in case a fire starts in your own home:

- Be sure there are *two* ways out of every room, especially every bedroom (this may require the purchase of a rope ladder so that you can use an upstairs window as an exit).

- Close your bedroom doors at night to hold back smoke in case a fire starts while you're asleep. If a fire does start, don't open the bedroom door unless you are sure the hallway is not filled with smoke.

- Have the family meet at a pre-arranged assembly point outside the home to be sure everyone is out.

- Know how to call the fire department.

- In general, concentrate on saving people, not possessions.

Bibliography

Crikelair, G.F., "Medical Aspects of Clothing Burns," *Textile Flammability and Consumer Safety,* Gottlieb Duttweiler Institute, Zurich, 1969.

"Fabric Flammability and Non-Phosphate Detergents," *Household and Personal Products Industry,* Nov.1972, 30-54.

Fourth Annual Report to the President and the Congress on the Studies of Deaths, Injuries, and Economic Losses Resulting from Accidental Burning of Products, Fabrics, or Related Materials, Fiscal Year 1972, Bureau of Product Safety, Food and Drug Administration, Department of Health, Education, and Welfare.

Oglesbay, Floyd B., "The Flammable Fabrics Problem," *Pediatrics,* vol.44, no.5, part II (Nov.1969), 827-832.

Slater, James A., "Fire Incidents Involving Sleepwear Worn by Children Ages 6-12," National Bureau of Standards Technical Note 810, December 1973.

U.S. Consumer Product Safety Commission, Fact Sheet No.9: Kitchen Ranges; No.23: Flammable Liquids; No.24: Laundering Procedures for Flame Retardant Fabrics; No.25: Federal Standards for Fabric Flammability; No. 28: Matches and Lighters.

White, William V., "Flammable Fabrics and the Burn Problem: A Status Report," *American Journal* of Public Health (Oct.1971), 2057-2064.

To report a product hazard or a product-related injury, Write to the U.S. Consumer Product Safety Commission, Washington, D.C. 20207. In the continental United States, call the toll-free safety hotline: 800-638-2666. Maryland residents only, call 800-492-2937.

Chapter 41

Children's Sleepwear

CPSC Product Safety Fact Sheet for Children's Sleepwear

Due to the tragic number of children who were severely burned when wearing sleepwear, the U.S. Consumer Product Safety Commission (CPSC) requires that all children's sleepwear through size 14 be made from flame-resistant material.

Before these requirements became effective, children under the age of 15 suffered one-third of all fabric burns, and sleepwear was the type of clothing most often ignited.

Under the Flammable Fabrics Act, two mandatory standards for the flame resistance of children's sleepwear sizes 0-6X and 7-14 (nightgowns, pajamas, robes, and similar clothing) exist. The standard for sleepwear sizes 0-6X (FF 3-71) went into effect July 29, 1972; for sizes 7-14 (FF 5-74), May 1, 1975. These flame-resistant fabrics must stop burning after the fire source is removed.

All children's sleepwear sizes 0-14 now on the market must comply with the standards, as well as all yard goods intended or promoted for use for children's sleepwear.

This chapter contains two documents: U.S. Consumer Product Safety Commission (CPSC), Publication #96: *Children's Sleepwear*, (Data collected from 1966-1973, in the First Annual Report, 1973, of the U.S. Consumer Product Safety Commission. Revised August 1981), and CPSC press release #98-087, dated March 25, 1998, "CPSC's Sleepwear Amendment to Help Reduce Burn Injuries to Children." Contact: Kathleen Begala (301) 504-0580 Ext. 1193.

Available data indicate a decrease in recent years in deaths and injuries involving sleep-wear ignition. While there may be several reasons for this reduction, the Commission believes that these sleepwear standards may have been a major factor.

The following points should help consumers buying children's sleepwear or sleep-wear fabric to understand how the standards affect what they will find in the stores:

Sleepwear

- Sleepwear is not required to carry a label stating it complies with the standards, although some manufacturers may voluntarily use such a label.

- Manufacturers **are** required by CPSC to label sleepwear with care instructions if the flame resistance is affected by laundering practices. (Consumers will see a care label in any case, because the Federal Trade Commission requires care instructions on all garments.)

- Virtually no U.S. manufacturers today add flame-retardant chemicals to sleepwear fabrics to make them resistant to fire. Instead, flame resistance is obtained through the use of inherently flame resistant fibers or by fabric construction. Some manufacturers may label sleepwear as being free from flame-retardant chemicals, though this labeling is not required.

- CPSC does not require daywear for infants and children, including diapers and underwear, to meet the children's sleepwear standards. If you are unsure whether a piece of clothing is sleepwear, look for a label indicating the manufacturer's intended use of the garment, for instance, as sleepwear or as underwear. The Commission encourages them to use of such labels, but does not require them on non-sleepwear garments that resemble sleepwear. If your child uses daywear (such as thermal underwear) for sleeping, he/she may be losing the protection afforded by flame resistant sleepwear.

Sleepwear Fabrics

- Any fabrics intended for children's sleepwear must meet the flammability standards.

- If you are uncertain which yard goods to use for sewing sleepwear, check the bolt for the manufacturer's voluntary label indicating the fabric complies with the standard.

Remember, flame resistant does not mean flame proof. Flame resistant fabrics will burn, but resist flames better than other fabrics do.

Additional Fire Protection Suggestions:

- Keep young children away from sources of fire, mainly stoves and ranges, matches and lighters.

- Do not store "goodies" above a range. They could tempt children to climb onto the range.

- Warn children about the dangers of these products, and those of space heaters, heating stoves, and fireplaces.

- Teach your children what to do if their clothing does catch fire:
  Never run.
  Drop down and roll.
  Smother the flames, when possible, with a blanket, coat, or rug.

Related CPSC Reading:

Fact Sheets

No.17	Flammable Fabrics
No. 23	Flammable Liquids
No. 24	Laundering Procedures for Flame Resistant Fabrics
No. 25	Fabric Flammability Standards
No. 25	Matches and Lighters
No. 34	Space Heaters
No. 44	Fireplaces
No. 92	Wood and Coal Burning Stoves.
Also	The *Guide to Fabric Flammability.*

To report a product hazard or a product-related injury, write to the U.S. Consumer Product Safety Commission, Washington, D.C. 20207. In the continental United States, call the toll-free hotline: 800-838-8326. Maryland residents only, call 800-492-8363. Alaska, Hawaii, Puerto Rico, virgin islands, 800-638-8333. A teletypewriter for the deaf is available on the following numbers: National (Including Alaska and Hawaii) 800-635-8270, Maryland resident, only 800-492-8104. During non-working hours, messages are recorded and answered on the following working day.

This document is in the public domain. It may be reproduced in part or in whole by an individual or organization without permission. If it is reproduced, however, the commission would appreciate knowing how it is used. Write to the U.S. Consumer Product Safety commission, Directorate for Communications, Washington, D.C. 20207.

CPSC's Sleepwear Amendment to Help Reduce Burn Injuries to Children

WASHINGTON, D.C. — To reduce burn injuries associated with oversize cotton garments such as T-shirts, sweats and other daywear garments used as sleepwear, CPSC amended the sleepwear standard under the Flammable Fabrics Act. Baggy or loose-fitting cotton or cotton blend garments ignite easily and burn quickly when they contact a flame. Loose-fitting daywear used as sleepwear is associated with 200 to 300 emergency room-treated burn injuries to children annually.

The amendment does not change the existing requirements for loose-fitting garments, which must continue to be flame-resistant. Parents can still choose polyester and other synthetic garments that are inherently flame-resistant. CPSC encourages parents not to put children to bed in loose-fitting cotton garments such as oversize T-shirts, but to choose safe sleepwear alternatives.

The Commission's amendment to the children's sleepwear standard under the Flammable Fabrics Act permits for sale as children's sleepwear:

1. natural fabric garments in sizes nine months or lower because infants who wear these sizes are insufficiently mobile to expose themselves to sources of fire, and

2. tight-fitting natural fabric garments in sizes above nine months because tight-fitting garments are less likely to be ignited and they burn slowly.

This amendment enables consumers who prefer to put their children to bed in cotton garments to choose safer, tight-fitting garments rather than loose-fitting daywear, such as T-shirts and sweats. The tight-fitting sleepwear contacts the skin at all points to protect children from burn injuries. Tight-fitting sleepwear is not easily ignited, and even if it ignites, it burns slowly and may self-extinguish because of a lack of oxygen to support the flame. CPSC has found no burn injuries associated with tight-fitting garments.

Retail stores are starting to carry the new tight-fitting garments in the sleepwear section of the store, along with the traditional flame-resistant sleepwear.

CPSC wants to work with fire fighters, pediatricians, retailers and manufacturers to make parents aware of the importance of putting their children to bed in tight-fitting or flame-resistant sleepwear to keep them safe from burn injuries.

The vote on amending the standard was two to one with Commissioners Thomas Moore and Mary Sheila Gall voting in the majority, and Chairman Ann Brown voting in the minority.

The U.S. Consumer Product Safety Commission protects the public from unreasonable risks of injury or death from 15,000 types of consumer products under the agency's jurisdiction. To report a dangerous product or a product-related injury and for information on CPSC's fax-on-demand service, call CPSC's hotline at (800) 638-2772 or CPSC's teletypewriter at (800) 638-8270. To order a press release through fax-on-demand, call (301) 504-0051 from the handset of your fax machine and enter the release number. Consumers can obtain this release and recall information at CPSC's web site at http://www.cpsc.gov or via Internet gopher services at gopher.cpsc.gov. Consumers can report product hazards to info@cpsc.gov. To establish a link from your web site to this press release on CPSC's web site, create a link to the following address: http://www.cpsc.gov/cpscpub/prerel/prhtml98/98087ml.

Chapter 42

How Safe Is Your Kitchen?

Children Are at Risk

Anyone who is responsible for a child's safety—including parents, grandparents, babysitters and older siblings—must have a basic understanding of the fire and burn risks in the kitchen.

- Keep children at a safe distance from hot liquids. A drink heated to 140 degrees F. can cause a burn in 5 seconds. At 160 degrees F., a burn will occur in 1 second. A child's quick movement could spill hot fluid and cause a serious burn.

- When toddlers are in the home, avoid using a tablecloth. If a child tries to pull himself up by the tablecloth, a heavy object or hot liquid on the table could fall on the child.

- Keep all hot items near the center of the table to prevent a young child from reaching them.

- While cooking, keep young children in a high chair or playpen, at a safe distance from hot surfaces, hot liquids and other kitchen hazards.

- Use extra caution if you use deep fat (oil) cookers/fryers when young children are present. The fat or oil may reach temperatures over 400 degrees F., hot enough to instantly cause a very serious burn.

- Install Ground Fault Circuit Interrupter receptacles near sinks and other wet areas.

- Keep appliance cords away from the edge of counters, and keep them unplugged and disconnected when not in use. A dangling cord is dangerous because it can get caught in a cabinet door or be pulled on by a curious child.

- Always use oven mitts or potholders to remove pots and pans from the stove.

- Keep pot handles turned in so the pots cannot be pulled off or knocked off the stove.

- Store cookies and other foods away from the stove area so no one will be tempted to reach across a hot burner. Store potholders, paper towels, seasonings and other cooking items at a safe distance from the stove.

- Establish a "SAFE AREA" in the kitchen where a child can be placed—away from risk, but under continuous supervision. Also, consider establishing a "NO ZONE" directly in front of the stove. Teach your child to avoid this area. You can mark the zone with yellow tape, a piece of bright carpet or other material.

- Use a fill-through-the-spout teapot to reduce the risk of hot water-associated scald burns. The central handle, the single, small opening, and a "spout whistle" are all safety features.

Adults Are at Risk, Too...

Burn injuries common to children are often observed in adults as well, especially older adults. While the injuries are similar, the cause may differ.

- Turn the pot handle toward the rear of the stove to reduce the risk of scald burns for all age groups.

- Keep clothing from coming into contact with a flame or heating element. Reaching over the stove could cause garments to catch fire, especially the sleeves of robes, dresses, housecoats, etc. Wear snug-fitting or short-sleeved clothing. Pure polyester, nylon and wool are reasonably flame resistant.

- Use an elastic band to hold long or loose sleeves out of the way. Slide the sleeve cuff up to the elbow.

- Turn off the heat or gas before reaching over the stove.

- If your sleeve should catch on fire, immediately cover the burning material with a potholder, mitt or towel, go to the sink and run cold water to put out the fire and cool the burn.

- If other parts of your clothing are on fire, immediately DROP and ROLL to put out the fire. Cool the burn with water.

Chemicals in the Kitchen

- Store all detergents, cleaning agents, bleach and other chemicals out of children's reach or in a locked cabinet.

- Before purchasing any household chemicals, read the contents label and the "caution" statement on the package. Whenever possible, purchase household chemicals that contain less dangerous substances.

Chapter 43

Burns Associated with Microwave Ovens

Information collected over the past two and a half years has indicated that burns associated with use or misuse of the microwave oven are increasing. The scald burn is the most common type of burn and most injuries involve the hands. The age distribution is rather broad, however, there continues to be a large number of young children who sustain the more serious burns. The single most common cause of injury is simply the fact that people do not expect items heated in the microwave oven to present the same risk as items heated by other more conventional means. Many people do not fully appreciate or understand how the microwave oven heats food. The fact that a food container may not be hot may mislead an individual to assume that the food itself is not really hot—thus a burn injury occurs.

As in the case with most burns, microwave oven associated burns are preventable and there are several ways to address the potential risk:

Behavior

- The single most important prevention measure is to read and FOLLOW THE DIRECTIONS. The directions associated with the operation of the microwave oven and the specific directions associated with heating prepared or packaged foods are equally important.

©1988. Shriners Burn Institute. Reprinted with permission.

- Test various foods and quantities of foods to determine what is the best and safest time/energy heating procedure or cycle.

- Stir foods to distribute the heat. Many microwave ovens have a tendency to heat from the outside edge toward the middle. This can produce very hot food on the edge and cold food in the middle.

- Use a pot holder or appropriate utensil to remove lids and coverings from heated containers to prevent steam or contact burns. This is also necessary when removing items which have been heated for extended periods of time—the container may be hot.

- Be sure there is enough moisture distributed in the food to allow proper heating and reduce the risk of "hot spots" or burning the food.

- Before giving any food to a child, test the food to see it ft is at a safe temperature.

- Be sure children are old enough to understand the safe use of the microwave oven before allowing them to heat foods. Children under the age of seven may not be able to read and follow directions and are at a higher injury risk potential than older children. Their height is, also, an important factor.

- In all cases, be sure an individual fully understands how to use the microwave oven before allowing them to heat foods. There are precautions to take before and after heating foods.

- Some manufacturers do NOT recommend that their products be heated in the microwave oven. Follow these recommendations (i.e., baby bottle liners and some baby foods).

- After heating moderate to large quantities of food, let the food and container remain in the microwave to allow vapor pressure to decrease—steam burns are very common when items are opened too quickly.

- Keep children at a safe distance from all hot foods and liquids no matter how the food or liquid was heated.

- Periodically check items which are to be heated for extended periods of time. Fires have developed when some foods were heated longer than necessary.

- Use caution when handling and cutting thick pieces of meat after heating, especially meats with considerable fat. Spattering of hot fat and meat juices may occur.

Environmental Control

- Puncture plastic pouches and plastic wrap covering before heating. This will reduce the risk of a vapor pressure build up and prevent steam burns.

- Put a cut in potato skins or other vegetables to reduce the risk of "bursting" when you cut into it after it is heated.

- Eggs should be removed from the shell before being cooked in the microwave oven. The egg in a shell may explode causing both mechanical and thermal injuries.

- Identity containers, dishes and utensils which are safe for use in the microwave oven. Some items are not "microwave safe" and may become very hot or even burst when heated in the microwave oven.

- When using very smooth vessels for heating liquids, place a plastic spoon in the vessel during the heating process. This will prevent the "super heated" phenomena which may result in liquid spattering and scald burns.

- Some paper products (i.e., paper towels) may have materials present which could cause them to become heated and even catch on fire. Only use appropriate paper products in the microwave oven. Check the product label.

- Check for the presence of metal when reheating some "fast food" items. Aluminum foil, staples in bags, twist-ties, etc. may become very hot and ignite combustible containers.

- Children who are permitted to operate the microwave oven should be tall enough to be able to safely remove items from the oven. One major risk is burns of the face which occur among children whose height puts their face at the level of the heating chamber of the microwave oven.

Design Intervention

- Purchase and use containers and utensils which are specifically designed for microwave cooking.

- Purchase containers with centrally located handles on lids to provide for safe removal after foods have been heated.

- Obtain lids which have "vent openings" to allow steam and pressure to escape. These lids will reduce the risk of steam burns (scald burns).

- Check with the dealer or manufacturer to determine it the microwave oven you choose can be installed where you wish to install it. Proper ventilation and control of moisture exposure may be important considerations for many microwave ovens.

- Purchase only microwave ovens which have a "fail safe" mechanism which will shut off the power when the door is opened or will prevent the door from opening when the oven is operating.

The microwave oven has become an essential appliance in many homes. It's proper and safe use can provide efficiency and convenience which may not be otherwise available in conventional heating appliances. Proper and safe use, however, is directly dependent on the knowledge and understanding of the user. Microwave ovens, as with any appliance, are as safe as the behavior of the user allows.

—by Matt Maley

Department of Risk Management, Shriners Burns Institute, Cincinnati, OH

Chapter 44

Electric Heating Pad Burns

Abstract

Patients with sensory deficits are especially prone to heating pad burns. Two cases are reported of patients with anesthetic skin who received partial and full-thickness burns of their feet from an electric heating pad. These burn injuries could have been prevented if the patients understood the potential hazard of heating pads.

Introduction

Certain populations are at a very high risk of suffering electric heating pad burns, which present a serious and preventable cause of thermal injury. Any patient with reduced sensitivity to heat is considered burn-prone and is especially susceptible to this type of injury (1). Moreover, patients with neurologic sensory deficits often face prolonged hospitalizations (2). It is the purpose of this report to describe two patients with neurologic disease who received significant burns while using a heating pad—one with congenital spina bifida with incomplete cord development and a second with insulin-dependent diabetes mellitus. Because a symptom associated with both spina bifida and diabetes mellitus is chronic pain, this population is predisposed to using a heating pad for therapeutic purposes (3,4). The frequency

©1994 *The Journal of Emergency Medicine*, Vol 12, No 6, pp 819-824, 1994

of these burns can be significantly reduced through prominent warning labels and injury-prevention education by physicians.

Case Report 1

A 32-year-old white female, with diminished sensation in her feet secondary to congenital spina bifida, sustained partial-thickness burns to her feet while using an electric heating pad (The Walker Co., Middleboro, Massachusetts; Model 204) to alleviate chronic foot and leg pain. The heating pad carried no warning label about the potential hazard that heating pads present to patients with anesthetic skin. The heating pad was draped over both feet for a period of 20 min, and the temperature was set on the medium setting. When the patient noticed red blisters on her feet the next morning, she went immediately to the emergency department.

The patient's diminished sensation that contributed to her burns was localized to the L5-S1 dermatomal distribution. She had a blister over the lateral aspect of the right heel and a blister lateral to the fifth metatarsal bone on the same foot. In addition, she had a blister on the left foot just inferior to the lateral malleolus. The patient's initial therapy in the burn center consisted of intravenous antibiotics for cellulitis in addition to hydrotherapy and topical wound care for the burns. Five days after admission to the burn center, the burn wounds failed to heal, requiring surgical debridement and the application of split thickness skin grafts to all three burn sites.

All grafts healed without infection, except the right lateral heel burn. This infection developed beneath the graft over the right lateral malleolus and extended eventually into the bone. At eight months postburn injury, the open wound and a portion of the right calcaneus were debrided. The wound was closed with a right lateral calcaneal artery fasciocutaneous flap, and the donor site was covered with a split-thickness skin graft. Two months later, both the wound and donor site were well healed.

Case Report 2

A 39-year-old white male, with insulin-dependent Type I diabetes, sustained a full-thickness burn over the right lateral malleolus after resting his foot on top of an electric heating pad (Sunbeam/Oster Co., Dallas, Texas; Model #734-8) for an entire night. The patient was attempting to alleviate chronic foot pain. The patient had diminished sensation of his feet in a stocking pattern. The heating pad had a specific warning label, indicating that it should not be used by a person with diabetes. The patient went to the emergency department eight days following the burn injury.

Past medical history included diabetic retinopathy, for which he had undergone multiple laser operations. To control his diabetes, the patient was administering 45-55 Units of NPH insulin each morning. On the day of admission, he underwent excision of the burn wound and split-thickness skin grafting. Six days later, the skin graft had failed to heal. The wound was debrided down to viable bleeding tissue, and a human cadaver allograft was placed on the wound. Two additional grafting procedures were attempted at four weeks and at six weeks postburn injury. The wound eventually healed by contraction after decortication of a necrotic portion of the right lateral malleolus.

Discussion

Electric heating pads are a type of resistance heater. They produce heat by passing an electric current through a series of resistance wires, which are embedded in insulating material. The wire acts as an obstacle, which impedes electrical current and causes it to emit heat. Both of the heating pads reported in this paper had switches for high, medium, and low settings. The maximum heat output of the pads is regulated by these switches, which control the wattage. The temperature is controlled by metal contactors, which open and close the circuit to the heating elements in response to temperature signals from thermostats in the body of the pad.

Since antiquity, patients have recognized the therapeutic value of the application of heat to areas of pain (5). Today, the use of heat for nonacute, painful disorders is commonly prescribed by health care professionals (6,7). The direct application of heat increases local blood flow by vasodilation and enhances the metabolic rate in the underlying tissue. These local factors appear to have a favorable influence on wound repair.

Thermal contact burns from electric heating pads secondary to sensory neuropathy have been previously reported. In 1982, Sandanam (8) described an 8-cm by 5-cm third-degree burn to the posterior aspect of the left arm in a 35-year-old patient with quadriplegia due to a demyelinating disorder. The patient was using the heating pad for therapeutic relief from painful shoulder capsulitis. Sandanam (8) noted that patients were more likely to receive burns from electric heating pads than from other conductive heating devices.

In particular, he warned against lying on top of a heating pad because of the decreased cutaneous blood flow due to the weight of the body, which interferes with temperature equilibration.

Stevenson et al. (9) presented three heating pad burn cases that occurred after flap reconstruction for surgical mastectomies. They found that patients requiring musculocutaneous flaps often have areas of anesthesia and are especially susceptible to burns by heating pads. For those patients who receive relief through heat application, the authors advised the use of a hot water bottle, which should be tested on normal skin prior to use. Formal et al. (10) described the problem of burns following spinal cord lesion. Of the 35 burns studied over a 6-year period, eight patients were burned by environmental heaters or therapeutic heating devices. Furthermore, all burns occurred below the level of the lesion, which implicated sensory deficit as a risk factor. They stressed the importance of injury prevention education for spinal cord injured patients. Katcher and Shapiro (11) reported 37 patients with diabetic peripheral neuropathy who sustained burns. Heating pads were the cause of two of the burn injuries. They also discussed the importance of an improved injury-prevention educational effort.

In 1991, Diller (12) described an elderly, institutionalized patient who sustained an extensive second-degree burn to the back after being left on an electric heating pad at the low power setting for 40 hours. He indicated that thermal injury is a function of both temperature and duration of exposure and demonstrated that, at the lowest power setting, heating pads are capable of producing second-degree thermal burns in 12 hours. Diller (12) recommended using extreme caution when using heating pads, especially where the skin is thin, where there is poor circulation, and when the patient is lying on top of the pad.

Human skin can tolerate temperatures up to 40°C (104°F) for relatively long periods of time before burn injury (13). Temperatures above this level cause a logarithmic increase in tissue damage. The degree of tissue injury can be correlated with both temperature and duration of exposure to the heat source. Consequently, the depth of burning is determined by multiple factors, which include the burning agent, the temperature, and the exposure time. If the temperatures generated by each heating pad were documented and reported, it would provide the physician and patient the opportunity to develop reasonable guidelines regarding recommended exposure times. Patients with sensate skin can safely judge the temperature of the heating pad. When the skin is anesthetic, the patient cannot reliably judge the temperature of the heating pad, which is an invitation to burn injury. Because some patients with anesthetic skin also have vascular ischemia, their skin is less able to dissipate heat than individuals with normal circulation.

Chronic pain in the lower extremities is reported for patients with diabetes mellitus and with spina bifida (3,4). For this reason, these patients would be likely to use a heating pad for therapeutic purposes. Unfortunately, it was not until 1976 that the Food and Drug Administration (FDA) recognized heating pads as a potential hazard for these and other patients with anesthetic skin. At that time, they required the placement of warning labels on these devices. The FDA's recommended label for infrared generators and heating pads states: "*Warning*—Use carefully. May cause serious burns. Do not use over insensitive skin areas or in the presence of poor circulation. The unattended use of infrared heat by children or incapacitated persons may be dangerous" (14). All heating pad models that were designed prior to 1976 were exempt from this regulation. Today, the prevalence of older model heating pads without any warning label contributes to the burn hazard of these devices.

The heating pad that caused the burns in the second case study had a detailed warning label. This is consistent with the safety instructions that Underwriters Laboratories (UL) requires for all of the electric heating pads that they test. This labeling system includes: "burns can occur regardless of control setting," which could have been useful information for the patient in the first case study whose heating pad had no such warning label, and who received her burns in a short duration on the medium setting (15).

In addition to a detailed labeling system, UL requires that all heating pads that they test uphold specific engineering standards and pass rigorous safety tests (15). For example, the insulation and covering are subjected to durability and flammability tests. Electrical components, such as thermostats and switches, are examined closely for sensitivity and reliability. In addition, all pads are required to be moisture resistant to minimize the risk of electrical shock. A durable pilot light must be readily visible to the user when the pad is on, providing an additional safety feature. It is recommended that all heating pads be tested by UL and carry a detailed warning label.

Unfortunately, patients with sensory deficits continue to use heating pads despite the presence of warning labels. The National Electronic Injury Surveillance System Report, which is issued annually by the U.S. Consumer Product Safety Commission, estimated that greater than 1,500 patients were treated in emergency departments in 1992 for electric heating pad burns (16). This high frequency of heating pad burns could be reduced by physician and patient education, UL testing of all heating pads, and comprehensive warning labels. On the basis of our clinical experience, we recommend that heating pads should not be used in patients with anesthetic skin. Because we realize that some patients with anesthetic skin will continue to use heating pads, the emergency physician must remember not to underestimate the severity of burn injuries caused by heating pads.

Conclusion

Two patients with sensory deficits who suffered severe burns due to exposure to a heating pad are reported. Both patients required multiple surgeries and prolonged hospitalizations. The potential burn hazard that heating pads present to patients with anesthetic skin could be prevented by physician and patient education, UL testing of all heating pads, and comprehensive warning labels.

Acknowledgment

This research was supported by a grant from the Texaco Foundation, White Plains, New York.

References

1. MacArthur J, Moore FD. Epidemiology of burns: the burn-prone patient. JAMA. 1975;231:259-63.

2. Brezel BS, Kassenbrock JM, Stein JM. Burns in substance abusers and in neurologically and mentally impaired patients. J Burn Care Rehabil. 1988;9:169-71.

3. Jelsma F, Ploetner EJ. Painful spina bifida occulta: with review of the literature. J Neurosurg. 195 3; 10: 19-27.

4. Ellenberg M. Neuropathy on long-standing insulin-dependent diabetic patients. Kidney Int Suppl. 1974;1:77-85.

5. Tepperman PS, Kekosz V. In: Webster JG, ed. Encyclopedia of medical devices and instrumentation, vol 3. New York: John Wiley & Sons; 1988:1484.

6. Delisa JA. Practical use of therapeutic physical modalities. Am Fam Physician. 1983;27(5):129-38.

7. Nanneman D. Thermal modalities: heat and cold; a review of physiologic effects with clinical applications. AAOHN J. 1991;39:70-5.

8. Sandanam J. Burns caused by heating pads. Med J Aust. 1982; 1:369.

9. Stevenson TR, Hammond DC, Keip D, Argenta LC. Heating pad burns in anesthetic skin. Ann Plast Surg. 1985;15:73-5.

10. Formal C, Goodman C, Jacobs B, McMonigle D. Burns after spinal cord injury. Arch Phys Med Rehabil. 1989;70:380-1.

11. Katcher ML, Shapiro MM. Lower extremity bums related to sensory loss in diabetes mellitus. J Fam Pract. 1987;24(2):149-5 1.

12. Diller KR. Analysis of burns caused by long-term exposure to a heating pad. J Burn Care Rehabil. 199 1; 12:214-7.

13. Robson MC, Kucan JO. The burn wound. Topics Emerg Med. 1981;3(3):59-67.

14. Code of Federal Regulations, vol 21, subpart H; April 1, 1992: 801.403.

15. UL 130 standards for safety: electric heating pads, 10th ed. Northbrook, Illinois: Underwriters Laboratories; revision May 12, 1993:33-4.

16. Product summary report. The National Electronic Injury Surveillance System. Washington, DC: U.S. Consumer Product Safety Commission-National Injury Information Clearinghouse, 1992.

by — Timothy J. Bill, BA,
Richard F. Edlich, M D, PhD,
and Harvey N. Himel, MD.

Department of Plastic Surgery and the DeCamp Burn Center, University of Virginia School of Medicine, Charlottesville, Virginia.

Chapter 45

Fireworks:
Playing with Fire—Safely

The American traditions of parades, cookouts, and fireworks help us celebrate the summer season especially our nation's birthday on the Fourth of July. However, fireworks can turn a joyful holiday into a painful memory when children and adults are injured while incorrectly using fireworks. Although most fireworks can be relatively safe with proper and careful usage, some fireworks, such as illegal fireworks, present substantial risks that can result in deaths, blindings, amputations, and severe burns.

- A 7-year-old boy lost half of his left hand including the fingers when he ignited an M-80 he found hidden in a family bedroom. The M-80 exploded in the boy's hand.

- An 8-year-old boy lost 3 fingers after igniting an M-80 on a kitchen stove. The victim was trying to exit his home when the device exploded in his hand.

- An 8-year-old girl received second and third degree burns to her leg when a spark from a sparkler she was holding ignited her dress.

To help prevent accidents like these, the federal government, under the Federal Hazardous Substances Act, prohibits the sale of the

U.S. CONSUMER PRODUCT SAFETY COMMISSION, Washington, D.C. 20207. FIREWORKS: Publication #12.

most dangerous types of fireworks to consumers. These banned fireworks include large reloadable shells, cherry bombs, aerial bombs, M-80 salutes and larger firecrackers containing more than two grains of powder. Also banned are mail-order kits designed to build the fireworks.

In a regulation that went into effect December 6, 1976, the U.S. Consumer Product Safety Commission lowered the permissible charge in firecrackers to no more than 50 milligrams of powder. In addition, the recently amended regulation provides performance specifications for fireworks other than firecrackers intended for consumer's use, including a requirement that fuses burn at lease 3 seconds, but no longer than 9 seconds. All fireworks must carry a warning label describing necessary safety precautions and instructions for safe use.

The Commission recently issued a new performance requirement to reduce the risk of potentially dangerous tip-over large multiple tube mine and shell devices. Tip-over of these devices has resulted in two fatalities. The new requirement went into effect on March 26, 1997.

The U.S. Consumer Product Safety Commission estimates that in 1996 about 7,600 people were treated in hospital emergency rooms for injuries associated with fireworks. Approximately 40 percent of the injuries were burns, and most of the injuries involved the hands, eyes and head. One-third of the victims were under 15 years of age.

Fireworks should be used only with extreme caution. Older children should be closely supervised, and younger children should not be allowed to play with fireworks.

Before using fireworks, make sure they are permitted in your state or local area. Many state and local governments prohibit or limit consumer fireworks, formerly known as class C fireworks, which are common fireworks and firecrackers sold for consumer use. Consumer fireworks include shells and mortars, multiple tube devices, Roman Candles, rockets, sparklers, firecrackers with no more than 50 milligrams of powder and novelty items such as snakes and airplanes.

The following is a summary of state regulations as of May 1, 1995.

- STATES THAT ALLOW SOME OR ALL TYPES OF CONSUMER FIREWORKS (formerly known as class C fireworks), APPROVED BY ENFORCING AUTHORITY, OR AS SPECIFIED IN LAW (32 states plus the District of Columbia): Alaska, Arkansas, Alabama, California, Colorado, District of Columbia, Florida, Idaho, Indiana, Kansas, Kentucky, Louisiana, Michigan, Mississippi, Missouri, Montana, Nebraska, New Hampshire, New Mexico, North Carolina, Oklahoma, Oregon, South Carolina, South Dakota, Tennessee, Texas, Utah, Virginia,

Washington, West Virginia, Wisconsin, Wyoming, (The above states enforce the federal regulations and applicable state restrictions).

- STATES HAVING NO FIREWORKS LAWS EXCEPT AT COUNTY LEVEL: Hawaii, Nevada (CPSC regulations are still applicable for these states).

- STATES THAT ALLOW ONLY SPARKLERS AND/OR OTHER NOVELTIES (total of 6 states): Illinois, Iowa, Maryland, Maine, Ohio, Pennsylvania

- STATES THAT BAN ALL CONSUMER FIREWORKS (including those which are allowed by CPSC regulations) (total 10 states): Arizona, Connecticut, Delaware, Georgia, Massachusetts, Minnesota, New Jersey, New York, Rhode Island, Vermont

To help consumers use fireworks more safely, the U.S. Consumer Product Safety Commission offers these recommendations:

- Do not allow young children to play with fireworks under any circumstances. Sparklers, considered by many the ideal "safe" firework for the young, burn at very high temperatures and can easily ignite clothing. Children cannot understand the danger involved and cannot act appropriately in case of emergency.

- Older children should only be permitted to use fireworks under close adult supervision. Do not allow any running or horseplay.

- Light fireworks outdoors in a clear area away from houses, dry leaves or grass and flammable materials.

- Keep a bucket of water nearby for emergencies and for pouring on fireworks that don't go off.

- Do not try to relight or handle malfunctioning fireworks. Douse and soak them with water and throw them away.

- Be sure other people are out of range before lighting fireworks.

- Never ignite fireworks in a container, especially a glass or metal container.

- Keep unused fireworks away from firing areas.

- Store fireworks in a dry, cool place. Check instructions for special storage directions.

- Parents should supervise the ordering and use of mail-order "make your own" firework kits.

To report a dangerous product or a product related injury and for information on CPSC's fax-on-demand service, call CPSC's hotline at 800-638-2772 or CPSC's teletypewriter at 800-638-8270. To order a press release through fax-on-demand, call 301-504-0051 from the handset of your fax machine and enter the release number. Consumers can obtain releases and recall information at CPSC's web site at www.cpsc.gov or via Internet gopher services at cpsc.gov. Consumers can report product safety hazards to info@cpsc.gov.

Chapter 46

Seven Steps to Safer Sunning

Put away the baby oil. Toss out that old metal sun reflector. Cancel your next appointment to the local tanning salon.

These are new days with new ways of sunning, and the practices that traditionally have gone into obtaining the so-called "healthy tanned" look are on the verge of fading into history.

In their place: safer sun practices that preserve people's natural skin color and condition.

That's what health experts are hoping for as the evidence against exposure to the sun and sunlamps continues to mount. Both emit harmful ultraviolet (UV) radiation that in the short term can cause painful sunburn and in the long term may lead to unsightly skin blemishes, premature aging of the skin, cataracts and other eye problems, skin cancer, and a weakened immune system.

The problems may become more prevalent, too, if, as some scientists predict, the Earth's ozone layer continues to be depleted. According to the Environmental Protection Agency, scientists began accumulating evidence in the 1980s that the ozone layer—a thin shield in the stratosphere that protects life from UV radiation—is being depleted by certain chemicals used on Earth. According to the most recent estimates from the National Aeronautics and Space Administration, the ozone layer is being depleted at a rate of 4 to 6 percent

FDA Consumer, Publication No. (FDA) 97-1252 This article originally appeared in the June 1996 *FDA Consumer*. The version below is from a reprint of the original article and contains revisions made in February 1997.

each decade. This means additional UV radiation reaching Earth's surface—and our bodies.

Although people with light skin are more susceptible to sun damage, darker skinned people, including African Americans and Hispanic Americans, also can be affected.

You may have already started to take precautions. But are you doing all you can?

The following recommendations come from various expert organizations, including the American Academy of Dermatology, American Cancer Society, American Academy of Ophthalmology, Skin Cancer Foundation, American Academy of Pediatrics, National Cancer Institute, National Weather Service, and Food and Drug Administration. FDA regulates many items related to sun safety, including sunscreens and sunblocks, sunglasses, and sun-protective clothing that makes medical claims. The agency also sets performance standards for sunlamps.

Here are seven steps to safer sunning:

1. **Avoid the sun.**

This is especially important between 10 a.m. and 3 p.m., when the sun's rays are strongest. Also avoid the sun when the UV Index is high in your area.

The UV Index is a number from 0 to 10+ that indicates the amount of UV radiation reaching the Earth's surface during the hour around noon. The higher the number, the greater your exposure to UV radiation if you go outdoors. The National Weather Service forecasts the UV Index daily in 58 U.S. cities, based on local predicted conditions. The index covers about a 30-mile radius from each city. Check the local newspaper or TV and radio news broadcasts to learn the UV Index in your area. It also may be available through your local phone company and is available on the Internet at the National Weather Service Climate Prediction Center's home page.

Don't be fooled by cloudy skies. Clouds block only as much as 20 percent of UV radiation. UV radiation also can pass through water, so don't assume you're safe from UV radiation if you're in the water and feeling cool. Also, be especially careful on the beach and in the snow because sand and snow reflect sunlight and increase the amount of UV radiation you receive.

People with darker skin will resist the sun's rays by tanning, which is actually an indication that the skin has been injured. Tanning occurs when ultraviolet radiation is absorbed by the skin, causing an increase in the activity and number of melanocytes, the cells that produce the pigment melanin. Melanin helps to block out damaging rays up to a point.

Those with lighter skin are more likely to burn. Too much sun exposure in a short period results in sunburn. A sunburn causes skin redness, tenderness, pain, swelling, and blistering. Although there is no quick cure, the American Academy of Dermatology recommends using wet compresses, cool baths, bland moisturizers, and over-the-counter hydrocortisone creams.

Sunburn becomes a more serious problem with fever, chills, upset stomach, and confusion. If these symptoms develop, see a doctor.

2. **Use sunscreen.**

With labels stating "sunscreen" or "sunblock," these lotions, creams, ointments, gels, or wax sticks, when applied to the skin, absorb, reflect or scatter some or all of the sun's rays.

Some sunscreen products, labeled "broad-spectrum," protect against two types of radiation: UVA and UVB. Scientists now believe that both UVA and UVB can damage the skin and lead to skin cancer.

Other products protect only against UVB, previously thought to be the only damaging type.

Some cosmetics, such as some lipsticks, also are considered sunscreen products if they contain sunscreen and their labels state they do.

Sunblock products block a large percentage of UV radiation.

FDA requires the labels of all sunscreen and sunblock products to state the product's sun protection factor, or "SPF," from 2 on up. The higher the number, the longer a person can stay in the sun before burning. In a 1993 tentative final monograph, FDA suggested 30 as the upper SPF limit because it was felt that anything above this offers little additional benefit and might expose people to dangerous levels of chemicals.

FDA also advised manufacturers that "water-resistant" or "sweat-resistant" products must list an SPF for both before and after being exposed to water or sweat. FDA also proposed that products claiming to be sunblocks have an SPF of at least 12 and contain titanium dioxide, the only opaque agent that blocks light. Also, any tanning product that doesn't contain a sunscreen would have to state on the label that the product does not contain a sunscreen, according to the tentative final monograph.

533

Manufacturers may already be following these recommendations.

Experts recommend broad-spectrum products with SPFs of at least 15. They also suggest applying the product liberally—about 30 milliliters (1 ounce) per application for the average-size person, according to The Skin Cancer Foundation—15 to 30 minutes every time before going outdoors. It should be applied evenly on all exposed skin, including lips, nose, ears, neck, scalp (if hair is thinning), hands, feet, and eyelids, although care should be taken not to get it in the eyes because it can irritate them. If contact occurs, rinse eyes thoroughly with water.

Sunscreens should not be used on babies younger than 6 months because their bodies may not be developed enough to handle sunscreen chemicals. Instead, use hats, clothing and shading to protect small babies from the sun. If you think your baby may need a sunscreen, check with your pediatrician.

For children 6 months to 2 years, use a sunscreen with at least an SPF of 4, although 15 or higher is best.

Use sunscreen products regularly on children, advises Stephen Katz, M.D., Ph.D., director of the National Institute of Arthritis and Musculoskeletal and Skin Diseases and chief of the National Cancer Institute's dermatology branch. "Get them used to it, so they can use it regularly like toothpaste," Katz says.

3. Wear a hat.

A hat with at least a 3-inch brim all around is ideal because it can protect areas often exposed to the sun, such as the neck, ears, eyes, and scalp. A shade cap (which looks like a baseball cap with about 7 inches of material draping down the sides and back) also is good. These are often sold in sports and outdoor clothing and supply stores.

A baseball cap or visor provides only limited protection but is better than nothing.

4. Wear sunglasses.

Sunglasses can help protect your eyes from sun damage.

The ideal sunglasses don't have to be expensive, but they should block 99 to 100 percent of UVA and UVB radiation. Check the label to see that they do. If there's no label, don't buy the glasses. And, don't go by how dark the glasses are because UV protection comes from an invisible chemical applied to the lenses, not from the color or darkness of the lenses.

Large-framed wraparound sunglasses are best because they can protect your eyes from all angles.

Children should wear sunglasses, too, starting as young as 1, advises Gerhard Cibis, a pediatric ophthalmologist in Kansas City, Mo. They need smaller versions of real, protective adult sunglasses—not toy sunglasses. Kids' sunglasses are available at many optical stores, Cibis says.

Ideally, says the American Academy of Ophthalmology, all types of eyewear, including prescription glasses, contact lenses, and intraocular lens implants used in cataract surgery, should absorb the entire UV spectrum.

You may want to put sunscreen on the eyelids and around the eyes, too, even if you're wearing sunglasses. According to Cibis, sunglasses prevent UV rays from getting into the eyes; they won't help protect the skin around them.

5. **Cover up.**

Wear lightweight, loose-fitting, long-sleeved shirts, pants or long skirts as much as possible when in the sun. Most materials and colors absorb or reflect UV rays. Tightly weaved cloth is best.

Avoid wearing wet clothes, such as a wet T-shirt, because when clothes get wet, the sun's rays can more easily pass through. If you see light through a fabric, UV rays can get through, too.

FDA's policy is that so-called "sun-protective" clothing will be regulated by the agency only if the clothing's label makes a medical claim, such as that it prevents skin cancer. As of early 1997, FDA had not approved any clothing for medical uses.

6. **Avoid artificial tanning.**

Many people believe that the UV rays of tanning beds are harmless because sunlamps in tanning beds emit primarily UVA and little, if any, UVB, the rays once thought to be the most hazardous. However, UVA can cause serious skin damage, too. According to some scientists, UVA may be linked to the most serious form of skin cancer, melanoma. A 1996 unpublished risk analysis by FDA scientists Sharon Miller, Scott Hamilton and Howard Cyr, Ph.D., concluded that people who use sunlamps about 100 times a year may be increasing their exposure to "melanoma-inducing" radiation by up to 24 times compared with the amount they would receive from the sun. This would depend on the type of sunlamp used and whether sunscreen is used regularly. The authors note that home users are a major concern because they may use their sunlamps as often as every day. But, Miller said, "This analysis was based on data from a non-mammalian animal model and the assumption that cumulative UV exposure—not just exposure that resulted in sunburns—contributes to the development of melanoma. The dose-response behavior of melanoma is not well understood, so our results must be regarded with caution."

Because of sunlamps' dangers, health experts advise people to avoid them for tanning.

Sunlamps remain on the market because, according to George Jan, Ph.D., a physicist in FDA's Center for Devices and Radiological Health, they represent an alternative to the sun, and unlike the sun, can be regulated to promote greater safety.

Under FDA regulations, sunlamp products must:

- have a timer to limit the amount of exposure a person can receive in one session

- have a label with recommended exposure position or distance from the sunlamp to reduce the risk of overexposure, even when the timer is set at its maximum limit

- limit the amount of short-wave UV radiation emitted from the product

- come with UV-blocking goggles, which the user should always wear

- carry a prominent warning about the dangers of overexposure, especially to those who are sensitive to UV radiation

- provide information on proper use.

Several products that claim to give a tan without UV radiation carry safety risks, too. These include so-called "tanning pills" containing carotenoid color additives derived from substances similar to beta-carotene, which gives carrots their orange color. The additives are distributed throughout the body, especially in skin, making it orange. Although FDA has approved some of these additives for coloring food, it has not approved them for use in tanning agents. And, at the high levels that are consumed in tanning pills, they may be harmful. According to John Bailey, Ph.D., acting director of FDA's Office of Cosmetics and Colors, the main ingredient in tanning pills, canthaxanthin, can deposit in the eyes as crystals, which may cause injury and impaired vision. There also has been one reported case of a woman who died from aplastic anemia, which her doctor attributed to her use of tanning pills.

Tanning accelerators, such as those formulated with the amino acid tyrosine or tyrosine derivatives, are ineffective and also may be dangerous. Marketers promote these products as substances that stimulate the body's own tanning process, although the evidence suggests they don't work, Bailey says. FDA considers them unapproved new drugs that have not been proved safe and effective.

Two other tanning products, bronzers and extenders, are considered cosmetics for external use. Bronzers, made from color additives approved by FDA for cosmetic use, stain the skin when applied and can be washed off with soap and water. Extenders, when applied to the skin, interact with protein on the surface of the skin to produce color. The color tends to wear off after a few days. The only color additive approved for extenders is dihydroxyacetone.

Although they give skin a golden color, these products do not offer sunscreen protection. Also, the chemicals in bronzers may react differently on various areas of your body, producing a tan of many shades.

7. **Check skin regularly.**

You can improve your chances of finding precancerous skin conditions, such as actinic keratosis—a dry, scaly, reddish, and slightly raised lesion—and skin cancer by performing simple skin self-exams regularly. The earlier you identify signs and see a doctor, the greater the chances for successful treatment.

The best time to do skin exams is after a shower or bath. Get used to your birthmarks, moles and blemishes so that you know what they usually look like and then can easily identify any changes they undergo. Signs to look for are changes in size, texture, shape, and color of blemishes or a sore that does not heal.

If you find any changes, see your doctor. Also, during regular checkups, ask your doctor to check your skin.

The more of these practices you can incorporate into your life, the greater your chances of reducing the damage sun can cause. And by teaching these same practices to your children, you can help them get off to a lifetime of safer sun practices.

Who's Most at Risk?

Take extra care to protect babies and children from the sun. Studies show that one or more severe, blistering sunburns as a child or teenager could increase the risk for melanoma, an often fatal form of skin cancer.

You need to be especially careful to play it safe in the sun if you:

• have fair skin; blond, red, or light brown hair; and blue green, or gray eyes

• have freckles and burn before tanning

• spend a lot of time outdoors

• were previously treated for skin cancer

• have a family history of skin cancer, especially melanoma

• work indoors all week and then try to catch up on your tan on weekends

• live or vacation at high altitudes (ultraviolet radiation from the sun increases 4 to 5 percent for every 1,000 feet above sea level)

• live or vacation close to the equator

• have certain diseases, such as lupus erythematosus

• take certain medicines, including:

• acne medicines
  — antibiotics, such as tetracyclines
  — antihistamines
  — oral contraceptives containing estrogen
  — nonsteroidal anti-inflammatory drugs, such as naproxen sodium
  — phenothiazines (major tranquilizers and anti-nausea drugs)
  — sulfa drugs
  — tricyclic antidepressants
  — thiazide diuretics
  — sulfonylureas, such as oral anti-diabetics.

Ask your doctor about the risk of any medicines you may be taking that could be harmful to you when you are in the sun. (See "Chemical Photosensitivity: Another Reason to Be Careful in the Sun" in the May 1996 *FDA Consumer,* reprinted as chapter 14 of this sourcebook.)

Which Sunscreen Product for You?

Sunburn and Tanning History	Recommended SPF (Sun Protection Factor)
Always burns easily; rarely tans	20 to 30
Always burns easily; tans minimally	12 to under 20
Burns moderately; tans gradually	8 to under 12
Burns minimally; always tans well	4 to under 8
Rarely burns, tans profusely	2 to under 4

Monthly Skin Self-examination

1. Examine your body, front and back, in the mirror, then the right and left sides with arms raised.

2. Examine back of neck and scalp with the help of a hand mirror—part hair or use blow dryer to lift hair and give you a close look.

3. Check back and buttocks with hand mirror.

4. Bend elbows and look carefully at forearms, upper underarms, and palms.

5. Look at backs of the legs and feet, including the soles and spaces between toes.

—by Paula Kurtzweil

Paula Kurtzweil is a member of FDA's public affairs staff.

Part Six

Emergency Procedures and First Aid

Chapter 47

Burn Care at the Fire Scene

New York City firefighters save countless lives every year, but we're always looking to make the number of lives lost smaller. In 1988, according to the FDNY annual report, 147 lives were lost to burns or a combination of burns and smoke inhalation. As firefighters, we're in a position to render immediate care to burn victims, so reviewing some basic guidelines will help us help others.

Burns are classified by how deeply they penetrate the epidermis (the outer layer of skin), the dermis (the inner layer of skin), and subcutaneous (beneath-the skin) tissue. (See figures 1-3.)

In almost all cases, firefighters will have time to provide only preliminary care before the Emergency Medical Service arrives. Based on the degree and size of the burn, one of the following will apply:

- For small-area first-or second-degree burns (generally less than 5 percent of the skin surface), immerse the burned area in cold water for 2 to 5 minutes. This should be no problem at the fire scene, since a hoseline or open discharge outlet can provide us with as much water as we need. After cooling the burn, cover it with a dry, sterile dressing to help prevent infection. After applying the dressing, continue to keep the area cool and wet, to prevent the heat of the burned area from causing additional damage.

- For large-area first-or second-degree burns and all third-degree burns, again cool the site and wrap it in a dry, sterile dressing.

©1989 WNYF. Reprinted with Permission. Although somewhat old, this article contains useful and current information on emergency burn first aid.

Figure 47.1. *lst DEGREE—RED AND SWOLLEN*

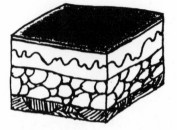

Penetration: Superficial-epidermis only

Pain: Some

Scarring: None

After dressing: Keep dry if burn is large, wet if it's small

Figure 47.2. *2nd DEGREE—EXTREMELY RED; BLISTERED AND SPOTTED*

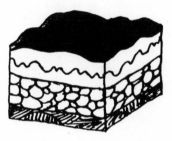

Penetration: Epidermis burned through; dermis partially destroyed

Pain: Severe

Scarring: None if the burn is properly treated

After dressing: Keep dry if burn is large, wet if it's small

Figure 47.3. *3rd DEGREE—CHARRED BLACK, OR DRY AND WHITE*

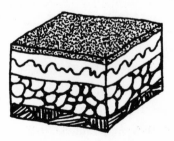

Penetration: Through both layers of skin

Pain: None, because the nerves are destroyed. Any pain is from accompanying 2nd-or 3rd-degree burns

Scarring: Heavy

After dressing: Keep dry

Then keep the area dry. This is necessary because burn victims tend to lose body heat and may suffer hypothermia.

Several situations might arise that require special instructions, regardless of the degree of burn:

- If fingers or toes have been burned, place folded or rolled gauze pads between the fingers or toes and wet with cold water. This is to prevent the burned digits from adhering to each other.

- If the eyelids have been burned, leave them closed. Place sterile pads over both eyes and wet them with cold water (sterile, if possible).

- When the burn has been caused by a semi-solid such as grease, tar, or wax, don't attempt to remove the substance. Doing so may tear skin from the burned area, or it may spread the hot substance and inflict even more burns. Apply cold water to the site to cool the substance and the burn, but don't cover the burn after cooling.

All burn victims should be treated for shock. This consists of checking their breathing, controlling bleeding, administering oxygen, maintaining body heat (without overheating), and slightly elevating the legs (only if there are no serious leg or chest injuries).

Only in rare instances will the Fire Department have to transport a burn victim to the hospital, and then only when the burns are life-threatening. These are the burns that emergency care texts classify as critical (life-threatening):

- Any burn that's accompanied by respiratory tract injuries, fractured bones, or subcutaneous tissue damage.

- Any second-or third-degree burn of the face, hands, feet, groin, or major joints. These areas are important because of the way burns heal; the skin will contract, which can limit motion.

- Third-degree burns affecting more than 10 percent of the total skin surface (but not located on the face, hands, feet, groin, or major joints).

- Second-degree burns affecting more than 30 percent of the total skin surface (but not located on the face, hands, feet, groin, or major joints).

- First-degree burns affecting more than 75 percent of the total skin surface.

"The Rule of Nines" is a quick way to assess the percentage of skin area involved. (See the figure 47.4.) For adults, it divides the body into 11 equivalent areas, each representing 9 percent of the skin surface, for a total of 99 percent. The groin accounts for the remaining 1 percent. Infants' and children's proportions are different from those of adults and therefore are assigned different percentages.

When the Fire Department does have to transport a burn victim, the unit should relay all the information it has about the victim to the hospital. This will help the medical staff prepare the proper medications and rooms for treatment.

Regardless of whether the Fire Department transports a patient, our knowledge of burn care will bring relief to the victim and help us serve the people of New York in the most important way possible: saving lives.

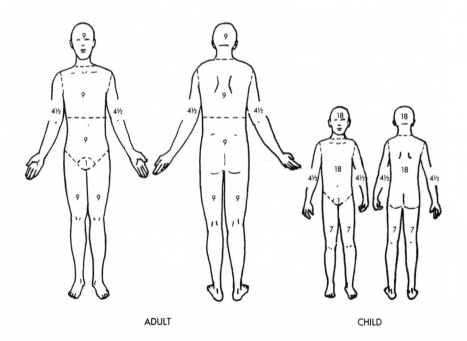

ADULT   CHILD

Figure 47.4. *The Rule of Nines for Field Use*

The information in this chapter is based on the following sources:

Emergency Care, 4th Edition, by Harvey D. Grant, Robert H. Murray, Jr., and J. David Bergeron (Prentice Hall Inc.: Englewood Cliffs, NJ, 1986)

City Wide Drill #12, "Basic First Aid"

Medical Surgical Nursing, by Wilma J. Phipps, R.N., Barbara C. Long, R.N., and Nancy Woods, R.N. (C.V. Mosby Co.: St. Louis, 1979)

Barbara Roth, R.N., head nurse, Burn Center at New York Hospital-Cornell Medical Center.

—by John Salka, EMT Lieutenant, Ladder Co. 18.

Chapter 48

Industrial Burns Don't Play Favorites: Burn Emergency Strategies

Do your employees know what to do in a burn emergency?

Burns are an equal-opportunity hazard. They happen in all industries. A recent survey of 23 states ranked retail trade, which includes restaurants and other food-related endeavors, at the top of the list for number of heat burns. It was followed by manufacturing; services, such as laundry and dry-cleaning plants, and automotive repair shops; and construction, which includes welding, roofing and plumbing.

Thermal burns, caused by contact with flames, a hot object or a hot liquid, are common in restaurants and other parts of the food industry (from water, grease, oil or steam), in the roofing industry (usually from melted tar), in factories (often from plastics and other molten materials), and in dry-cleaning establishments (from steam and hot equipment). Burns from fires, although especially hazardous for fire fighters, can affect any worker who comes near flames. And welders often experience burns of the eye from radiation exposure.

Chemical burns commonly occur in laboratories, coal mines, tanneries, automotive repair shops and any other of the thousands of industries that use chemicals to manufacture products or perform services.

Electrical burns occur in plants of all kinds, in hospitals and even on farms.

©1992 *Safety and Health*. September 1992. Reprinted with permission.

Dr. Charles Drueck, trauma-unit director at Evanston (Ill.) Hospital, has seen his share of industrial burns. The following are just a few:

• A dry-cleaning-plant worker caught his hand in a mangle with a defective release mechanism and suffered a critical burn that penetrated all the way to his tendons.

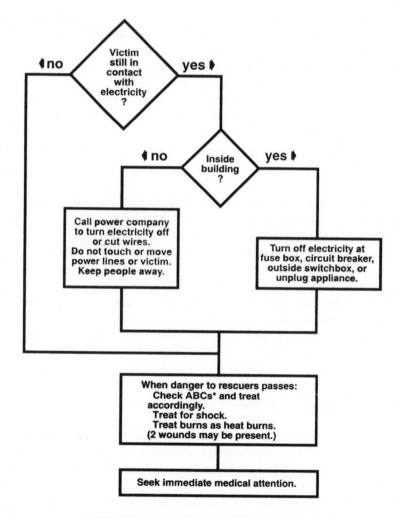

*ABC=Airway, Breathing and Circulation

Figure 48.1. *Electrical Injuries*

- A restaurant cook suffered a seizure as he loaded potato strips into a french fryer and plunged both his hands into the hot grease.

- A glass etcher donned a pair of protective gloves before he dipped a pane into a solution of hydrochloric acid. The acid leaked through a small hole in the glove, and the worker suffered a chemical burn on his hand.

All of these burns, and others like them, are preventable, says Drueck. Keep machinery in proper working order. Consider a worker's medical problems in job placement. Check protective clothing for defects and replace pieces regularly.

Although no concrete figures are available for the number of companies that offer burn prevention or first-aid programs, many industries do attempt to prevent accidents. For example, the National Restaurant Association, in Washington, D.C., offers all restaurant owners a manual that includes material on burn prevention and treatment. And Jim Brown, director of public health and safety for the association, reports that most major restaurant chains establish their own safety practices to protect employees against burns.

But research shows that burns occur on the job even when workers take preventive measures. An OSHA study of industrial burns in 1985 found that most of those injured wore some type of protective gear at the time of their accident, but that the burn area was not covered by the clothing.

Peggy Gutman, director of occupational health services at Grant Hospital in Chicago, manages a group of nurses who are contracted by industry. She believes that workers who get burned while wearing protective clothing either do not wear the clothing correctly or don't wear correct clothing. Data collected by the U.S. Bureau of Statistics support her belief.

Quick Action Is Essential

Since industrial burns do occur, even when preventive steps are taken, it is important to remember that first-aid measures, immediately applied, can lessen the impact of burns. But before you administer first aid to a burn victim, you must determine the injury's severity. How deep is the burn? How large an area of the body is burned? Where on the body is the burn?

Burns are classified as superficial, partial-thickness and full-thickness wounds depending on how deep the burn penetrates the victim's

551

body. Trauma medic Drueck says, "I still like to refer to burns as first, second and third degree, but superficial, partial and full thickness are more descriptive if you think of the layers of skin and how a burn progresses through them."

Superficial burns are first-degree burns. First-degree burns, which include sunburn, affect the epidermis or outer layer of the skin. They usually cause minor pain, mild swelling and redness of the skin. Drueck says that first-degree burns tend to peel and heal themselves in about five days. They seldom require the attention of a physician.

Partial-thickness, or second-degree burns, damage the epidermis and the dermis, the secondary layer of the skin. These burns produce blisters, usually quite painful to touch, air or liquid and are prone to infection. Drueck divides them into superficial (healing in seven to 10 days) and deep (taking up to three weeks to heal). Second-degree burns often call for medical treatment.

Full-thickness wounds, or third-degree burns, destroy the dermis and epidermis and extend into the subcutaneous fat, muscle and bone. The burned area of skin may appear charred or whitish; its texture usually is dry and hard. Often the patient feels no pain, because his or her nerve endings have been destroyed. Third-degree burns always require medical attention. Most will need skin grafts to heal.

In general, a burn is considered more critical if it affects a larger area of the body. For instance, a second-degree burn that affects 15 percent of an adult's body is considered a minor burn. If that same burn involves up to 25 percent of the body, the burn is upgraded to moderate. And if it covers more than 25 percent of the body, it becomes critical. (See "The Rule of Nines" and Burn Severity Table 48.1 and Figure 48.4.)

Dr. Cathryn Pajak, also associated with Chicago's Grant Hospital as medical director of occupational health services, notes that burns of the hands, feet and genitals always call for medical attention in a hospital. Even more critical are burns to the face or eyes. "All companies that work with chemicals should have eye-wash fountains available," says Pajak. "if an eye burn occurs, the victim's eye should be washed for 15 to 20 minutes before being taken to a medical facility where more specialized equipment is available."

First, Stop the Burning

You have several objectives when you apply first aid:

1. relieve pain,

2.   prevent infection,
3.   prevent or treat for shock,
4.   soothe the patient and
5.   call for help.

First and foremost, Drueck emphasizes, "You must stop the burning process. Put out the fire. Pull the victim away from the flame or the hot liquid. If clothes are burning, have the victim drop and roll, or wrap him or her in a blanket."

Remove any smoldering clothing or clothing that's been contaminated by a burning chemical, or soak it with water. Don't try to remove clothing that is stuck to the skin—cut it away or let it alone. Also, remove all jewelry, such as rings. They retain heat and are hard to remove if body parts swell.

If it's an electrical burn, turn off the power before you offer assistance. Use a blanket or protective clothing before touching the person, so that you don't become a second victim. In any burn accident, you must be careful not to become a victim too.

Next, treat any bleeding and check the victim's vital signs. If breathing has stopped, you may have to administer rescue breathing or CPR before you proceed. Specific steps for treating thermal burns are as follows. Chemical and electrical burns require somewhat different treatment.

First-degree burns. Hold the burned area under cold running water, submerge it in comfortably cold water or apply a cold-water compress until the pain decreases. Cover the burned area with a sterile, clean bandage. Give the victim aspirin to help alleviate pain.

Second-degree burns. Put the burned area in cool (no ice) water until the pain eases. Many experts advise tepid water since cold water may actually aggravate the patient's condition by causing hypothermia (shock).

Gently blot the area dry with a clean cloth. Cover with a dry, clean protective bandage to prevent infection. Do not place a wet dressing over a burn, since it dries out quickly and sticks to the burn. Also, wet dressings can induce hypothermia.

If the arms or legs are burned, elevate them to prevent swelling. Call a doctor.

Do not try to break blisters, since that might cause infection. And do not use antiseptic preparations.

Third-degree burns. Check immediately to see that the victim is breathing. Give rescue breathing or CPR if necessary. Elevate the victim's legs eight to 12 inches to keep warm and treat for shock.

Cover the burned area with sterile dressings or clean cloths. Elevate burned arms and legs to reduce swelling and pain. Call a doctor.

Do not apply cold compresses or water to a third-degree burn. It may induce hypothermia.

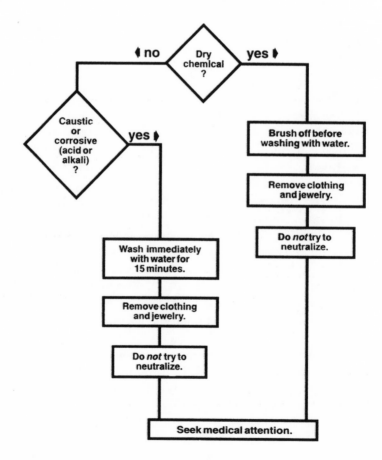

Figure 48.2. Chemical Burns

Use Water for Chemical Burns

"With most chemical burns, you must wash the chemical off the body as quickly as possible," says Drueck. "Don't look for a neutralizing agent, just get the victim under the nearest shower, hose or other water source. And take off all contaminated clothing and jewelry while you are washing away the chemical."

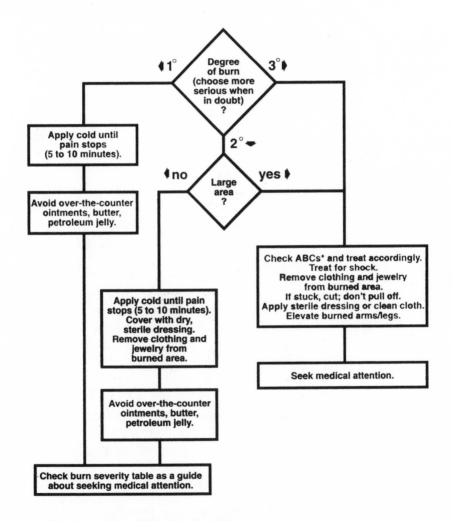

*ABC=Airway, Breathing and Circulation

Figure 48.3. *Heat Burns*

Table 48.1. Burn Severity

Burn classification	Characteristics	Burn Surface Area (BSA)
Minor burn	first-degree burn	
	second-degree burn	15 percent BSA in adults
	second-degree burn	<5 percent BSA in children/elderly persons
	third-degree burn	<2 percent BSA
Moderate burn	second-degree burn	15 percent-25 percent BSA in adults
	second-degree burn	10 percent-20 percent BSA in children/elderly persons
	third-degree burn	<10 percent BSA
Critical burn	second-degree burn	>25 percent BSA in adults
	second-degree burn	>20 percent BSA in children/elderly person
	third-degree burn	>10 percent BSA Burns of hands, face, eyes, feet or perineum. Most victims with inhalation injury, electrical injury, major trauma or pre-existing diseases.

If the chemical is a dry one, however, Drueck emphasizes that you must, "brush the powder off the clothing or body part before flushing with water, even though the chemical may not seem like it's burning. Sometimes water will activate a dry chemical."

In all cases of chemical burns, flush with water for at least 15 minutes. Do not apply the water with any type of pressure, because the pressure could drive the chemical deeper into the skin.

Chemicals can continue burning through successive layers of skin, so it is essential that you get the victim to a medical facility as soon as possible for evaluation and treatment.

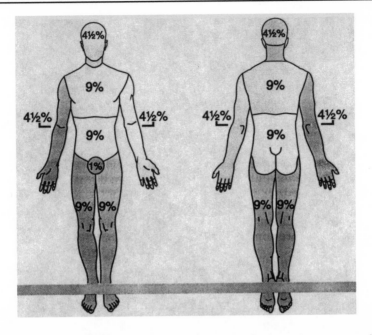

Figure 48.4. The Rule of Nines. *The extent of a burn is expressed as a percentage of the total body surface. The Rule of Nines is accurate for adults but does not make allowances for the different proportions of a child. See chapter 16, "A Simple Guide to Burn Treatment."*

Check the Power First

The most important rule in the case of electrical burns is not to go near the victim until the power is off or the victim is no longer touching the source of electricity. Then check for vital signs. If the victim is not breathing, administer rescue breathing or CPR. If the victim is unconscious, cover him or her for warmth, and call for medical attention immediately.

Surface electrical burns occur where the current enters and exits the body. They are usually third-degree burns and should be treated accordingly. "But a lot of the burn damage occurs inside the body where the electrical current passes through and heats the muscles and tissue that it touches," says Drueck. "This should be treated by paramedics or doctors at a hospital."

Drueck says he sees few electrical burns among employees of power companies, because the industry has educated its work force about burn prevention. He believes many other industries are just as con-scientious.

Unfortunately, however, experience and statistics show that there still is a need to know more about burns in many work settings. A combination of preventive techniques and accident management are the best tactics to reduce the number of these painful incidents.

For further reading:

First Aid and CPR, Level 2, National Safety Council, 1991.

The American Medical Association Handbook of First Aid and Emergency Care, developed by American Medical Association editors, Stanley M. Zydlo Jr., M.D. and James A. Hill, M.D. (1990). Random House, N.Y.

"Thermal Injuries in the Workplace," *AAOHN Journal*, Oct. 1990, pp. 492-496.

"Heat Burns Sustained in the Work-place," Martin E. Personick, *Monthly Labor Review*, July 1990, pp. 37-38.

Accident Facts, 1990 edition, National Safety Council, pp. 40-41.

Charts from the National Safety Council's First Aid and CPR, Level 2 manual.

Sources:

Jim Brown, director of public health and safety, National Restaurant Association; Dr. Charles Drueck, trauma unit director, Evanston Hospital, Evanston, Ill.; Peggy Gutman, director of occupational health services, Grant Hospital, Chicago; Alan F. Hoskin, manager of statistics department, National Safety Council; Dr. Cathryn Pajak, medical director of occupational health services, Grant Hospital, Chicago.

—by David Murray

Chapter 49

Dos and Don'ts for Minor Burns

- **Do cool the burn**—Hold the burned area under cold running water for 15 minutes. If impractical, immerse the burn in cold water or cover it with cold compresses. Cooling the burn reduces swelling by carrying heat away from your skin.

- **Don't use ice**—Putting ice directly on a burn can cause frostbite and further damage your skin.

- **Do consider a lotion**—Once a burn is completely cooled, you may find a lotion or moisturizer prevents drying and increases your comfort. For sunburn try 1 percent hydrocortisone cream.

- **Don't use butter**—Immediately putting butter on burned skin holds heat in the tissue and causes more damage. Applying butter also increases your chance of infection.

- **Do bandage a burn** —Cover the burn with a sterile gauze bandage. (Fluffy cotton may be irritating.) Wrap loosely to avoid putting pressure on burned skin. Bandaging keeps air off the area and reduces pain.

- **Don't break blisters**—Fluid-filled blisters protect against infection, if blisters break, wash area with mild soap and water, then apply an antibiotic ointment and gauze bandage.

Chapter 50

Emergency Treatment of Burns by Type

Thermal Burns

Thermal burns are caused by contact with open flames, hot liquids, hot surfaces and other sources of high heat.

1. Stop the burning. Remove the victim from the heat source.
2. Cool the burn with cold water.
3. Check breathing. Stop bleeding.
4. Cover the burn with a sterile pad or clean sheet.
5. Maintain body temperature and take victim to the nearest medical facility.

Note: Do not apply oils, sprays or ointments to a serious burn.

- Sunburn may also be cooled with water. If the sunburn is severe or is very extensive, seek medical attention.

Chemical Burns

1. Flush skin with water for at least 20 minutes.

©1998 Shriners Hospital for Children. "Emergency treatment of burns." [http:www.shrinershq.org/Prevention/BurnTips/treatment.html] You can request a free printed copy of this chapter as a booklet. Write to International Shrine Headquarters, 2900 Rocky Point Dr., Tampa, Fl 33607-1460. Reprinted with permission.

2. Remove contaminated clothing, but avoid spreading the chemical to unaffected areas.

3. If the victim's eyes are involved, flush the eyes continuously with water until medical help is obtained. Remove contact lenses.

4. Follow steps 3 to 5 for thermal burns (check breathing, stop bleeding, cover burn, maintain body temperature and transport to medical facility).

Note: In cases involving some powdered or dry chemicals, it may not be appropriate to flush with water. If a dry chemical is involved, carefully brush the chemical off the skin and check the package or package insert for emergency information.

Electrical Burns

1. Pull the plug at the wall or shut off the current. Do not touch the victim while they are in contact with electricity.

2. Follow steps 3 to 5 for thermal burns.

3. All electrical injuries should receive medical attention.

- In homes where young children are present, consider using "tamper-proof" or child-proof receptacles or receptacle covers.

- Limit your use of extension cords.

General Considerations

- Remove rings, belts, shoes and tight clothing before swelling occurs.

- If clothing is stuck to the burn, DO NOT REMOVE IT.

- Carefully cut around the stuck fabric to remove loose fabric.

- Burns on the face, hands and feet should always be considered serious and should receive prompt medical attention.

For Further Information

International Shriners Headquarters
2900 Rocky Point Dr.
Tampa, Fl 33607-1460
813-281-0300

Chapter 51

Over-the-Counter Options: Help for Cuts, Scrapes, and Burns

A half-inch scar on my left knee is a graphic reminder of a painful scrape at age 7. Also painful was the burn of Merthiolate antiseptic, applied as first aid to ward off infection.

Today's approved over-the-counter (OTC) topical (used on the skin) first-aid antimicrobials are less irritating and more effective than Merthiolate, which contains the mercury drug thimerosal. The Food and Drug Administration has approved seven topical OTC antibiotics (see "OTC Antibiotics below") and is evaluating OTC topical antiseptics under a proposed rule. The proposal would ban numerous antiseptics, including mercurials, as ineffective and some, including thimerosal, as also unsafe.

Antibiotics are also available by prescription as injectable and oral medicines and medicines for the eye and ear. They are used to treat infections. While some can kill a limited number of bacteria, other varieties affect many bacteria.

Antiseptics weaken microbes, but don't usually kill them. Health-care antiseptics in soaps and other products help prevent the spread of infection in medical facilities.

OTC first-aid antibiotics and antiseptics are applied to the skin to help prevent infection in minor cuts, scrapes and burns.

"Used topically, OTC antimicrobials inhibit the growth of bacteria, but don't necessarily kill them all," says Audrey Love, a microbiologist with the division of OTC drug evaluation in FDA's Center for

FDA Consumer, May 1996.

Drug Evaluation and Research. "If an injury is extensive," Love says, "it should be taken care of by a doctor. But consumers have to consider for themselves, based on reading the labeling, whether a product is something they should use."

FDA has published rules (monographs) establishing adequate labeling for OTC antimicrobials, and conditions under which products would be generally recognized as safe and effective for use without medical supervision. The final antibiotics rule (1987) and proposed antiseptics rule (1991) specify active ingredients and concentrations, as well as labeling information such as product identification, indications for use, warnings, and directions for use. All drugs must meet the agency's good manufacturing practice requirements for product identity, strength, quality, and purity.

Some Restrictions

OTC first-aid antimicrobials are for use only up to one week. If an injury persists or worsens after this time, the label warns consumers to stop use and consult a doctor.

The products are not for existing infections, animal bites, sunburn, punctures, or eye injuries. Nor should they be used for cuts, scrapes or burns needing medical care, such as:

- cuts that are deep, continue bleeding, or may require stitches
- scrapes with imbedded particles that can't be flushed away
- large wounds
- burns more serious than a small reddened area.

Use of an antibiotic or antiseptic does not in itself constitute first-aid treatment of a minor wound.

A panel of experts convened by FDA defined first aid as "a process that includes initial adequate cleansing which may or may not be followed by application of a safe, non-irritating product which does not interfere with normal wound healing and which may reduce the bacterial numbers and help prevent infection." (From 1972 to 1981, at FDA's request, 16 outside panels evaluated marketed OTC drugs. Their charge completed, the panels no longer meet.)

FDA requires that labels for antibiotics advise users to first "clean the affected area." Antiseptics also would be labeled with the advice.

Because topical antimicrobials are not totally effective in killing bacteria, FDA does not allow firms to place the claim "Helps kill bacteria" in the same area as the required information. FDA believes the term "kill" implies the product will eliminate all bacteria and could be misleading if appearing with the required term "infection" (or alternate term "bacterial contamination") in the label's indications section. The claim may be used, though, as additional information elsewhere in the label.

More about Antibiotics

In its final rule, FDA listed these antibiotic active ingredients as safe and effective: bacitracin, bacitracin zinc, chlortetracycline hydrochloride, tetracycline hydrochloride, neomycin sulfate, oxytetracycline hydrochloride, and polymyxin B sulfate—the latter two only for combination products because of their limited effectiveness against certain microorganisms when used alone.

The rule does not allow the previously marketed antibiotic gramicidin, because it has the potential to break down red blood cells when absorbed through fresh wounds. The agency called for a well-designed, double-blind study (where neither patient nor doctor knows who gets the drug) to show gramicidin's effects.

The data on which FDA based its approval of the other antibiotics included a well-controlled study of minor skin injuries or insect bites in 59 children. Streptococcal infection developed in 15 of the 32 receiving a topical placebo and in three of the 27 receiving a topical antibiotic. Twelve of the 15 receiving placebos eventually needed oral antibiotics, and one of the three using antibiotics did as well.

The agency agreed with comments that many such injuries are self-healing, but that some do not heal without treatment and it is impossible to make this distinction at the time of injury.

Also, says FDA's Love, there's always a chance someone can be allergic to a drug—prescription or OTC. "People who tend to be allergic," she says, "should talk to their doctor or pharmacist before trying any OTC medicine for the first time."

About 1 in 20 people is allergic to neomycin, according to an article in the August 1995 *Harvard Health Letter*. If a reaction such as redness, itching or burning occurs, the article advises, "Stop using the preparation immediately, and consult a physician if symptoms worsen or persist for more than 48 hours."

Hypersensitivity reactions may also occur with bacitracin, according to the *Handbook of Nonprescription Drugs* (10th edition), published by the American Pharmaceutical Association and The National Professional Society of Pharmacists, Washington, D.C. The handbook also states that tetracycline products may trigger reactions in allergic

565

patients, "some of whom may have severe reactions even if exposure is by topical application only."

With repeated use on large areas, neomycin also fosters development of neomycin-resistant strains of Staphylococci bacteria. Neomycin products that include polymyxin B and bacitracin guard against this.

To prevent neomycin overuse, FDA limits the drug to ointments and creams, the most likely dosage forms for small wounds. Also, all OTC antimicrobials must be labeled for short-term use. The agency believes short-term use of neomycin ointments or creams on small wounds would not risk overuse. To reduce the risk even further, FDA requires labels for ointments and creams to identify a dose as "an amount equal to the surface area of the tip of a finger."

Another issue is the combination of a product with a local "caine" anesthetic, such as benzocaine, as is allowed for bacitracin ointment or a combination ointment of bacitracin, neomycin, or polymyxin B. The review panel was concerned an anesthetic might mask symptoms of infection, delaying treatment by a doctor. But FDA believes the required warnings on the label adequately inform consumers when to consult a doctor. (See "Labeling Final Rule below.")

OTC Antibiotics

The following antibiotic products have been approved by FDA for use without a prescription. They are ointments unless otherwise noted:

Single-ingredient Products

- bacitracin—Baciguent
- bacitracin zinc—Bacitracin Zinc
- chlortetracycline hydrochloride—Aureomycin
- neomycin sulfate—Neomycin, Myciguent Cream
- tetracycline hydrochloride—Achromycin

Combination Products

- Bacitracin-neomycin—none currently marketed

- bacitracin-polymyxin B aerosol—none currently marketed

- bacitracin-neomycin-polymyxin B—Lanabiotic, Medi-Quik Triple Antibiotic, Clomycin Cream (with lidocaine anesthetic), Mycitracin Plus Pain Reliever (with lidocaine)

- bacitracin zinc-neomycin—none currently marketed

- bacitracin zinc-polymyxin B ointment, aerosol or powder—Polysporin, Polysporin Powder

- bacitracin zinc-neomycin-polymyxin B—Neomixin, Neosporin Original

- neomycin-polymyxin B ointment or cream—Neosporin Plus Maximum Strength Cream (with lidocaine)

- oxytetracycline-polymyxin B ointment or powder—none currently marketed.

More about Antiseptics

In its proposed rule, FDA listed these active antiseptic ingredients as tentatively safe and effective: ethyl alcohol (48 to 95 percent), isopropyl alcohol, benzalkonium chloride, benzethonium chloride, camphorated metacresol, camphorated phenol, phenol, hexylresorcinol, hydrogen peroxide solution, iodine tincture, iodine topical solution, povidone-iodine, and methylbenzethonium. Five ingredients listed as tentatively effective only in combination products are ethyl alcohol (26.9 percent), eucalyptol, menthol, methyl salicylate, and thymol.

The proposal would ban numerous mercury ingredients and cloflucarban, fluorosalan and tribromsalan antiseptics as not generally recognized as safe and effective for OTC use.

FDA had requested study data on whether use of topical povidone-iodine affected thyroid function. In submitted data, iodine blood levels did increase after two weeks' use, but returned to normal when use was stopped. There was no effect on thyroid function.

Antiseptics would be labeled similarly to antibiotics, but with some differences.

Labels on camphorated metacresol, camphorated phenol, and phenol, for example, would warn, "Do not bandage."

"The drugs can be hard on the skin," says Debbie Lumpkins, a microbiologist in FDA's division of OTC drug evaluation. She explains that "when bandaged, the skin gets damp, increasing absorption. Therefore, more drug enters the skin and may cause more damage than if you just left the wound uncovered."

Labels for ethyl alcohol (48 to 95 percent) and isopropyl alcohol (50 to 91.3 percent) would warn: "Flammable, keep away from fire or flame."

For liquid antiseptics, labels would direct users to let the product dry before bandaging.

567

Comments on the proposal were minimal, Lumpkins says, emphasizing that FDA's evaluation of the ingredients is still very much an evolving process.

"Frequently," she says, "we find that one study or one article says one thing, and there's another study or article on the other side. We have to determine the facts. Literature searches that we can now do so easily help, but we won't find everything. We rely on people to bring things to our attention."

Recent publications advise against two currently marketed antiseptics. The National Safety Council's *1996 First Aid Pocket Guide* states: "DO NOT use hydrogen peroxide. It does not kill bacteria, and it adversely affects capillary blood flow and wound healing." And the *Handbook on Nonprescription Drugs* states ethyl alcohol "is not a desirable wound antiseptic because it irritates already damaged tissue. The coagulum [crust] formed may, in fact, protect the bacteria."

The final rule will reflect FDA's evaluation of all the data, Lumpkins says. Thus, antiseptic ingredients proposed as safe and effective could be found unsafe or ineffective, or new ingredients could be added, depending on new information.

Whether using an OTC antibiotic or antiseptic, consumers should realize "there are limits to what the products can do," Lumpkins says. "People should read the label, and use the product appropriately. If they notice a change in their condition, or if there's redness or swelling, they shouldn't continue to try to treat it. They should see a doctor."

Labelling Final Rule

Under the final rule, labels for topical antibiotics must:

- state the established name of the drug

- identify the drug as a "first-aid antibiotic"

- state the drug's approved use—for example: "First aid to help protect against infection in minor cuts, scrapes, and burns." (Allowed alternative wording includes "help prevent skin infection" or "help reduce the risk of bacterial contamination." Other descriptive statements may be added, provided they are truthful and not misleading)

- warn:

568

— *"For external use only. Do not use in the eyes or apply over large areas of the body. In case of deep or puncture wounds, animal bites, or serious burns, consult a doctor."*

— *"Stop use and consult a doctor if the condition persists or gets worse. Do not use longer than one week unless directed by a doctor."*

• advise to clean the area, to use a small amount one to three times daily, and to cover with a sterile bandage if desired

• specify on ointments and creams to use *"an amount equal to the surface area of the tip of a finger."* Combination products must give the established name of each active ingredient. Labels must identify any added anesthetic as such, include the directions and warnings in its monograph, and state: *"First aid for the temporary relief of pain* [or other approved alternative] *in minor cuts, scrapes, and burns."*

—by Dixie Farley

Dixie Farley is a staff writer for *FDA Consumer*.

Part Seven

Additional Help and Information

Chapter 52

Burns Terminology

A

Acute Period: The second phase of burn care, beginning with the end of successful fluid resuscitation. The acute period ends with the completion of autografting and/or spontaneous healing of all wounds.

Allograft: A graft taken from another member of the same species. In The case of burns, the top layers of skin are removed from donors who have died. The removal of this thin slice of skin does not disfigure the body.

Autograft: Often referred to as a skin graft. The patient's own skin is used. The upper layers of skin are taken from an unburned body area and applied to a clean burn wound. That way both the donor skin site and the deep burn can heal, Ap autograft is a permanent skin covering.

B

Bacteria: Also called germs. The cause of most burn infections.

Burn Depth: One of the factors used to classify burn severity, ranging from superficial to deep. Often designated as degree of burn: first, second, third, or fourth. Current terminology classifies using "superficial," "full-thickness," and "partial thickness."

Burn Surface Area (BSA): One of the factors used to classify burn severity, refers to the percentage of body area affected. Usually measured using the rule of nines.

C

Circumferential Burn: One that goes around the neck, trunk or extremities.

Contracture: A tightening of tissue between two joints, resulting from "shrinkage" of scar tissue. This results in impairment of joint function.

Culture: A laboratory test procedure used to evaluate a body area for growth of bacteria.

D

Debridement: Removal of dead tissue from the wound surface, either in the operating room or in the treatment room.

Dermis: The second (deeper) layer of skin.

Donor Site: The place on the patient from which unburned skin is taken for grafting.

E

Edema: Swelling caused by the collection of fluid in the tissues. Immediately after a burn, considerable swelling takes place; This is normal, but can be so severe that it can be frightening to family members.

Epidermis: Outermost layer of skin.

Eschar: The dead tissue on the surface of the wound which must be removed for healing to occur and for prevention of infection.

Escharotomy: The process of cutting through the dead tissue (eschar) on the surface of the wound to relieve pressure caused by swelling.

Excision: Sharp surgical removal of tissue.
exceedingly rich in tiny blood vessels; provides a base of support for skin grafts.

F

First-Degree Burn: A superficial burn in which the epidermis is partially destroyed but the basal layer remains intace. Initially appears red, swollen and painful (e.g., a sunburn). Usually heals spontaneously.

Full Thickness Burn: A burn which cannot readily heal by itself because all of the layers of skin have been destroyed. These areas are usually grafted. (Often referred to as third-degree burn).

G

Graft: Non-burned skin which is placed on the burn. These can be allografts, autografts or xenografts.

Granulation Tissue: A specialized tissue created by the body as a defense against invading bacteria,

H

Hyperalimentation: Administration of more than usual amounts of required nutrients, via the intestine or through a central venous catheter.

Hyperthermia: Abnormally high body temperature.

Hypertrophic Scar: The enlargement of the skin tissue. The overgrowth of skin cells that form raised, thick scars which appear after the initial healing.

Hypothermia: Abnormally low body temperature.

I

Isolation: Techniques used to decrease transmission of bacteria between patients and care-givers.

IV—Intravenous tube: A mode for delivery of fluids through a catheter into a vein.

K

Keloid: A severe type of hypertrophic scar tissue.

N

NPO: An abbreviation of the Latin words meaning "nothing by mouth." This order is prior to surgery to prevent vomiting of food from the stomach into the lungs while under anesthesia.

O

O.R.: Operating Room.

O.T.: Occupational Therapy.

P

Partial Thickness Burn: A burn in which damage does not extend through the entire thickness of the skin (dermis). Enough of the deeper layers remain to permit spontaneous healing of the skin with time (often referred to as second-degree burn).

Percent of Burn: Measurement of body surface injured.

PT: Physical Therapy

S

Second-Degree Burn: A burn in which damage does not extend through the entire thickness of the skin (dermis). Enough of the deeper layers remain to permit spontaneous healing of the skin with time (often referred to as partial-thickness burn).

Sepsis: Presence of bacteria in the bloodstream resulting in acute changes (usually severe) in bodily functions.

Skin Graft: A method of repairing areas of lost or damaged skin by detaching a piece of healthy skin from one part of the body and placing it surgically over the affected area. Donor skin can be stretched from six to ten times its area to cover. New cells grow from the graft and cover the damaged area with fresh skin. Skin from a donor is usually rejected within a few days and needs to be replaced with artificial skin or the patient's own skin. Two types of grafts are "split-thickness" and "full-thickness." Split thickness grafts take less than the full thickness of the graft in order to allow the donor site to regenerate quickly. Full-thickness grafts are preferred for visible areas like the face because they result in a cosmetically superior result. They use the full thickness of skin and require stitching in the donor site.

Skin Tags: A small, brown or flesh-colored protruding flap of skin caused by unsatisfactory healing of a wound or occurring spontaneously. Skin tags can be removed usually.

Superficial Burn: Often referred to as a first-degree burn. Affects superficial layer of skin tissue (epidermis). Initially appears red, swollen and painful (e.g., a sunburn). Heals spontaneously.

T

Thermal Injury: A wound caused by heat (e.g., fire, hot surface of a stove, hot liquids, etc.)

Tracheostomy: A surgical opening into the trachea (windpipe) below the larynx (voice box) which helps supply air to the lungs.

Tubbing: Immersion of the patient in a bathtub to cleanse the wound, soak off dressings and allow for range of motion exercises.

X

Xenografts: A graft taken from another species (e.g., a pig), usually considered a biologic dressing rather than a true skin graft. It temporarily provides some of the functions of skin and promotes healing.

Chapter 53

Resources for Burn Patients

American Board of Professional Disability Consultants
1350 Beverly Road Suite 115-327 McLean, VA 22101
703/709-8644 703/709-8644 (fax)
email abpdc@erols.com
Disabilities served: All disabilities
Users served: Professionals in the disability field

Description: The American Board of Professional Disability
Consultants certifies attorneys, physicians, psychologists, and
counselors as specialists in disability and personal injury consultation.

Information services: The board publishes a newsletter and the
National Register of Professional Disability Consultants and
Guide to Disability and Health-Related Organizations.

**American Society of Plastic and Reconstructive Surgery
(ASPRS),**
444 East Algonquin Road Arlington Heights, IL 60005 800/635-0635
(Plastic Surgeons Referral Service)
847/228-9900
web page: www.plasticsurgery.org
Disabilities served: Abnormalities caused by birth defect, disease, or
trauma
Users served: The public, plastic surgery patients, and plastic surgeons certified by the American Board of Plastic Surgery

Description: Founded in 1931, the American Society of Plastic and Reconstructive Surgeons (ASPRS) is comprised of about 4,500 plastic surgeons certified by the American Board of Plastic Surgery. ASPRS seeks to educate the public on the specialty of plastic surgery, and to assist individuals in selecting a properly trained physician. The society promotes high professional standards of care through scientific education and research coordinated by its Plastic Surgery Educational Foundation (PSEF).

It also assists board-certified plastic surgeons in fulfilling their professional needs by acting as an advocate with the government and insurance industry, offering practice-management services and coordinating similar activities.

Information services: ASPRS offers a toll-free, 24-hour referral service to assist prospective patients in selecting a qualified plastic surgeon and to verify that a physician is certified in plastic surgery. The service also offers detailed educational brochures on various plastic surgery procedures. In conjunction with the Plastic Surgery Educational Foundation, ASPRS publishes a monthly scientific journal, Plastic and Reconstructive Surgery, and a monthly socioeconomic newspaper for members, Plastic Surgery News. For general information, ASPRS can be contacted at the above address, or by phone (communications department) at 847/228-9900, ext. 349.

American Camping Association (ACA)

Bradford Woods 5000 State Road 67 North Martinsville, IN 46151-7902
765/342-8456 765/342-2065 (fax)
email: customerservice@aca-camps.org
web page: www.aca-camps.org
Disabilities served: All disabilities
Users served: People with disabilities

Description: The American Camping Association (ACA) accredits camps throughout the country when they meet standards for health, safety, personnel, and program. Included in its annual guide are camps that serve children with physical or mental disabilities in general; others that serve children with epilepsy, diabetes, asthma, and learning disabilities; and those for children, youths, and adults who are deaf, blind, and have physical, emotional, or mental disabilities.

American Burn Association
625 N Michigan Ave, Suite 1630 Chicago IL 60611
800/548-2876 312-642-9130 (fax)
email: aba@ameriburn.org
web page: www.ameriburn.org
Disabilities served: Burn injuries
Users served: Physicians, nurses, therapists, educators, health administrators, and other professionals with a demonstrated interest in burn injury

> Description: The American Burn Association was founded in 1967, as an outgrowth of a series of annual seminars sponsored by leading institutions in the field of burn treatment. Standing committees are maintained in such areas as burn prevention, organization and delivery of burn care, and education.

> It is an organization of health care professionals interested in the care of burned patients, education of burn team members, prevention of burn injuries, and research.

> The association's objectives are to stimulate and sponsor study and research in the treatment and prevention of burns, provide a forum for the presentation of such knowledge, foster training opportunities for individuals interested in burns, and encourage publications pertaining to these activities.

> Information services: Association communications include a membership directory published every other year, three to four newsletters a year, and an annual directory of educational programs and materials. Members also receive the Journal of Burn Care and Rehabilitation, six issues a year.

> Burn Care Resources in North America, listing approximately 210 hospitals in the United States and Canada, is published every two years.

Burn Care Resources in North America. (1993)
American Burn Association, 625 N Michigan Ave Suite 1630 Chicago IL 548-2876; 312/642-9130 (fax).
email: aba@ameriburn.org
web page: www.ameriburn.org

> This directory lists approximately 210 hospitals in the United States and Canada.

International Shriners Headquarters
2900 N Rocky Point Dr., Tampa, FL 33607
813/281-0300 813/281-8113 (fax)
http:www.shrinershq.org
Disabilities served: Children's orthopaedic or burn disabilities
Users served: Children with disabilities, up to age 18

Description: The Shriners' first children's orthopaedic hospital opened in 1922 as the official philanthropy of the fraternal order. There are now 19 orthopaedic hospitals and 3 burn institutes serving children up to age 18 in the United States, Mexico, and Canada. Diagnosis and treatment are offered solely on the basis of medical and financial need, at no charge to the patient's family. The burn institutes accept children who need immediate care or those needing plastic surgery and rehabilitation ("healed" burns). Research on the causes of crippling and scarring and on methods of treatment is conducted at each Shrine hospital. Members' assessments, charitable bequests, and a variety of fundraising activities support this network of patient care and research facilities.

Information services: Application forms for hospital admission, brochures on the hospitals and burn institutes, and donation and bequest forms are available from local Shrine temples or from the international headquarters. Eligibility for treatment is determined on the basis of applications, which are completed by parents or guardians, the referring physician, and a local Shrine sponsor. The Shriners Hospital for Crippled Children in Tampa, Florida should be called for emergency admission to burn institutes or hospitals, 813/281-0300.Toll-free numbers are: 800/237-5055; for Florida, 800/282-9161.

Mayo Clinic Health Letter
Mayo Foundation for Medical Education and Research
Rochester, Minnesota 55905.
For Subscription information, please call 1-800-333-9038.
web page: www.mayohealth.org

National Burn Victim Foundation (NBVF)
246A Madisonville Rd PO Box 409 Basking Ridge NJ 07920
908/953-9091 908/953-9099 (fax)
email: natl@aol.com

web page: www.nbvf.org
Disabilities served: Individuals with burn injury
Users served: Medical professionals, criminal justice personnel, child
welfare workers, social workers

Description: The National Burn Victim Foundation (NBVF) is a
nonprofit agency providing advocacy and services to burn victims and their families free of charge. On a national basis the
NBVF is a resource for burn-related information and referrals.

Programs include a support system for disaster response, evaluation service for child burns suspected of being the result of
abuse or neglect, community burn-prevention education, and
commitment to finding new methods of burn treatment. Professional seminars on child-abuse evaluation are conducted several
times a year.

Information services: The NBVF issues a quarterly newsletter, Update, which reports on the activities and programs of
the National Burn Victim Foundation and on new methods of
treating burn victims. It is available free of charge to those
requesting to be on the mailing list. Membership in the
NBVT is available at various levels. NBVF may be contacted
for further information. The NBVF offers brochures and pam-
phlets on its programs and services and on burn prevention
on request. A fee is required to cover costs for large quantities of the brochures.

North Texas Burn Rehabilitation Model System (NTBRMS)
University of Texas Southwestern Medical Center at Dallas (UT
Southwestern) Department of Physical Medicine and Rehabilitation
(PMR) 5323 Harry Hines Boulevard Dallas, TX 75235-9055
214/648-2288 214/648-8828 (fax)
Disabilities served: Burn injury
Users served: Patients with burn injuries, burn specialists

Description: The goal of the North-Texas Burn Rehabilitation
Model System is to establish a coordinated, comprehensive,
multidisciplinary system of rehabilitation services for adults
who have sustained severe burn injury, evaluate the service
demonstration program, and conduct site-specific and collaboration research. This project is funded by the National Institute
on Disability and Rehabilitation Research(NMRR).

One hundred fifty to two hundred adults with severe burn injury from a 70,000 to 80,000 square-mile area in northeast Texas are studied per year. These people receive inpatient medical-surgical and rehabilitation treatment at the regional burn center at Parkland Memorial Hospital (PMH) in Dallas, Texas. Outpatient rehabilitation treatment is provided at PMH, UT Southwestern Medical Center, and, in some cases, near the patient's home. The project conducts an annual educational seminar, is producing a syllabus, a brochure to distribute to professionals in the region, and a newsletter for patients and professionals. Site-specific and collaborative research is being conducted and results will be published on the study of functional outcome of severe hand burns and the course of psychosocial recovery from severe burn injury.

Information services: This project provides information and referral services, develops model programs, conducts training seminars and evaluates technology.

Phoenix Society for Burn Survivors, Inc.

National Headquarters
33 Main Street, Suite 403
Nashua, New Hampshire   03060
(603) 889-3000* (603) 889-4688 Fax
888-BURN (2876) (toll free for burn survivors)
email: information@burns-phoenix-society.org
web page: www.burns-phoenix-society.org
Disabilities served: Disabilities caused by burn injuries
Users served: Burn survivors and their families

Description: A worldwide self-help organization established in 1977 for burn survivors and their families, the Phoenix Society for Burn Survivors, Inc. works to ease the psychosocial adjustment of people with severe burns during and after hospitalization so that they can return to normal lives within their communities. While anyone with an interest in the goals of the society is free to join, members are in large part burn survivors. Members cooperate with members of the hospital staff, help the survivor return to work or school, and arrange support group meetings in their community.

Information services: Burn survivors and their families who would like to get in touch with other burn survivors for counseling or help may contact the Phoenix Society for referral to the nearest area coordinator.

The society publishes a quarterly newsletter, The Icarus File, which is included with membership. Nonmembers may sub- scribe for a nominal charge. In addition, a list of audiovisual materials on fire prevention, burn care, true life stories of burn survivors, and other topics are available from the society. Information assistance is available in Spanish; the society is prepared to make arrangements, for other languages as necessary.

Phoenix Society Burn Camps:
Penny Pearl, RN, BA. Linda French, PT.   Beth Franzen, OTR.
UC Davis Regional Burn Center 2315 Stockton Blvd., Sacramento CA 95817 (916)
734-3636
Firefighters Pacific Burn Institute 3101 Stockton Blvd. Sacramento, CA 95820
(916) 739-8525

U.S. Consumer Product Safety Commission
Washington, D.C. 20207
http://www.cpsc.gov

University of Washington Burn Injury Rehabilitation Model System
University of Washington Burn Center Harborview Medical Center 325 Ninth Avenue Seattle, WA 98104
206/731-3140 206/223-3656 (fax)
Disabilities served: Burn injuries
Users served: Burn survivors, health care providers, vocational rehabilitation specialists

Description: This model system, with support from the National Institute on Disabilities and Rehabilitation Research (NIDRR), provides state-of-the-art rehabilitation to burn survivors; gathers data related to burn rehabilitation; participates in a national database; conducts research on burn rehabilitation; and disseminates information to burn survivors, their families, and health care providers.

The University of Washington Burn Rehabilitation Model System includes seven projects: (1) complete burn care from injury to discharge; (2) a research program in burn rehabilitation through a protocol to study the effects of pressure garments on burn wound healing; (3) a study of the effect of various interventions on burn rehabilitation through a self-care system, a provider system, and a research protocol designed to improve the compliance with splints and pressure garments; (4) a study of the effect of various interventions on independent living and vocational rehabilitation through two interventions; (5) longitudinal data on burn survivors; (6) participation in a national database; and (7) dissemination of the information from this research and demonstration project to burn survivors, their families, and health care providers.

Information services: This project publishes journal articles and provides audiovisuals; develops curricula/training materials, develops technology and provides technical assistance; and provides information and referral services.

Western Pennsylvania Hospital Foundation.
Department P.
4818 Liberty Ave.
Pittsburgh, Pa. 15224

Index

Index

Page numbers in *italics* refer to illustrations or tables; the letter 'n' refers to a note.

A

acanthosis, ultraviolet radiation 147
acetaminophen 274
acetic acid 288, 296–97
acid burns, described 177–78
  see also chemical burns
actinic prurigo, light susceptibility 151
actinic reticuloid, light susceptibility 151
acute care period
  burn statistics 38
  defined 573
adolescents, nutrition measurement 333, 337
adults
  burn injury statistics 8, 10
  kitchen safety 512–13
  rule of nines *546, 557*
Advanced Tissue Sciences, cultured skin 354
age factor
  burn injury 176
  burn mortality 64

age factor, continued
  burn statistics 8–9, 37, 489
  residential fires 17, 499
  ultraviolet radiation susceptibility 151–52
  work-related burn injury 95
  work-related burns 93
agriculture, electrical burns 56
aircraft crashes
  burn deaths 20, 34
  burn statistics 3
airway, emergency care 182–83, 209, 550
  children 245–46
alcohol use
  burn victims 176
  house fires 24, 54
alkali burns
  see also chemical burns
  described 178
  workplace 169
allantoin, burn treatment 208
allografts
  children 251
  defined 573
  described 351
  electrical burns 134
  types, described 201
  wound dressings 358, 362

589

body image, hidden burns 429–32
Boeckx, Willy 441
Bogaerts, Frida 441
Bradley, T. 138
Brandt, Christopher P. 172
Breslau, Alan J. 428, 432
Brigham, Peter 12
Brigham, Peter A. 51
Bronaugh, Robert L. 354, 355
Brown, Ann 509
Brown, Jim 551, 558
BSA *see* body (burn) surface area (BSA)
Budget Reconciliation Act (1987) 73
Bureau of Standards, National 24
Burgess, Molly C. 244
Burn Association, American
  artificial skin 349
  burn care needs 61
  burn center admissions 38
  burn center referral 233
  burned patients care 581
  burn injury incidence 46
  burn injury statistics 31
  facts and figures 4, 5
  fire-safe cigarettes 24
  major burn injuries 58
  transport to burn center 185
  trends in burn center admissions 40
burn camps 459–62
burn care facilities 53–74
  see also hospitals
  economic factors 66–74
  locations *60*
  staffing considerations 65
  statistics 29–46
Burn Care Resources in North America 581
burn centers 214, 233–34
  intensive care units 59, 67, 259
  rehabilitation 407–9
  statistics 4, 5, 38–39, 55, 102–3
burn codes 31–32
burn degrees *see* first degree burns; second degree burns; third degree burns
burn depth
  classification system 189–91, 280, 543–45
  defined 573

burn depth, continued
  described 180, 184, 223–25
  tissue removal 199–201
burn extent, described 184–85
  see also total body surface area (TBSA)
Burn Foundation
  burn center admissions 41
  burn injuries databases 12
  burn injury statistics 31
  regional data 37
Burn Information Exchange, National (NBIE)
  burn trauma information 407
  facts and figures 5
burn injuries
  body surface area 57–59
    see also body (burn) surface area
  categories 9
  cause of death 19
    statistics 84
  complications 132–33
  degrees *see* first degree burns; second degree burns; third degree burns
  delayed deaths 14
  described 176–77
  dressings 210–11
    see also wound dressings
  insurance reimbursement 69–74
  multi-system effects 57, 59
  outcome assessments 64–66
  statistics 31–33, 53–54, 86, 245, 487–89
  severity information,488 4–5
  thickness *see* full thickness burns; partial thickness burns
  treatment 108, 213–20
    emergency care 179–86, 231–33
    guide 189–204
    phases, described 221, 402–5, 446–49, 467
    phases, plans 235–38
    research 205–12
    types, described 227–30
    zones, described 225
Burn Medicine, National Institute for (NIBM)
  burn rehabilitation 399–400, 404
  model rehabilitation program 407

591

O

occupational hazards
see also industrial sector
see also workplace injuries
electrical burns 56
hot tar burns 57, 98
welding burns 57
Occupational Safety and Health Administration
burn prevention programs 170
industrial burns study 551
Oceanic and Atmospheric Administration, National
lightning deaths and injuries 140
ozone layer depletion 531
Office of Medical Applications of Research 144
ointments, described 289
Ophthalmology, American Academy of
eye protection 535
safer sunning recommendations 532
organ donation, skin 351
Organogenesis, Inc., Apligraf developer 355–56
Original BioBrane 352
outside fires, statistics 82
oxycodone 272
oxytetracycline hydrochloride
burn treatment 208, 565, 567

P

pain, chronic 261
pain behavior, described 160
see also pain perception factors
pain management 259–75
factors, described 264
heating pads 519
medications
burn treatment 201–2, 208
chemical burns 120
lightning injury 141
nursing care 240–41
ultraviolet radiation susceptibility 158
work-related burns 165
phases, described 267–74, 447

pain perception by individual, described 260
see also pain perception factors
pain perception factors 259
Pajak, Cathryn 552, 558
Pappert, Amy 161
parakeratosis, ultraviolet radiation 147
Park-Davis, itching remedies 426
Parkland Memorial Hospital (Dallas, TX) 584
partial thickness burns 551–52
see also second degree burns
chemicals 120–21
defined 576
itching 425
patient transfers, burn injuries 61–64, 233–34
Peacock, Richard D. 92
Pearl, Penny 585
Pediatrics, American Academy of 532
pentazocine 272
percent of burn, defined 576
persistent light reaction, light susceptibility 151
Peters, W. J. 104
petrolatum, burn treatment 208, 228
Pfizer, Inc., itching remedies 426
Pharmaceutical Association, American 565
Pharmacists, National Professional Society of 565
Phenergan (promethazine) 161
phenol, burn treatment 204, 208, 567
phenolate sodium, burn treatment 208
phenylketonuria, ultraviolet radiation susceptibility 151
Phoenix Society Burn Camps 585
Phoenix Society for Burn Survivors, Inc.
burn camp 460–61
burn camp information 462
burn scars 371
burn survivors 584–85
itching remedies 427, 428
phosphorus burns
see also chemical burns
treatment 204
workplace 170

Contagious & Non-Contagious Infectious Diseases Sourcebook

Basic Information about Contagious Diseases like Measles, Polio, Hepatitis B, and Infectious Mononucleosis, and Non-Contagious Infectious Diseases like Tetanus and Toxic Shock Syndrome, and Diseases Occurring as Secondary Infections Such as Shingles and Reye Syndrome, Along with Vaccination, Prevention, and Treatment Information, and a Section Describing Emerging Infectious Disease Threats

Edited by Karen Bellenir and Peter D. Dresser. 566 pages. 1996. 0-7808-0075-3. $78.

Death & Dying Sourcebook

Basic Information for the Layperson about End-of-Life Care and Related Ethical and Legal Issues, Including Chief Causes of Death, Autopsies, Pain Management for the Terminally Ill, Life Support Systems, Coma, Euthanasia, Assisted Suicide, Hospice Programs, Living Wills, Near-Death Experiences, Counseling, Mourning, Organ Donation, Cryogenics and Physician Training and Liability, Along with Statistical Data, a Glossary, and Listings of Sources for Additional Help and Information

Edited by Annemarie Muth. 600 pages. 1999. 0-7808-0230-6. $78.

Diabetes Sourcebook, 1st Edition

Basic Information about Insulin-Dependent and Noninsulin-Dependent Diabetes Mellitus, Gestational Diabetes, and Diabetic Complications, Symptoms, Treatment, and Research Results, Including Statistics on Prevalence, Morbidity, and Mortality, Along with Source Listings for Further Help and Information

Edited by Karen Bellenir and Peter D. Dresser. 827 pages. 1994. 1-55888-751-2. $78.

"...very informative and understandable for the layperson without being simplistic. It provides a comprehensive overview for laypersons who want a general understanding of the disease or who want to focus on various aspects of the disease." — *Bulletin of the MLA, Jan '96*

Diabetes Sourcebook, 2nd Edition

Basic Consumer Health Information about Type 1 Diabetes (Insulin-Dependent or Juvenile-Onset Diabetes), Type 2 (Noninsulin-Dependent or Adult-Onset Diabetes), Gestational Diabetes, and Related Disorders, Including Diabetes Prevalence Data, Management Issues, the Role of Diet and Exercise in Controlling Diabetes, Insulin and Other Diabetes Medicines, and Complications of Diabetes Such as Eye Diseases, Periodontal Disease, Amputation, and End-Stage Renal Disease; Along with Reports on Current Research Initiatives, a Glossary, and Resource Listings for Further Help and Information

Edited by Karen Bellenir. 725 pages. 1998. 0-7808-0224-1. $78.

Diet & Nutrition Sourcebook, 1st Edition

Basic Information about Nutrition, Including the Dietary Guidelines for Americans, the Food Guide Pyramid, and Their Applications in Daily Diet, Nutritional Advice for Specific Age Groups, Current Nutritional Issues and Controversies, the New Food Label and How to Use It to Promote Healthy Eating, and Recent Developments in Nutritional Research

Edited by Dan R. Harris. 662 pages. 1996. 0-7808-0084-2. $78.

"Useful reference as a food and nutrition sourcebook for the general consumer."
— *Booklist Health Sciences Supplement, Oct '97*

"Recommended for public libraries and medical libraries that receive general information requests on nutrition. It is readable and will appeal to those interested in learning more about healthy dietary practices."
— *Medical Reference Services Quarterly, Fall '97*

"With dozens of questionable diet books on the market, it is so refreshing to find a reliable and factual reference book. Recommended to aspiring professionals, librarians, and others seeking and giving reliable dietary advice. An excellent compilation." — *Choice, Feb '97*

Diet & Nutrition Sourcebook, 2nd Edition

Basic Consumer Health Information about Dietary Guidelines, Recommended Daily Intake Values, Vitamins, Minerals, Fiber, Fat, Weight Control, Dietary Supplements, and Food Additives; Along with Special Sections on Nutrition Needs throughout Life and Nutrition for People with Such Specific Medical Concerns as Allergies, High Blood Cholesterol, Hypertension, Diabetes, Celiac Disease, Seizure Disorders, Phenylketonuria (PKU), Cancer, and Eating Disorders, and Including Reports on Current Nutrition Research and Source Listings for Additional Help and Information

Edited by Karen Bellenir. 600 pages. 1999. 0-7808-0228-4. $78.

Domestic Violence Sourcebook

Basic Information about the Physical, Emotional and Sexual Abuse of Partners, Children, and Elders, Including Information about Hotlines, Safe Houses, Safety Plans, Resources for Support and Assistance, Community Initiatives, and Reports on Current Directions in Research and Treatment; Along with a Glossary, Sources for Further Reading, and Listings of Governmental and Non-Governmental Organizations

Edited by Helene Henderson. 600 pages. 1999. 0-7808-0235-7. $78.

Ear, Nose & Throat Disorders Sourcebook

Basic Information about Disorders of the Ears, Nose, Sinus Cavities, Pharynx, and Larynx, Including Ear Infections, Tinnitus, Vestibular Disorders, Allergic and Non-Allergic Rhinitis, Sore Throats, Tonsillitis, and Cancers That Affect the Ears, Nose, Sinuses, and Throat, Along with Reports on Current Research Initiatives, a Glossary of Related Medical Terms, and a Directory of Sources for Further Help and Information

Edited by Karen Bellenir and Linda M. Shin. 592 pages. 1998. 0-7808-0206-3. $78.

Endocrine & Metabolic Disorders Sourcebook

Basic Information for the Layperson about Pancreatic and Insulin-Related Disorders Such as Pancreatitis, Diabetes, and Hypoglycemia; Adrenal Gland Disorders Such as Cushing's Syndrome, Addison's Disease, and Congenital Adrenal Hyperplasia; Pituitary Gland Disorders Such as Growth Hormone Deficiency, Acromegaly, and Pituitary Tumors; Thyroid Disorders Such as Hypothyroidism, Graves' Disease, Hashimoto's Disease, and Goiter; Hyperparathyroidism; and Other Diseases and Syndromes of Hormone Imbalance or Metabolic Dysfunction, Along with Reports on Current Research Initiatives

Edited by Linda M. Shin. 632 pages. 1998. 0-7808-0207-1. $78.

Environmentally Induced Disorders Sourcebook

Basic Information about Diseases and Syndromes Linked to Exposure to Pollutants and Other Substances in Outdoor and Indoor Environments Such as Lead, Asbestos, Formaldehyde, Mercury, Emissions, Noise, and More

Edited by Allan R. Cook. 620 pages. 1997. 0-7808-0083-4. $78.

". . . a good survey of numerous environmentally induced physical disorders . . . a useful addition to anyone's library."
— *Doody's Health Science Book Reviews, Jan '98*

". . . provide[s] introductory information from the best authorities around. Since this volume covers topics that potentially affect everyone, it will surely be one of the most frequently consulted volumes in the *Health Reference Series*." — *Rettig on Reference, Nov '97*

"Recommended reference source."
— *Booklist, Oct '97*

Ethical Issues in Medicine Sourcebook

Basic Information about Controversial Treatment Issues, Genetic Research, Reproductive Technologies, and End-of-Life Decisions, Including Topics Such as Cloning, Abortion, Fertility Management, Organ Transplantation, Health Care Rationing, Advance Directives, Living Wills, Physician-Assisted Suicide, Euthanasia, and More; Along with a Glossary and Resources for Additional Information

Edited by Helene Henderson. 600 pages. 1999. 0-7808-0237-3. $78.

Fitness & Exercise Sourcebook

Basic Information on Fitness and Exercise, Including Fitness Activities for Specific Age Groups, Exercise for People with Specific Medical Conditions, How to Begin a Fitness Program in Running, Walking, Swimming, Cycling, and Other Athletic Activities, and Recent Research in Fitness and Exercise

Edited by Dan R. Harris. 663 pages. 1996. 0-7808-0186-5. $78.

"A good resource for general readers."
— *Choice, Nov '97*

"The perennial popularity of the topic . . . make this an appealing selection for public libraries."
— *Rettig on Reference, Jun/Jul '97*

Food & Animal Borne Diseases Sourcebook

Basic Information about Diseases That Can Be Spread to Humans through the Ingestion of Contaminated Food or Water or by Contact with Infected Animals and Insects, Such as Botulism, E. Coli, Hepatitis A, Trichinosis, Lyme Disease, and Rabies, Along with Information Regarding Prevention and Treatment Methods, and a Special Section for International Travelers Describing Diseases Such as Cholera, Malaria, Travelers' Diarrhea, and Yellow Fever, and Offering Recommendations for Avoiding Illness

Edited by Karen Bellenir and Peter D. Dresser. 535 pages. 1995. 0-7808-0033-8. $78.

"Targeting general readers and providing them with a single, comprehensive source of information on selected topics, this book continues, with the excellent caliber of its predecessors, to catalog topical information on health matters of general interest. Readable and thorough, this valuable resource is highly recommended for all libraries."
— *Academic Library Book Review, Summer '96*

"A comprehensive collection of authoritative information." — *Emergency Medical Services, Oct '95*

Continues next page

Gastrointestinal Diseases & Disorders Sourcebook

Basic Information about Gastroesophageal Reflux Disease (Heartburn), Ulcers, Diverticulosis, Irritable Bowel Syndrome, Crohn's Disease, Ulcerative Colitis, Diarrhea, Constipation, Lactose Intolerance, Hemorrhoids, Hepatitis, Cirrhosis, and Other Digestive Problems, Featuring Statistics, Descriptions of Symptoms, and Current Treatment Methods of Interest for Persons Living with Upper and Lower Gastrointestinal Maladies

Edited by Linda M. Ross. 413 pages. 1996. 0-7808-0078-8. $78.

". . . very readable form. The successful editorial work that brought this material together into a useful and understandable reference makes accessible to all readers information that can help them more effectively understand and obtain help for digestive tract problems." — *Choice, Feb '97*

Genetic Disorders Sourcebook

Basic Information about Heritable Diseases and Disorders Such as Down Syndrome, PKU, Hemophilia, Von Willebrand Disease, Gaucher Disease, Tay-Sachs Disease, and Sickle-Cell Disease, Along with Information about Genetic Screening, Gene Therapy, Home Care, and Including Source Listings for Further Help and Information on More Than 300 Disorders

Edited by Karen Bellenir. 642 pages. 1996. 0-7808-0034-6. $78.

"Provides essential medical information to both the general public and those diagnosed with a serious or fatal genetic disease or disorder." — *Choice, Jan '97*

"Geared toward the lay public. It would be well placed in all public libraries and in those hospital and medical libraries in which access to genetic references is limited." — *Doody's Health Sciences Book Review, Oct '96*

Head Trauma Sourcebook

Basic Information for the Layperson about Open-Head and Closed-Head Injuries, Treatment Advances, Recovery, and Rehabilitation, Along with Reports on Current Research Initiatives

Edited by Karen Bellenir. 414 pages. 1997. 0-7808-0208-X. $78.

Health Insurance Sourcebook

Basic Information about Managed Care Organizations, Traditional Fee-for-Service Insurance, Insurance Portability and Pre-Existing Conditions Clauses, Medicare, Medicaid, Social Security, and Military Health Care, Along with Information about Insurance Fraud

Edited by Wendy Wilcox. 530 pages. 1997. 0-7808-0222-5. $78.

"The layout of the book is particularly helpful as it provides easy access to reference material. A most useful addition to the vast amount of information about health insurance. The use of data from U.S. government agencies is most commendable. Useful in a library or learning center for healthcare professional students." — *Doody's Health Sciences Book Reviews, Nov '97*

Healthy Aging Sourcebook

Basic Consumer Health Information about Maintaining Health through the Aging Process, Including Advice on Nutrition, Exercise, and Sleep, Along with Help in Making Decisions about Midlife Issues and Retirement, Practical and Informed Choices in Health Consumerism, and Data Concerning the Theories of Aging, Aging Now, and Aging in the Future, Including a Glossary and Practical Resource Directory

Edited by Jenifer Swanson. 500 pages. 1999. 0-7808-0390-6. $78.

Immune System Disorders Sourcebook

Basic Information about Lupus, Multiple Sclerosis, Guillain-Barré Syndrome, Chronic Granulomatous Disease, and More, Along with Statistical and Demographic Data and Reports on Current Research Initiatives

Edited by Allan R. Cook. 608 pages. 1997. 0-7808-0209-8. $78.

Kidney & Urinary Tract Diseases & Disorders Sourcebook

Basic Information about Kidney Stones, Urinary Incontinence, Bladder Disease, End Stage Renal Disease, Dialysis, and More, Along with Statistical and Demographic Data and Reports on Current Research Initiatives

Edited by Linda M. Ross. 602 pages. 1997. 0-7808-0079-6. $78.

Learning Disabilities Sourcebook

Basic Information about Disorders Such as Dyslexia, Visual and Auditory Processing Deficits, Attention Deficit/Hyperactivity Disorder, and Autism, Along with Statistical and Demographic Data, Reports on Current Research Initiatives, an Explanation of the Assessment Process, and a Special Section for Adults with Learning Disabilities

Edited by Linda M. Shin. 579 pages. 1998. 0-7808-0210-1. $78.

Medical Tests Sourcebook

Basic Consumer Health Information about Medical Tests, Including Periodic Health Exams, General Screening Tests, X-ray and Radiology Tests, Electrical Tests, Tests of Body Fluids and Tissues, Scope Tests, Lung Tests, Gene Tests, Pregnancy Tests, Newborn Screening Tests, Sexually Transmitted Disease Tests, and Computer Aided Diagnoses; Along with a Section on Paying for Medical Tests, a Glossary, and Resource Listings

Edited by Joyce B. Shannon. 600 pages. 1999. 0-7808-0243-8. $78.

Men's Health Concerns Sourcebook

Basic Information about Health Issues That Affect Men, Featuring Facts about the Top Causes of Death in Men, Including Heart Disease, Stroke, Cancers, Prostate Disorders, Chronic Obstructive Pulmonary Disease, Pneumonia and Influenza, Human Immunodeficiency Virus and Acquired Immune Deficiency Syndrome, Diabetes Mellitus, Stress, Suicide, Accidents and Homicides; and Facts about Common Concerns for Men, Including Impotence, Contraception, Circumcision, Sleep Disorders, Snoring, Hair Loss, Diet, Nutrition, Exercise, Kidney and Urological Disorders, and Backaches

Edited by Allan R. Cook. 760 pages. 1998. 0-7808-0212-8. $78.

Mental Health Disorders Sourcebook

Basic Information about Schizophrenia, Depression, Bipolar Disorder, Panic Disorder, Obsessive-Compulsive Disorder, Phobias and Other Anxiety Disorders, Paranoia and Other Personality Disorders, Eating Disorders, and Sleep Disorders, Along with Information about Treatment and Therapies

Edited by Karen Bellenir. 548 pages. 1995. 0-7808-0040-0. $78.

"This is an excellent new book . . . written in easy-to-understand language."
— *Booklist Health Science Supplement, Oct '97*

". . . useful for public and academic libraries and consumer health collections."
— *Medical Reference Services Quarterly, Spring '97*

"The great strengths of the book are its readability and its inclusion of places to find more information. Especially recommended." — *RQ, Winter '96*

". . . a good resource for a consumer health library."
— *Bulletin of the MLA, Oct '96*

"The information is data-based and couched in brief, concise language that avoids jargon. . . . a useful reference source." — *Readings, Sept '96*

"The text is well organized and adequately written for its target audience." — *Choice, Jun '96*

". . . provides information on a wide range of mental disorders, presented in nontechnical language."
— *Exceptional Child Education Resources, Spring '96*

"Recommended for public and academic libraries."
— *Reference Book Review, '96*

Ophthalmic Disorders Sourcebook

Basic Information about Glaucoma, Cataracts, Macular Degeneration, Strabismus, Refractive Disorders, and More, Along with Statistical and Demographic Data and Reports on Current Research Initiatives

Edited by Linda M. Ross. 631 pages. 1996. 0-7808-0081-8. $78.

Oral Health Sourcebook

Basic Information about Diseases and Conditions Affecting Oral Health, Including Cavities, Gum Disease, Dry Mouth, Oral Cancers, Fever Blisters, Canker Sores, Oral Thrush, Bad Breath, Temporomandibular Disorders, and other Craniofacial Syndromes, Along with Statistical Data on the Oral Health of Americans, Oral Hygiene, Emergency First Aid, Information on Treatment Procedures and Methods of Replacing Lost Teeth

Edited by Allan R. Cook. 558 pages. 1997. 0-7808-0082-6. $78.

"Recommended reference source." — *Booklist, Dec '97*

Pain Sourcebook

Basic Information about Specific Forms of Acute and Chronic Pain, Including Headaches, Back Pain, Muscular Pain, Neuralgia, Surgical Pain, and Cancer Pain, Along with Pain Relief Options Such as Analgesics, Narcotics, Nerve Blocks, Transcutaneous Nerve Stimulation, and Alternative Forms of Pain Control, Including Biofeedback, Imaging, Behavior Modification, and Relaxation Techniques

Edited by Allan R. Cook. 667 pages. 1997. 0-7808-0213-6. $78.

"The information is basic in terms of scholarship and is appropriate for general readers. Written in journalistic style . . . intended for non-professionals. Quite thorough in its coverage of different pain conditions and summarizes the latest clinical information regarding pain treatment." — *Choice, Jun '98*

"Recommended reference source."
— *Booklist, Mar '98*

Continues next page

Physical & Mental Issues in Aging Sourcebook

Basic Consumer Health Information on Physical and Mental Disorders Associated with the Aging Process, Including Concerns about Cardiovascular Disease, Pulmonary Disease, Oral Health, Digestive Disorders, Musculoskeletal and Skin Disorders, Metabolic Changes, Sexual and Reproductive Issues, and Changes in Vision, Hearing, and Other Senses; Along with Data about Longevity and Causes of Death, Information on Acute and Chronic Pain, Descriptions of Mental Concerns, a Glossary of Terms, and Resource Listings for Additional Help

Edited by Heather E. Aldred. 625 pages. 1999. 0-7808-0233-0. $78.

Pregnancy & Birth Sourcebook

Basic Information about Planning for Pregnancy, Maternal Health, Fetal Growth and Development, Labor and Delivery, Postpartum and Perinatal Care, Pregnancy in Mothers with Special Concerns, and Disorders of Pregnancy, Including Genetic Counseling, Nutrition and Exercise, Obstetrical Tests, Pregnancy Discomfort, Multiple Births, Cesarean Sections, Medical Testing of Newborns, Breastfeeding, Gestational Diabetes, and Ectopic Pregnancy

Edited by Heather E. Aldred. 737 pages. 1997. 0-7808-0216-0. $78.

". . . for the layperson. A well-organized handbook. Recommended for college libraries . . . general readers."
— Choice, Apr '98

"Recommended reference source."
— Booklist, Mar '98

"This resource is recommended for public libraries to have on hand."
— American Reference Books Annual, '98

Public Health Sourcebook

Basic Information about Government Health Agencies, Including National Health Statistics and Trends, Healthy People 2000 Program Goals and Objectives, the Centers for Disease Control and Prevention, the Food and Drug Administration, and the National Institutes of Health, Along with Full Contact Information for Each Agency

Edited by Wendy Wilcox. 698 pages. 1998. 0-7808-0220-9. $78.

Rehabilitation Sourcebook

Basic Information for the Layperson about Physical Medicine (Physiatry) and Rehabilitative Therapies, Including Physical, Occupational, Recreational, Speech, and Vocational Therapy; Along with Descriptions of Devices and Equipment Such as Orthotics, Gait Aids, Prostheses, and Adaptive Systems Used during Rehabilitation and for Activities of Daily Living, and Featuring a Glossary and Source Listings for Further Help and Information

Edited by Theresa K. Murray. 600 pages. 1999. 0-7808-0236-5. $78.

Respiratory Diseases & Disorders Sourcebook

Basic Information about Respiratory Diseases and Disorders, Including Asthma, Cystic Fibrosis, Pneumonia, the Common Cold, Influenza, and Others, Featuring Facts about the Respiratory System, Statistical and Demographic Data, Treatments, Self-Help Management Suggestions, and Current Research Initiatives

Edited by Allan R. Cook and Peter D. Dresser. 771 pages. 1995. 0-7808-0037-0. $78.

"Designed for the layperson and for patients and their families coping with respiratory illness. . . . an extensive array of information on diagnosis, treatment, management, and prevention of respiratory illnesses for the general reader."
— Choice, Jun '96

"A highly recommended text for all collections. It is a comforting reminder of the power of knowledge that good books carry between their covers."
— Academic Library Book Review, Spring '96

"This sourcebook offers a comprehensive collection of authoritative information presented in a nontechnical, humanitarian style for patients, families, and caregivers."
— Association of Operating Room Nurses, Sept/Oct '95

Sexually Transmitted Diseases Sourcebook

Basic Information about Herpes, Chlamydia, Gonorrhea, Hepatitis, Nongonoccocal Urethritis, Pelvic Inflammatory Disease, Syphilis, AIDS, and More, Along with Current Data on Treatments and Preventions

Edited by Linda M. Ross. 550 pages. 1997. 0-7808-0217-9. $78.